Hepatitis C: Symptoms, Diagnosis and Treatment

Hepatitis C: Symptoms, Diagnosis and Treatment

Editor: Matt Henry

hayle
medical

New York

Hayle Medical,
750 Third Avenue, 9th Floor,
New York, NY 10017, USA

Visit us on the World Wide Web at:
www.haylemedical.com

ISBN 978-1-64647-562-9 (Hardback)

Cataloging-in-Publication Data

Hepatitis C : symptoms, diagnosis and treatment / edited by Matt Henry.
p. cm.
Includes bibliographical references and index.
ISBN 978-1-64647-562-9
1. Hepatitis C. 2. Symptoms. 3. Hepatitis C--Diagnosis. 4. Hepatitis C--Treatment.
5. Hepatitis, Viral. 6. Flaviviral diseases. I. Henry, Matt.
RC848.H425 H47 2023
616.362 3--dc23

Contents

Preface

Hepatitis C refers to a type of viral infection that causes damage and inflammation in the liver. It is caused by the hepatitis C virus. The virus spreads through the body fluids or blood of an infected person. There are various stages of hepatitis C such as the incubation period, acute hepatitis C, chronic hepatitis C, cirrhosis and liver cancer. The signs and symptoms of infection include yellow discoloration of the eyes and skin, fatigue, dark-colored urine, weight loss, loss of appetite, and itchy skin. The polymerase chain reaction (PCR) test and antibody test are typically used to diagnose hepatitis C. There is no vaccine available to protect against infection from the hepatitis C virus. However, the majority of cases of chronic and acute hepatitis C can be treated with direct-acting antiviral medications (DAAs). This book contains a detailed explanation of the symptoms, diagnosis and treatment of hepatitis C. It aims to shed light on some of the unexplored aspects of this disease. A number of latest researches have been included to keep the readers up-to-date with the global concepts in this medical condition.

All of the data presented henceforth, was collaborated in the wake of recent advancements in the field. The aim of this book is to present the diversified developments from across the globe in a comprehensible manner. The opinions expressed in each chapter belong solely to the contributing authors. Their interpretations of the topics are the integral part of this book, which I have carefully compiled for a better understanding of the readers.

At the end, I would like to thank all those who dedicated their time and efforts for the successful completion of this book. I also wish to convey my gratitude towards my friends and family who supported me at every step.

Editor

1

Could insulin receptor H1085H C > T single nucleotide polymorphism predict insulin resistance in type 2 diabetic and chronic hepatitis C virus patients in Egypt?

Rania Nabil Bedair[1], Gehan M. Magour[1], Said Ahmed Ooda[2], Eman M. Amar[1] and Ahmed Mostafa Awad[1*]

Abstract

Background: Insulin-receptor (INSR) is an $\alpha_2\beta_2$ heterotetramer disulfide-linked trans-membrane glycoprotein and a family member of tyrosine kinase receptors. It mediates the pleiotropic actions of insulin regulating glucose homeostasis. It is encoded by a single gene: INSR gene. The INSR gene comprises 22 exons. Exons 17–22 encode the tyrosine kinase domain, and mutations in this region impair the function of the insulin receptor that may cause insulin resistance and hyperinsulinemia. Single nucleotide polymorphism with C > T substitution at His 1058 position of INSR (rs 1799817) located in exon 17 was considered to be involved in insulin resistance. Insulin receptor might be counter-regulated by degradation, differential expression, or modification by phosphorylation in cells expressing HCV core protein. HCV infection eventually leads to liver steatosis and fibrosis, increased oxidative stress, and peroxidation, all of which trigger a cascade of inflammatory responses, thus contributing to the development of insulin resistance. The present retrospective case-control aimed to study INSR H1085H C > T (rs 1799817) SNP in Egyptian patients suffering from chronic HCV infection with DM. The current study was conducted on two hundred and two participants of 100 males and 102 females, divided as follows: the control group (group I) included 50 apparently healthy volunteers of comparable age, sex, and socioeconomic status as patients groups, group II included 50 type 2 DM patients without HCV infection, group III included 52 chronic HCV infected patients without DM, and group IV included 50 HCV patients with DM.

Results: HOMA-IR and QUICKI index was significantly higher in the patient groups (groups II, III, and IV) than in controls ($P < 0.001$, $P = 0.019$, and $P < 0.001$, respectively). It was significantly lower in patients of group III than in patients of groups II and IV with $P < 0.001$ for both. DM patient group without HCV infection (group II) and HCV with DM (group IV) showed a significant decrease in CC genotypes and a significant increase in TT genotypes than the controls ($P < 0.001$, $P = 0.018$, respectively). HCV patients with DM (group IV) had the highest frequency of heterozygous genotype (CT) (50%). HCV-infected patients with T2DM (group IV) also showed a significantly higher frequency of minor allele (T) (35%) than controls (20%), and a lower frequency of the wild allele (C) (65%) than controls (80%).

Conclusion: The mutant allele "T" of INSR H1085H C > T (rs 1799817) SNP might be associated with an increased risk of developing insulin resistance and T2DM.

Keywords: Hepatitis C virus, Type 2 diabetes mellitus, INSR H1085H C > T SNP

* Correspondence: dr_amawad@hotmail.com
[1]Chemical Pathology Department, Medical Research Institute, Alexandria University, Alexandria, Egypt
Full list of author information is available at the end of the article

Background

Hepatitis C virus (HCV) infection, a common chronic liver disease, is a major public health problem. It was estimated that more than 185 million persons (2–3% of the world population) are HCV infected; of them, around 71 million are chronically infected individuals and 34 million are chronically infected with HCV genotype 4. Before the era of directly acting antiviral agents (DAAS), Egypt had the highest prevalence of HCV worldwide and ranked 5th among all countries for the burden of disease from viral hepatitis. Genotype 4 represents over 90% of HCV cases in Egypt [1, 2].

Hepatitis C viral eradication after antiviral treatment can lead to an improvement in insulin resistance and a reduction in the incidence of diabetes mellitus after the end of therapy. This offers a strong argument in favor of a causal relationship between HCV and DM [3].

Several hypotheses have been proposed to the mechanisms underlying HCV-mediated insulin resistance. HCV infection eventually leads to liver steatosis and fibrosis, increased oxidative stress, and peroxidation, all of which trigger a cascade of inflammatory responses, thus contributing to the development of insulin resistance [4].

Insulin receptor (INSR) is an $\alpha_2\beta_2$ heterotetramer disulfide-linked trans-membrane glycoprotein and a family member of tyrosine kinase receptors. It mediates the pleiotropic actions of insulin regulating glucose homeostasis [5, 6].

The insulin receptor is encoded by a single gene: INSR gene. The INSR gene is located on the short (p) arm of chromosome 19 and comprises 22 exons. Exons 17–22 encode the tyrosine kinase domain, and mutations in this region impair the function of the insulin receptor that may cause insulin resistance and hyperinsulinemia. Single nucleotide polymorphism (SNP) with C > T substitution at His 1058 position of INSR (rs 1799817) located in exon 17 was considered to be involved in insulin resistance [7, 8]. Insulin receptor might be counter-regulated by degradation, differential expression, or modification by phosphorylation in cells expressing HCV core protein [9].

SNP in the INSR was among the most frequently studied candidate genes in DM. To the best of our knowledge, no much data are available on INSR H1085H SNP in HCV-infected populations with DM.

Methods

The present research is a retrospective case-control study aimed to study INSR H1085H C > T (rs 1799817) SNP in Egyptian patients suffering from chronic HCV infection with DM. Our study was conducted on two hundred and two participants of 100 males and 102 females, divided as follows: the control group (group I) included 50 apparently healthy volunteers of comparable age, sex, and socioeconomic status as patients groups, group II included 50 type 2 DM patients without HCV infection, group III included 52 chronic HCV infected patients without DM, and group IV included 50 HCV patients with DM.

Exclusion criteria include patients with hepatocellular carcinoma (HCC) or any other malignancy, coexisting viral infection like hepatitis B surface antigen-positive patients, renal failure, liver failure, chronic pancreatitis, polycystic ovarian disease (PCOD), pregnant females, and those taking medications that affect insulin resistance including glucocorticoids were excluded from the study.

1. Full history was taken from all subjects.
2. Full physical examination and anthropometric measurements including body mass index [10] and waist to hip ratio (WHR) [11] were done.
3. Ultrasound abdomen [12]
4. The following laboratory investigations were done including determination of fasting and postprandial serum glucose, glycated hemoglobin (HbA_1C), triglycerides, cholesterol (total, high-, and low-density lipoprotein fractions), urea, creatinine, uric acid levels, alanine aminotransferase (ALT), aspartate aminotransferase (AST), and gamma-glutamyl transferase (GGT) activities [13]. Insulin level was determined [14], and then the Homeostatic Model Assessment of Insulin Resistance (HOMA IR) [15] and Quantitative Insulin Sensitivity Check (QUICKI) index [16] were calculated. Polymerase chain reaction (PCR) [17] for HCV for groups III and IV, HCV antibodies [17] for groups I and II, and hepatitis B surface antigen [18] for all groups were done.
5. Genomic DNA was extracted from peripheral blood leukocytes by using ion-exchange column chromatography. Genotyping of INSR H1085H (rs 1799817) using polymerase chain reaction (PCR-RFLP) technique with restriction enzyme PmlI was done [19]. The details of molecular studies which had been done in the current study are as follows:

DNA extraction from peripheral blood leucocytes [19]

The genomic DNA extraction from peripheral blood leukocytes was carried out using column-based commercial genomic DNA extraction kits Thermo Scientific Gene JET^{TM} Whole Blood Genomic DNA Purification Mini Kit #K0781 (Fermentas-Thermo, USA).

Then assessing the integrity of the extracted genomic DNA by agarose gel electrophoresis (AGE), the eppendorf containing the checked purified DNA in the elution buffer was tightly capped and stored till the time of PCR at − 20 °C.

Polymerase chain reaction amplification using specific primers [19]

A set of primers flanking the SNP region were used for the detection of insulin receptor H1085H C > T (rs 1799817) single nucleotide polymorphisms using the following reagent:

1) DreamTaq PCR Master Mix (2X) # K1071 (200 runs of 50 µl) Thermo Scientific™
2) DNA gel Loading Dye (6X) # R0611: Thermo Scientific™
3) Primers: A pair of primers for each gene H1085H C > T (rs 1799817) was used. The lyophilized primers were supplied by Invitrogen, UK, which were reconstituted by addition of sterile nuclease-free water as follow:

Insulin receptor H1085H C > T (rs 1799817)

For the forward sense sequence, 195 µl was added and 225 µl for the reverse sense sequence to give a final concentration of 100 pmoles/µl for each and stored at − 20 °C. It was diluted to give a final concentration of 10 pmoles/µl.

Primers for insulin receptor H1085H C > T (rs 1799817) Forward sense sequence: (INSR-G01)

5′-CCA AGG ATG CTG TGT AGA TAA G-3 (Tm (thermodynamic) = 64 °C)

Reverse antisense sequence: (INSR-F12)

5′-TCA GGA AAG CCA GCC CAT GTC-3 (Tm (thermodynamic) = 66 °C)

Protocol of amplification

In a 0.2-ml eppendorf tube placed on ice, the following reagents were added and mixed.

DreamTaq PCR Master Mix (2X)	12.5 µl
Forward primer	0.5 µl (10 pmol)
Reverse primer	0.5 µl (10 pmol)
Extracted DNA	1 µl
Water nuclease-free	10.5 µl

The total volume was 25 µl, and then the tubes were transferred to the thermal cycler (Quanta Biotech, UK) where the PCR conditions were adjusted (Table 1).

The amplified products were separated on 2% agarose gel electrophoresis after adding a loading dye as follows: 2 µl loading dye added to 10 µl of amplified DNA.

Table 1 Thermal cycler condition of insulin receptor H1085H C > T (rs 1799817)

Phases	Cycle number	Temperature (°C)	Time
Amplification			
• Denaturation		93	45 s
• Annealing	35	56	30 s
• Extension		72	45 s
Final extension	1	72	7 min

Restriction digestion of PCR products using PmlI for insulin receptor H1085H C > T (rs 1799817) [19]

Restriction includes endonuclease enzymes, PmlI enzyme for insulin receptor H1085H C > T (rs 1799817), targeting specific sequence of the amplified DNA product for detection of INSR H1085H C > T (rs 1799817) gene polymorphisms.

Reagents

For *INSR* H1085H C > T (rs 1799817)

- Eco72I (PmlI) (10 U/µl) # ER0361: restriction enzyme recognized CAC^GTG sites and cut best at 37 °C in Tango buffer. PmlI was used for insulin receptor H1085H C > T (rs 1799817) polymorphism.
- 10× buffer tango for Pm1I containing 33 mM tris-acetate (PH7.9), 10 mM magnesium acetate, 66 mM potassium acetate, and 0.1 mg/ml BSA.

Protocol for restriction enzymes

Eco72I (PmlI) for insulin receptor H1085H C > T (rs 1799817) polymorphism In an eppendorf tube, the following reagents were mixed.

Water (nuclease-free)	18 µl
10× tango buffer	2 µl
Amplified PCR product	10 µl
Restriction enzyme, PmlI	2 UI

Thus, the total volume was 32 µl. They were mixed gently, spin down for few seconds, and incubated at 37 °C for 2 h then the digested products were separated on agarose gel electrophoresis after adding loading dye as follows: 2 µl of loading dye was added to 10 µl of restricted DNA products.

Agarose gel electrophoresis for the amplified and digested PCR products using

1) Gene Ruler ™ 50 bp DNA ladder (Thermo Fisher Scientific), the DNA fragments ranged from 50 to 1000 bp. It contains two reference bands: 250 and 500 bp.
2) Tris borate EDTA (TBE) buffer (10×) stock solution: working TBE (1×) buffer was prepared by measuring 100 ml stock solution and completed to 1 l of distilled water.
3) Agarose gel (wt/vol) 2.5% then 100 volts was applied for about 45 min till the loading dye had migrated to near the end of the plate. The DNA will migrate towards the anode.

- A negative control, water (nuclease-free) and positive control, and previous read samples were allowed to run in case of amplified product detection.
- In the case of pm1I INSR-restricted products, a PCR product was allowed to separate with each run to identify unrestricted products.
- Ultraviolet transillumination (302 nm) was used for the visualization of the DNA bands.

Results

For insulin receptor H1085H C > T (rs 1799817) polymorphism

The amplified DNA leads to the formation of 317 bp amplicon. When a C allele was present in PmlI SNP (rs1799817) within the exon 17 of the *INSR* gene, the PmlI enzyme yielded 274 and 43 bp fragments on the agarose gel. The PCR products remained uncut (317 bp) in the presence of the restriction enzyme (PmlI), confirming the presence of a T allele in this locus.

So, in the amplified product of H1085H, CC genotype appears as two bands of 274 bp and 43 bp fragments and CT genotype appears as 317 bp, 274 bp, and 43 bp fragments while TT genotype appears as a single uncut 317 bp fragment (Figs. 1 and 2)

There was no significant difference in both age (P = 0.183) and sex (P = 0.101) between the four studied groups.

Regarding BMI, it was significantly higher in diabetic patients without HCV infection (group II) and in HCV patients with DM (group IV) than controls, and group IV than group III (P < 0.001 for all).

Regarding WHR, it was significantly higher in group II and group IV than controls, in group III and group IV than group II, and in group IV than group III (P < 0.001 for all).

Serum levels of AST, ALT, and GGT were significantly higher in groups III and IV than controls and group II (P < 0.001 for all). There was no significant difference between serum activities of AST and GGT in group II and controls (P = 0.063 and P = 0.703, respectively). Serum activity of ALT was significantly increased in group II than controls (P = 0.032), but this was of no significance as the serum level of ALT was within the normal range in both groups. There was no significant difference as regard AST, ALT, and GGT activities between group IV and group III.

Fasting serum (FSG), postprandial serum glucose (PPSG), and glycosylated hemoglobin (HbA_1C%) were significantly higher in diabetes mellitus patients in groups II and IV than in controls with P < 0.001 (Table 2).

There was no significant difference between patients of group III and controls regarding FSG, PPSG, and HbA_1C%. HbA_1C% was significantly higher in patients of group II than in patients of group IV (P = 0.005) (Table 2).

Also, fasting insulin was significantly higher in groups II, III, and IV than in controls with P < 0.001. And it was significantly lower in patients of group III than in patients of group II and group IV with P = 0.002 and P < 0.001, respectively. And it was significantly higher in patients of group IV than in patients of group II with P < 0.001 (Table 2).

Regarding HOMA-IR, it was significantly higher in groups II, III, and IV than in controls with P < 0.001, P = 0.019, and P < 0.001, respectively. And it was significantly lower in patients of group III than in patients of groups II and IV with P < 0.001 for both (Table 2).

Regarding QUICKI index, it was significantly lower in patient groups II, III, and IV than in controls with P < 0.001. And it was significantly higher in patients of group III than in diabetic patients in groups II and IV with P < 0.001. It was significantly lower in patients of group IV than in patients of group II with P = 0.009 (Table 2).

It was noticed that the observed frequencies of the different genotypes of INSR H1085H C > T polymorphism were compared to the expected frequencies, according to the Hardy-Weinberg equilibrium, in each of the studied groups. All the studied groups showed P > 0.05 (after performing chi-square test) indicating an agreement with Hardy-Weinberg equilibrium.

The INSR H1085 C > T genotype distribution was significantly different between the four studied groups (P < 0.001). DM patient group without HCV infection (group II) and HCV with DM (group IV) showed a significant decrease in CC genotypes and a significant increase in TT genotypes than the controls (P < 0.001, P = 0.018, respectively). There was a significant increase in

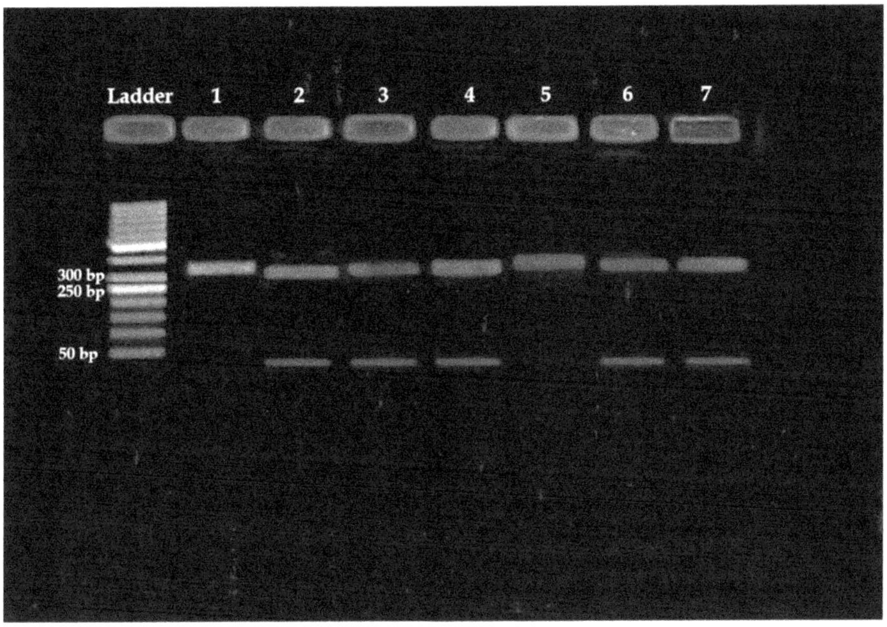

Fig. 1 Agarose gel electrophoresis (2.5 %) of PmlI-digested PCR product for *INSR* H1085 C > T SNP (rs 1799817). DNA ladder of 50 bp interval (50–1000 bp), lane 1: 317 bp DNA amplicon of *INSR* C > T; lanes 2–4 and lanes 6 and 7: CC; lane 5: TT

TT genotypes in DM patients without HCV infection (group II) than HCV patients (groups III and IV) ($P < 0.001$ for both). On the contrary, there was no significant difference in genotype distribution between HCV-infected patients without DM (group III) and controls or between HCV-infected patients without DM (group III) and HCV-infected patients with DM (group IV) ($P = 0.131$ and $P = 0.658$, respectively). It was noticed that the highest frequency of wild genotype of INSR polymorphism (CC) was in controls (60%), while the lowest one was in DM patients without HCV infection (group II) (10%). The highest frequency of homozygous mutant genotype (TT) was in DM patients without HCV (62%), whereas the mutant genotype was absent in controls. HCV patients with DM (group IV) had the highest frequency of heterozygous genotype (CT) (50%) (Table 3, Fig. 3).

The allelic frequency was significantly different between the four studied groups ($P < 0.001$). Groups II and IV showed a significant increase in T allele than

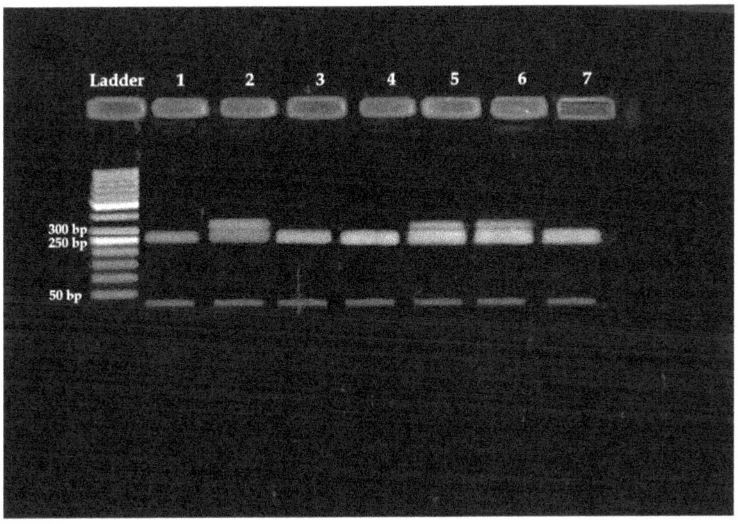

Fig. 2 Agarose gel electrophoresis (2.5 %) of PmlI-digested PCR product for *INSR* H1085 C > T SNP (rs 1799817). DNA ladder of 50 bp interval (50–1000 bp), lanes 1, 3, 4, and 7: CC; lanes 2, 5, and 6: CT

Table 2 Statistical significance of fasting serum glucose level (FSG) (mg/dl), postprandial serum glucose (PPSG) (mg/dl), HbA_1C (%), fasting insulin (μIU/ml), and HOMA-IR and QUICKI index in the studied groups

	Group I (n = 50)	Group II (n = 50)	Group III (n = 52)	Group IV (n = 50)	Test of sig.	P
FSG (mg/dl)						
Min.–Max.	75.0–99.0	129.0–322.0	59.0–100.0	83.0–766.0	H = 143.378	< 0.001*
Mean ± SD	86.3 ± 5.62	195.2 ± 51.82	82.31 ± 11.46	182.68 ± 106.6		
Median	87.0	189.0	80.0	168.50		
$p_{Group\ I}$		< 0.001*	0.239	<0.001*		
Sig. bet. Grps		p_1 < 0.001*, p_2 = 0.132, p_3 < 0.001*				
PPSG (mg/dl)						
Min.–Max.	85.0–130.0	108.0–391.0	77.0–145.0	85.0–540.0	F = 72.836	< 0.001*
Mean ± SD	102.3 ± 12.9	207.3 ± 70.44	101.6 ± 17.87	223.62 ± 81.85		
Median	99.0	201.0	95.0	210.0		
$p_{Group\ I}$		< 0.001*	1.000	< 0.001*		
Sig. bet. Grps		p_1 < 0.001*, p_2 = 0.447, p_3 < 0.001*				
HbA_1C (%)						
Min.–Max.	3.80–5.50	6.20–13.70	3.80–5.40	5.40–12.20	F = 145.963	< 0.001*
Mean ± SD	4.68 ± 0.49	8.75 ± 2.01	4.58 ± 0.47	7.89 ± 1.42		
Median	4.80	8.10	4.50	7.75		
$p_{Group\ I}$		< 0.001*	0.974	< 0.001*		
Sig. bet. Grps		p_1 < 0.001*, p_2 = 0.005*, p_3 < 0.001*				
Fasting insulin (μIU/ml)						
Min.–Max.	1.20–10.10	5.40–77.0	2.40–25.30	10.0–514.2	H = 121.986	< 0.001*
Mean ± SD	5.75 ± 2.65	17.09 ± 16.22	9.19 ± 3.65	40.68 ± 72.89		
Median	5.65	11.0	9.30	18.65		
$p_{Group\ I}$		< 0.001*	< 0.001*	< 0.001*		
Sig. bet. Grps		p_1 = 0.002*, p_2 < 0.001*, p_3 < 0.001*				
HOMA-IR						
Min.–Max.	0.30–2.20	2.70–49.0	0.50–5.30	4.60–65.10	H = 157.864	< 0.001*
Mean ± SD	1.23 ± 0.55	9.14 ± 11.09	1.81 ± 0.73	12.76 ± 11.04		
Median	1.30	5.10	1.95	7.40		
$p_{Group\ I}$		< 0.001*	0.019*	< 0.001*		
Sig. bet. Grps		p_1 < 0.001*, p_2 = 0.055, p_3 < 0.001*				
QUICKI index						
Min.–Max.	0.34–0.49	0.23–0.33	0.30–0.43	0.21–0.31	F = 150.524	< 0.001*
Mean ± SD	0.38 ± 0.04	0.30 ± 0.03	0.35 ± 0.02	0.28 ± 0.02		
Median	0.37	0.30	0.35	0.29		
$p_{Group\ I}$		< 0.001*	< 0.001*	< 0.001*		
Sig. bet. Grps		p_1 < 0.001*, p_2 = 0.009*, p_3 < 0.001*				

controls (P < 0.001, P = 0.018, respectively). There was no significant difference in allelic frequency between HCV-infected patients without DM (group III) and controls (P = 0.106) or between group III and group IV (P = 0.428) (Table 3, Fig. 4).

Testing the dominant model of inheritance revealed a statistically higher frequency of exposed genotypes "CT&TT" among the diabetics (group II) when compared to the control group (90% vs 40%, respectively; P < 0.001), with a substantial increase in insulin resistance and DM risk among the exposed group (CT and TT), with a crude odds ratio of 13.5 (95% confidence interval, 4.569–39.889) when compared to unexposed group (CC). After logistic regression analysis, the odds ratio was adjusted for BMI, age, and sex to be 12.238 (95% confidence interval, 3.041–49.239) (P < 0.001).

Table 3 Comparison between the four studied groups according to genotype distribution of INSR H1085H C > T (rs 1799817) polymorphism

Parameters	Group I (*n* = 50)		Group II (*n* = 50)		Group III (*n* = 52)		Group IV (*n* = 50)		χ^2	*P*
	N	%	*N*	%	*N*	%	*N*	%		
INSR H1085H C > T										
CC homo wild	30	60.0	5	10.0	24	46.2	20	40.0	84.746*	< 0.001*
CT hetero	20	40.0	14	28.0	25	48.1	25	50.0		
TT homo mutant	0	0.0	31	62.0	3	5.8	5	10.0		
Sig. bet. Grps	$p_1 < 0.001^*$, ${}^{MC}p_2 = 0.131$, $p_3 = 0.018^*$, $p_4 < 0.001^*$, $p_5 < 0.001^*$, ${}^{MC}p_6 = 0.658$									
C	80	80.0	24	24.0	73	70.2	65	65.0	76.146*	< 0.001*
T	20	20.0	76	76.0	31	29.8	35	35.0		
Sig. bet. Grps	$p_1 < 0.001^*$, $p_2 = 0.106$, $p_3 = 0.018^*$, $p_4 < 0.001^*$, $p_5 < 0.001^*$, $p_6 = 0.428$									

χ^2 chi-square test, *MC* Monte Carlo, *p p* value for comparing between the different groups, common letters are not significant (i.e., different letters are significant), p_1 *p* value for comparing between group I and group II, p_2 *p* value for comparing between group I and group III, p_3 *p* value for comparing between group I and group IV, p_4 *p* value for comparing between group II and group III, p_5 *p* value for comparing between group II and group IV, p_6 *p* value for comparing between group III and group IV, *Sig. bet. Grps* significance between groups
*Statistically significant at $p \leq 0.05$

Testing the recessive model, where the exposed group was considered to be composed of only subjects with the homo-mutant TT genotype, was not applicable as the odds ratio cannot be estimated because of the absence of (TT) genotype among the control subjects.

Comparing between groups I and III, no statistically significant difference was found in the risk of development of IR and DM according to INSR H1085H C > T genotypes between exposed and unexposed groups in both dominant and recessive modes of inheritance.

Testing the dominant model of inheritance revealed a statistically higher frequency of exposed genotypes "CT&TT" among the HCV-infected patients with DM (group IV) than the control group (60% vs 40%, respectively; *P* = 0.046) with an apparently increase in insulin resistance and DM risk among the exposed group (CT and TT) with a crude odds ratio of 2.250 (95% confidence interval, 1.011–5.008) than unexposed group (CC). After logistic regression analysis, the odds ratio was adjusted for BMI, age, and sex to be insignificant, 15.120 (95% confidence interval, 0.841–271.824) (*P* = 0.065), meaning that genotype exposure by itself was insignificant, but with other confounders like BMI, the risk of IR and DM increased.

Testing the recessive model, where the exposed group was composed of only subjects with the homo-mutant

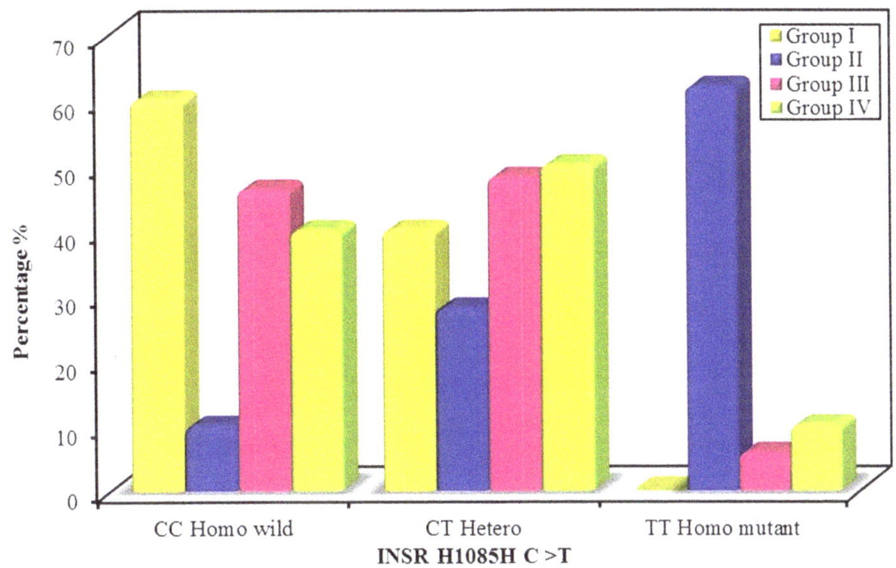

Fig. 3 Comparison between the four studied groups according to INSR H1085H C > T genotype distribution

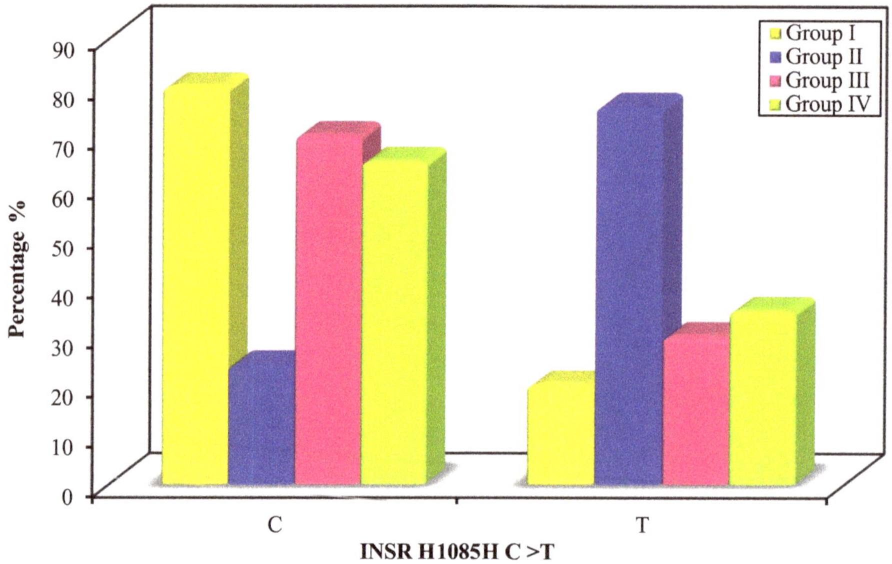

Fig. 4 Comparison between the four studied groups according to INSR H1085H C > T allele frequency

TT genotype, was not applicable, and odds ratio cannot be estimated because of the absence of (TT) genotype among the control subjects.

Diabetic patients (groups II and IV) were divided into controlled (with HA1c ≤ 7), fairly controlled (with HA1c = 7.1–9), and uncontrolled (with HA1c > 9). In group II, 20% of patients were controlled, 44% were fairly controlled, and 36% were uncontrolled. In group IV, 34% of patients were controlled, 44% were fairly controlled, and 22% were uncontrolled. We studied INSR H1085 C > T genotype distribution in controlled versus uncontrolled DM patients. There was no statistically significant difference regarding INSR H1085 C > T genotype distribution between controlled and uncontrolled DM patients in group II (P = 0.774) and group IV (P = 0.572).

Discussion

Type 2 diabetes mellitus is found to be 1.8- to 2.5-fold higher in patients with chronic HCV infection and two- to threefolds more prevalent in HCV than in HBV infection worldwide. HCV eradication after antiviral treatment could lead to an improvement in insulin resistance and a reduction in the incidence of diabetes mellitus after the end of therapy. This offers a strong argument in favor of a causal relationship between HCV and DM [3].

Several hypotheses have been proposed to explain the mechanisms underlying HCV-mediated insulin resistance. Insulin receptor (INSR), a family member of tyrosine kinase receptors, mediates pleiotropic actions of insulin regulating glucose homeostasis. The main action of its activation is inducing glucose uptake. The decrease in insulin receptor signaling leads to hyperglycemia and all the sequelae of type 2DM [4–6].

Insulin receptor might be counter-regulated in cells expressing HCV core protein which may contribute, at least in part, to the induction of insulin resistance in hepatocytes expressing HCV core protein [9].

The study of INSR H1085H C > T SNP and its effect on insulin resistance is important. Unfortunately, it was not studied frequently. Moreover, it was studied mainly on females with polycystic ovary syndrome (PCOS) giving importance to the current study.

From the current study, it could be concluded that the mutant allele "T" was associated with a statistically significant increased risk of developing insulin resistance and DM.

Also, results of the present study revealed a statistically significant higher frequency of exposed genotypes (TT and CT) among patients of DM without HCV infection (group II) 90% than the control group 40% with a substantial increase in insulin resistance and DM risk among the exposed group (CT and TT) than the unexposed group (CC).

This association between INSR H1085H (rs 1799817) SNP, insulin resistance, and DM risk among diabetic patients without HCV infection (group II) remained after performing logistic regression analysis to adjust for some important insulin resistance confounding factors.

On the contrary, HCV-infected patients with DM (group IV) showed a statistically higher frequency of exposed genotypes (TT and CT) among them than the control group. After logistic regression analysis, the odds ratio was adjusted for BMI, age, and sex to be insignificant.

In accordance with the present work, Mukherjee et al. [20] studied INSR H1085 H C > T polymorphism on Indian females by direct sequencing and found that the polymorphic genotype (CT and TT) was significantly associated with PCOS in lean women ($P = 0.004$).

Tucci et al. on Canadian population and Tucci et al. [21] on Caucasian population had found an association between rs1799817 and PCOS.

Siegel et al. [22] on Americans argued for the first time that the INSR gene itself took part in the development of insulin resistance as the main cause of PCOS.

Two genome-wide studies (GWAS) by Chen et al. [23] and Shi et al. [24] reported an association of rs1799817 of INSR gene in PCOS women with an increase in the frequency of uncommon T allele in lean PCOS women with body mass index [(BMI) < 27 kg/m^2] than lean controls.

Kumar et al. [25] found an increased frequency of INSR H1085H T allele in PCOS patients from China and India.

Moreover, to overcome small sample sizes, two meta-analysis studies were done: Ioannidis et al. [26] and Feng et al. [8]. They showed no significant association between INSR H1085H polymorphism and PCOS.

Mutib et al. [27] had also found an association of INSR H1085H polymorphism and PCOS, indices of insulin resistance, and dyslipidemia in Iraqi women using restriction fragment length polymorphism (RFLP-PCR) but unlike the current study, they found that CC genotype frequency was higher in PCOS patients whereas TT genotype was higher in control women. These differences in phenotypic expression could be due to the frequency of distribution of genotypes TT, CT, and CC across the population where the effect of genotype influences suppression or increased expression of phenotypic change.

Unlike the current work, some studies reported no association of PmlI (rs1799817) polymorphism in the INSR gene, insulin resistance, and PCOS risk including Urbanek et al. [28], Tehrani et al. [29], Bagheri et al. [19], and Xu et al. [30] on Han Chinese. Moreover, Thangavelu et al. [31] showed also a negative association between polymorphism and PCOS women, but the genotypes influenced the phenotypic expression as women with TT genotype of H1085H showed an increase in insulin level. Zhu et al. [32] showed also no association with INSR H1085 polymorphism and DM or diabetic nephropathy in Chinese Han population. On the contrary to the current study, Bodhini et al. [33] found that "T" allele was significantly lower in the DM subjects with temporary significant protection against diabetes as it became insignificant after adjustment of P value by other confounders.

The discrepancy between the current work and these studies may be caused by population stratification; using the classic case-control design would have the limitation of associations between allelic variants in candidate genes and disease might have arisen on account of population stratification by ethnicity or environmental factors. Also, most of the studies were conducted on females only. Another reason may be using different techniques to determine the SNP that differs in method performance.

Although HCV infection is an important risk factor for insulin resistance and diabetes mellitus, the current work found no significant association between INSR H1085H C > T polymorphism and HCV-induced IR and DM. However, no previous studies regarding the INSR H1085H SNP and the risk of insulin resistance and DM or even the risk of HCV-induced DM in Egyptians were done, giving importance to the current study.

Conclusions

From this study, it could be concluded that the INSR H1085H (rs 1799817) polymorphism might be a contributing risk factor for the development of type 2 diabetes mellitus as established by the high frequency of minor allele (T) in type 2 diabetic patients without HCV infection. We could also conclude that increased frequency of mutant allele (T) than wild allele (C) in INSR H1085H polymorphism in type 2 diabetic patients with BMI < 25 kg/m^2 might be risk factors for type 2 diabetes mellitus even in subjects with normal body weight. Finally, we were able to assure that BMI has its role as an independent risk factor for the development of type 2 diabetes mellitus as in our study, there was a significant increase of body mass index in type 2 diabetics without HCV infection and HCV-infected patients with type 2 diabetes mellitus.

In the light of the current study conclusion and its limitation, we are recommending the study of other related gene polymorphisms that might contribute to the development of type 2 diabetes in HCV patients, to study the relation of INSR H1085H to the response of different antidiabetic drugs, to assess of gene expression of INSR in HCV infected patients which may be useful for early detection of type 2 diabetes in these patients, and to conduct the study on larger sample size and in other ethnic HCV cohorts are needed to validate the present study. Finally, we are recommending regular screening for type 2 diabetes mellitus in HCV patients.

Abbreviations

ATP: Adenosine triphosphate; BMI: Body mass index; BUN: Blood urea nitrogen; CHC: Chronic hepatitis C virus; CKD: Chronic kidney disease; DAAS: Directly acting antiviral agents; DGGE: Denaturing gradient gel electrophoresis; DM: Diabetes mellitus; DNA: Deoxyribonucleic acid; ER: Endoplasmic reticulum; FSG: Fasting serum glucose; FSH: Follicular stimulating hormone; G6P: Glucose 6 phosphate; HbA_1C: Hemoglobin A_1C;

HBV: Hepatitis B virus; HCV: Hepatitis C virus; HOMA-IR: Homeostatic model assessment for insulin resistance; IL-6: Interleukin-6; INSR: Insulin receptor; IR: Insulin resistance; Kb: Kilo bite; KDa: Kilo Dalton; KRLB: Kinase regulatory loop binding domain; LH: Luteinizing hormone; MFA: Minor frequency allele; mRNA: Messenger RNA; NGS: Next-generation sequencing; NO: Nitric oxide; NTR: Non-translated region; PCOS: Polycystic ovarian syndrome; PI-3 kinase: Phosphoinositide-3 kinase; PIP-3: Phosphatidylinositol (3, 4, 5)-trisphosphate; PKC: Protein kinase C; PPSG: Postprandial serum glucose; QUICKI: Quantitative insulin sensitivity check index; RER: Rough endoplasmic reticulum; RFLP: Restriction fragment length polymorphism; RNA: Ribonucleic acid; ROS: Reactive oxygen species; Rpm: Revolutions per minute; Rs: Reference SNPs (ID); RSP: Residue signal peptide; RT-qPCR: Real-time quantitative polymerase chain reaction; RTK: Receptor tyrosine kinase; SH2: Src homology 2; SNPs: Single nucleotide polymorphisms; T2DM: Type 2 diabetes mellitus; TC: Total cholesterol; TGN: Trans-Golgi network; TNF-α: Tumor necrotizing factor-α; WHR: Waist hip ratio; β-cell: Beta-cell

Acknowledgements
Not applicable

Authors' contributions
SO analyzed and interpreted the patient data regarding the liver disease, EA performed the laboratory and molecular studies and was a major contributor in writing the manuscript, AW supervised the laboratory studies and subject selections, RB shared in research idea formulation and study design, and GM validated the data and managed and supervised the whole work. All authors read and approved the final manuscript.

Ethics approval and consent to participate
The study was conducted after approval of Medical Research Institute, Alexandria University Ethical Committee, no available reference number, and according to the Helsinki Declaration. The study was explained to all participating subjects and written informed consents were taken from all of them.

Competing interests
The authors declare that they have no competing interests.

Author details
[1]Chemical Pathology Department, Medical Research Institute, Alexandria University, Alexandria, Egypt. [2]Experimental and Clinical Internal Medicine, Medical Research Institute, Alexandria University, Alexandria, Egypt.

References

1. Messina JP, Humphreys I, Flaxman A, Brown A, Cooke GS et al (2015) Global distribution and prevalence of hepatitis C virus genotypes. Hepatology. 61: 77–87
2. Nouroz F, Shaheen S, Mujtaba G, Noreen S (2015) An overview on hepatitis C virus genotypes and its control. Egypt J Med Hum Genetics. 16:207–286
3. Negro F (2012) Steatosis and insulin resistance in response to treatment of chronic hepatitis C. J Viral Hepat. 19:42–47
4. Gao TT, Qin ZL, Ren H, Zhao P, Qi ZT (2015) Inhibition of IRS-1 by hepatitis C virus infection leads to insulin resistance in a PTEN-dependent manner. Virol J. 12:12
5. González-Sánchez JL, Serrano-Ríos M (2007) Molecular basis of insulin action. Drug News Perspect. 20:527–531
6. Belfiore A, Frasca F (2009) Insulin receptor isoforms and insulin receptor/insulin-like growth factor receptor hybrids in physiology and disease. Endocr Rev. 30:586 623
7. Hubbard SR (2013) Structural biology: Insulin meets its receptor. Nature. 493: 171–172
8. Feng C, Lv PP, Yu TT, Jin M, Shen JM, Wang X et al (2015) The association between polymorphism of INSR and polycystic ovary syndrome: a meta-analysis. Int J. Mol. 16:2403–2425
9. Banerjee S, Saito K, Goughoulte MA, Meyer K, Ray RB et al (2008) Hepatitis C virus core protein upregulates serine phosphorylation of insulin receptor substrate-1 and impairs the downstream Akt/ProteinKinase B signaling pathway for insulin resistance. J Virol 82:2606–2612
10. Daud S, Javaid F (2012) Estimation of body mass index (BMI) in medical students. PJMHS. 5:702–705
11. Wang C, Wang B, He H, Li X, Wei D, Zhang J et al (2012) Association between insulin receptor gene polymorphism and the metabolic syndrome in Han and Yi Chinese. Asia Pac J Clin Nutr. 21:457–463
12. Gerstenmaier JF, Gibson RN (2014) Ultrasound in chronic liver disease. Insights Imaging 5(4):441–455
13. Burtis CA, Ashwood ER, Bruns DE (2012) Tietz textbook of clinical chemistry and molecular diagnostics. 5th Ed. Elsevier Saunders Company, St Louis, pp 676–679 (albumin creatinine ratio), 718-22(glucose), 771-8 (lipid profile), 680-4(creatinine), 690 (uric acid), 143-6 (ALT, AST and GGT)
14. Guojun Z, Yanguo T, Ranxing Z, Yan Z, Tao K et al (2013) Analysis of current status of serum insulin determination by different chemiluminescence immunoassay systems. J Capital Med Univ 34:545–549
15. Matthews DR, Hosker JP, Rudenski AS, Naylor BA, Treacher DF, Turner RC (1985) Homeostasis model assessment: insulin resistance and beta-cell function from fasting plasma glucose and insulin concentrations in man. Diabetologia. 28:412–419
16. Rabasa-Lhoret R, Bastard JP, Jan V (2003) Modified quantitative insulin sensitivity check index is better correlated to hyperinsulinemic glucose clamp than other fasting-based index of insulin sensitivity in different insulin-resistant states. J Clin Endocrinol Metab. 88:4917–4923
17. Chakravarti A, Charhan MS, Dogra G, Banerjee S (2013) Hepatitis C virus core antigen assay: can we think beyond convention in resource limited settings? Braz J Infect Dis 17:369–374
18. Dufour R (2006) Hepatitis B surface antigen (HBs Ag) assays- Are they good enough for their current uses? Clin Chem 52:1457–1459
19. Bagheri M, Abdi-Rad I, Jazani NH, Zarrin R, Nanbakhsh F et al (2015) Association study between INSR/Nsil (rs2059806) and INSR/PmlI (rs1799817) SNPs in women with polycystic ovary syndrome from West Azerbaijan Province. Iran. J Reprod Infertil. 16:109–112
20. Mukherjee S, Shaikh N, Khavale S, Shinde G, Meherji P, Shah N et al (2009) Genetic variation in exon 17 of INSR is associated with insulin resistance and hyperandrogenemia among lean Indian women with polycystic ovary syndrome. Eur J Endocrinol 160(5):855–862
21. Tucci S, Futterweit W, Concepcion ES, Greenberg DA, Villanueva R, Davies TF et al (2001) Evidence for association of polycystic ovary syndrome in Caucasian women with a marker at the insulin receptor gene locus. J Clin Endocrinol Metab 86:446–449
22. Siegel S, Futterweit W, Davies TF, Concepcion ES, Greenberg DA, Villanueva R et al (2002) A C/T single nucleotide polymorphism at the tyrosine kinase domain of the insulin receptor gene is associated with polycystic ovary syndrome. Fertil Steril 78(6):1240–1243
23. Chen ZJ, Zhao H, He L, Shi Y, Qin Y, Shi Y et al (2011) Genome-wide association study identifies susceptibility loci for polycystic ovary syndrome on chromosome 2p16.3, 2p21 and 9q33.3. Nat Genet 43:55–59
24. Shi Y, Zhao H, Shi Y, Cao Y, Yang D, Li Z et al (2012) Genome-wide association study identifies eight new risk loci forpolycystic ovary syndrome. Nat Genet 44(9):1020–1025
25. Kumar AN, Naidu JN, Stayanarayana U, Anitha M (2014) Past, Present and future of insulin gene and its related genes in relation to polycystic ovary syndrome. J Mol Genet Med 8:107
26. Ioannidis A, Ikonomi E, Dimou NL, Douma L, Bagos PG (2010) Polymorphisms of the insulin receptor and the insulin receptor substrates genes in polycystic ovary syndrome: a Mendelian randomization meta-analysis. Mol Genet Metable 99:174–183
27. Mutib MT, Hamd FB, Al-Salihi AR (2014) INSR gene variation is associated with decreased insulin sensitivity in Iraqi women with PCOS. Iran J Reprod Med 12(7):499–506

28. Urbanek M, Legro RS, Driscoll D, Strauss JF, Dunaif A, Spielman RS (2000) Searching for the polycystic ovary syndrome genes. J Pediatr Endocrinol Metab 13:1311–1313
29. Tehrani FR, Daneshpour M, Hashemi S, Zarkesh M, Azizi F (2013) Relationship between polymorphism of insulin receptor gene, and adiponectin gene with PCOS. Iran J Reprod Med 11(3):185–194
30. Xu X, Zhao H, Shi Y, You L, Bian Y, Zhao Y, Chen Z (2011) Family association study between INSR gene polymorphisms and PCOS in Han Chinese. Reprod Biol Endocrinol 9:76
31. Thangavelu M, Godla UR, Paul SFD, Ravi M (2017) Single-nucleotide polymorphism of INS, INSR, IRS1, IRS2, PPAR-G andCAPN10 genes in the pathogenesis of polycystic ovary syndrome. J Genet 96(1):87–96
32. Zhu AN, Yang XX, Sun MY, Zhang ZX, Li M (2015) Associations between INSR and MTOR polymorphisms in type 2 diabetes mellitus and diabetic nephropathy in a Northeast Chinese Han population. Genet Mol Res 14(1): 1808–1818
33. Bodhini D, Sandhiya M, Ghosh S, Majumder PP, Rao MR, Mohan V, Radha V (2012) Association of His1085His INSR gene polymorphism with type 2 diabetes in South Indians. Diabetes Technol Ther 14(8):696–700

2

Insulin receptor substrate-1 G972R single nucleotide polymorphism in Egyptian patients with chronic hepatitis C virus infection and type 2 diabetes mellitus

Rania Nabil Bedair[1], Gehan M. Magour[1], Said Ahmed Ooda[2], Eman M. Amar[1] and Ahmed M. Awad[1*]

Abstract

Background: Insulin receptor substrate-1 (IRS1) plays a critical role in insulin signaling. IRS-1 gene polymorphism with glycine to arginine substitution (GGG ↔ AGG substitutions) in codon 972 (G972R) (rs1801278) is a common polymorphism of the IRS-1 gene, which may have a pathogenic role in the development of type 2 diabetes mellitus (type 2 DM) due to insulin resistance and impaired insulin secretion. In hepatitis C virus infection (HCV), the IRS proteins might be counter-regulated by degradation, differential expression, or modification by phosphorylation in cells expressing HCV core protein, which inhibits the interactions of IRS-1 with both the insulin receptor and the downstream effectors of IRS-1. The present retrospective case–control study aimed to evaluate IRS-1 G972R (rs 1801278) SNP in Egyptian patients with HCV and type 2 DM, two hundred and two subjects including 100 males and 102 females The present work is a retrospective case–control study aimed to detect IRS-1 G972R (rs 1801278) SNP in Egyptian patients with chronic HCV infection and DM. The subjects were divided into the control group (group I) which included 50 apparently healthy volunteers of comparable age, gender, and socioeconomic status to patients; group II included 50 type 2 diabetic patients without chronic hepatitis C infection; group III included 52 chronic HCV-infected patients without type 2 diabetes mellitus; and group IV included 50 chronic hepatitis C-infected patients with type 2 diabetes mellitus. IRS-1 G972R (rs 1801278) genotyping was done by using polymerase chain reaction (PCR-RFLP) technique with restriction enzymes BstNI.

Results: HOMA-IR and QUICKI index was significantly higher in the patient groups (groups II, III, and IV) than controls ($P < 0.001$, $P = 0.019$, and $P < 0.001$ respectively). There was a significant increase in minor allele (A) in groups II, III, and IV than controls ($P = 0.007$, $P = 0.017$, and $P = 0.007$ respectively). There was increased frequency of mutant allele (A) than wild allele (G) of IRS-1 G972R polymorphism in type 2 diabetic patients with BMI < 25 kg/m^2. The DM patients without HCV infection (group II), HCV patients without DM (group III), and HCV patients with DM (group IV) showed a significant decrease in GG genotypes and a significant increase in AA genotypes than the controls ($P = 0.017$, $P = 0.019$, and $P = 0.009$ respectively). Body mass index and waist to hip ratio were significantly higher in DM patients without chronic hepatitis C infection (group II) and in HCV patients with type 2 diabetes (group IV) than controls, in hepatitis C patients with type 2 diabetes (group IV) than controls, and in group IV than group III ($P < 0.001$).

(Continued on next page)

* Correspondence: dr_amawad@hotmail.com
[1]Chemical Pathology Department, Medical Research Institute, Alexandria University, Alexandria, Egypt
Full list of author information is available at the end of the article

(Continued from previous page)
Conclusion: IRS-1 G972R (rs 1801278) polymorphism might be a contributing risk factor for the development of type 2 DM. The mutant allele (A) of IRS-1 suggests the role of this SNP as risk factors for type 2 diabetes mellitus even in subjects with normal body weight. The increase of body mass index may be an independent risk factor for the development of type 2 diabetes mellitus.

Keywords: Hepatitis C virus, Type 2 diabetes mellitus, Insulin receptor substrate-1 gene polymorphism

Background

Approximately 399,000 people die each year from hepatitis C, mostly from cirrhosis, hepatocellular carcinoma, and liver failure. HCV has been classified into six major genotypes; HCV genotype 4 is common in the Middle East and in Africa including Egypt [1, 2].

Type 2 diabetes mellitus (DM) is 1.8- to 2.5-fold higher in patients with chronic HCV infection and two- to three-folds more prevalent in HCV than in HBV infection [3–5].

During HCV infection, the tumor necrosis factor-α system is activated and interleukin-6 levels are increased, which disturb tyrosine phosphorylation of insulin receptor substrate-1 (IRS-1) [6].

Insulin receptor phosphorylates tyrosine residues of an intracellular cytoplasmic adaptor protein, the IRS. The IRS-1 is the first member of the family to be identified. The IRS-1 binding and phosphorylation leads to an increase in the high-affinity glucose transporter-4 (GLUT4) molecules on the outer membrane of insulin-responsive tissues, including muscle cells and adipose tissue causing an increase in the uptake of glucose from the blood into these tissues. Defects in muscle IRS-1 expression and function lead to impairment in the insulin signaling pathway resulting in insulin resistance and DM [7–9].

The IRS-1 gene contains the entire 5′-untranslated region and protein coding region in a single exon and is localized on chromosome 2. A glycine to arginine substitution (GGG ↔ AGG substitutions) in codon 972 (G972R) (rs 1801278) is the common polymorphism of the IRS-1 gene, which may have a pathogenic role in the development of type 2 DM due to insulin resistance and impaired insulin secretion [10–12]. IRS proteins might be counter-regulated by degradation, differential expression, or modification by phosphorylation in cells expressing HCV core protein which inhibits the interactions of IRS-1 with both the insulin receptor and the downstream effectors of IRS-1 [13].

Single nucleotide polymorphism in the IRS-1 gene has been frequently studied as a candidate gene in DM. To the best of our knowledge, no much data are available on IRS-1 G972R SNPs in HCV-infected populations with DM.

Methods

The present work is a retrospective case–control study aimed to detect IRS-1 G972R (rs 1801278) SNP in Egyptian patients with chronic HCV infection and DM. We conducted the current study on two hundred and two subjects consisted of 100 males and 102 females, divided into the control group (group I) which included 50 apparently healthy volunteers of comparable age, gender, and socioeconomic status to patients; group II included 50 type 2 diabetic patients without chronic hepatitis C infection; group III included 52 chronic HCV-infected patients without type 2 diabetes mellitus; and group IV included 50 chronic hepatitis C-infected patients with type 2 diabetes mellitus.

Any patient with hepatocellular carcinoma or any other malignancy, coexisting chronic viral infection like chronic hepatitis B (HBV), chronic kidney disease, liver cell failure, chronic pancreatitis, polycystic ovarian disease (PCOD), pregnant females, and those on treatment affecting insulin resistance were excluded from the study. All HCV-infected cases were active with positive PCR results during the time of the study.

The study was explained to all subjects, and written informed consents were taken from all of them. The study was conducted after approval of the Medical Research Institute, Alexandria University Ethical committee, no available reference number, and according to the Helsinki Declaration. The study was explained to all participating subjects, and written informed consents were taken from all of them.

Full history was taken from all subjects, full physical examination and anthropometric measurements including body mass index [14] and waist to hip ratio (WHR) [15] were done, and abdomen ultrasound was done to all subjects. Moreover, Child–Pugh classification [16] was done for the patient group only.

Child–Pugh scoring			
	1	2	3
Encephalopathy	None	Grades 1–2	Grades 3–4
Ascites	None	Mild/moderate	Severe
Serum albumin (g/dl)	> 3.5	2.8–3.5	< 2.8
Serum total bilirubin (mg/dl)	< 2	2–3	> 3
INR	< 1.7	1.7–2.3	> 2.3

Child–Pugh classification	
Risk group	Numerical score

Methods *(Continued)*

1- Child-Pugh class A	5–6 points
2- Child-Pugh class B	7–9 points
3- Child-Pugh class C	10–15 points

Also, there were some laboratory investigations performed on the participating subjects including fasting and postprandial serum glucose, glycated hemoglobin (HbA_1C), lipid profile, renal function tests, and liver enzymes [17]. Serum insulin was included [18], for the determination of Homeostatic Model Assessment of Insulin Resistance (HOMA-IR) [19] and Quantitative Insulin Sensitivity Check (QUICKI) index [20].

HCV polymerase chain reaction (PCR) [21], for groups III and IV only; antibodies for HCV [21], for groups I and II only; and lastly surface antigen for hepatitis B [22] were assayed for all groups. We have performed some molecular studies as follows: extraction of genomic DNA was done from peripheral blood leukocytes by using ion-exchange column chromatography. IRS-1 G972R (rs 1801278) genotyping by using polymerase chain reaction (PCR-RFLP) technique with restriction enzymes BstNI was done [23].

The molecular studies which had been done in the current study included the following.

DNA extraction from peripheral blood leucocytes [23]

The genomic DNA extraction from peripheral blood leukocytes was carried out using column-based commercial genomic DNA extraction kits Thermo Scientific Gene JET^{TM} Whole Blood Genomic DNA Purification Mini Kit #K0781 (Fermentas, Thermo, USA).

Then assessment of the integrity of the extracted genomic DNA was done by agarose gel electrophoresis (AGE). The Eppendorf containing the checked purified DNA in the elution buffer was tightly capped and stored till the time of PCR at – 20 °C.

Polymerase chain reaction amplification using specific primers [23]

A set of primers flanking the SNP region were used for the detection of insulin receptor substrate-1 G972R (rs 1801278) single nucleotide polymorphisms using the following reagent:

1. DreamTaq PCR Master Mix (2X) # K1071(200 runs of 50 µl) Thermo Scientific™
2. DNA gel Loading Dye (6X) # R0611: Thermo Scientific™
3. Primers: A pair of primers G972R (rs 1801278) polymorphisms were used. The lyophilized primers were supplied by Invitrogen, UK, which were reconstituted by addition of sterile nuclease-free water as follows:
   (a) Insulin receptor substrate-1 G972R (rs 1801278)

For the forward sense sequence, 165 µl was added and 126 µl for the reverse sense sequence to give a final concentration of 100 pmoles/µl for each and stored at – 20 °C. It was diluted to give a final concentration of 10 pmoles/µl.

I Primers for insulin receptor substrate-1 G972R (rs 1801278)

Forward sense sequence: (IRS-1- G02)

5′CTT CTG TCA GGT GTC CAT CC 3′ (Tm (thermodynamic) = 62 °C)

Reverse antisense sequence: (IRS-1- G03)

5′-TGG CGA GGT GTC CAC GTA GC 3 (Tm (thermodynamic) = 66 °C)

Protocol of amplification

In a 0.2-ml Eppendorf tube placed on ice, the following reagents were added and mixed:

DreamTaq PCR Master Mix (2X)	12.5 µl
Forward primer	0.5 µl (10 pmol)
Reverse primer	0.5 µl (10 pmol)
Extracted DNA	1 µl
Water nuclease free	10.5 µl

The total volume was 25 µl, and then the tubes were transferred to the thermal cycler (Quanta Biotech, UK) where the PCR conditions were adjusted (Table 1).

The amplified products were separated on 2% agarose gel electrophoresis after adding loading dye as follows: 2 µl loading dye added to 10 µl of amplified DNA.

Restriction digestion of PCR products using MvaI (BstNI) for insulin receptor substrate-1 G972R (rs 1801278) [23]

Restriction endonuclease enzymes, MvaI (BstNI) enzyme for insulin receptor substrate-1 G972R (rs 1801278) targeting specific sequence of the amplified DNA product for detection *IRS-1* G972R (rs 1801278) gene polymorphisms.

Reagents

- MvaI (BstNI) (10 U/µl) restriction enzyme recognized CC^WGG sites and cut best at 37 °C in R buffer. It is used for insulin receptor substrate-1 G972R (rs 1801278) polymorphism.

- 10 x buffer R for MvaI containing 10 mM Tris–HCl (pH 7.4 at 25 °C), 400 mM KCl, 0.1 mM EDTA, 1 mM DTT, 0.2 mg/ml BSA, and 50% glycerol.

Reagents were supplied by ThermoFisher Scientific, stored at − 20 °C.

Protocol for restriction enzymes

In an Eppendorf tube, the following reagents were mixed:

Water (nuclease free)	18 µl
10 x R buffer	2 µ
Amplified PCR product	10 µ
Restriction enzyme, BstNI	2 µ

Thus, the total volume was 32 µl. They were mixed gently, spin down for a few seconds, and incubated at 37 °C for 16 h, and then the digested products were separated on agarose gel electrophoresis after adding loading dye as follows: 2 µl of loading dye was added to 10 µl of restricted DNA products.

Agarose gel electrophoresis for the amplified and digested PCR products

1) Gene Ruler TM 50 bp DNA ladder (Thermo Fisher Scientific), the DNA fragments range from 50 to 1000 bp. It contains two reference bands: 250 and 500 bp.
2) Tris borate EDTA (TBE) buffer (10x) stock solution: working TBE (1x) buffer was prepared by measuring 100 ml stock solution and completed to 1 l of distilled water.
3) Agarose gel (wt/vol) 2.5% then 100 volts was applied for about 45 min till the loading dye had migrated to near the end of the plate. The DNA will migrate towards the anode.
   - A negative control, water (nuclease free), and a positive control, previous read samples, were allowed to run in case of amplified product detection.
   - Ultraviolet transillumination (302 nm) was used for visualization of the DNA bands.

Table 1 Thermal cycler condition of insulin receptor substrate-1 G972R (rs 1801278)

Phases	Cycle number	Temperature (°C)	Time
Initial denaturation	1	95	1 min
Amplification			
• Denaturation	35	95	1 min
• Annealing		61	45 s
• Extension		72	1 min
Final extension	1	72	7 min

Results

The amplified DNA leads to the formation of 263-bp amplicon. In the presence of the restriction enzyme MvaI (BstNI), allele G was digested to 159- and 81-bp fragments, whereas allele A yielded 108-bp, 81-bp, and 51-bp fragments, and the results were photographed.

So, in the amplified product G972R, the GG genotype appeared as two bands of 159 and 81 bp; the genotype GA appeared as four bands at 159, 108, 81, and 51 bp; and the AA genotype was expected to show three bands on 108, 81, and 51 bp (Figs. 1 and 2).

A missing 23-bp band did not appear. According to previous studies which used restriction enzyme MvaI (BstNI), GG genotype gives 159, 81, and 23 bp bands, and the AA genotype gives 108, 81, 51, and 23 bp. This band did not appear on our gel.

Results

There was no significant difference in both sex and age between the four studied groups (P = 0.101, 0.183) respectively.

BMI was significantly higher in DM patients without chronic hepatitis C infection (group II) and in HCV patients with type 2 diabetes (group IV) than controls and in group IV than group III ($P < 0.001$). The highest BMI was observed in HCV-infected patients with T2DM (group IV).

WHR was significantly higher in group II and group IV than in controls, in group III and group IV than in group II, and in group IV than in group III ($P < 0.001$).

Serum levels of liver enzymes (AST, ALT, and GGT) were significantly higher in patients of groups III and IV than in controls and in patients of group II with $P < 0.001$ for all. There was no significant difference between serum activities of AST and GGT in group II and in controls. By the reverse, serum activity of ALT was significantly increased in group II than in controls ($P = 0.032$). There was no significant difference between group IV and group III.

Serum cholesterol levels were significantly higher in patients of group II and significantly lower in patients of group III than in controls with $P < 0.001$. Serum cholesterol level was significantly increased in patients of group II than in patients of group IV with $P < 0.001$. There was no significant difference between group IV and controls ($P = 0.835$).

Serum triglyceride level was significantly higher in group II than in controls and group IV ($P < 0.001$ for both), but there was no significant difference between HCV patients (groups III and IV) and controls.

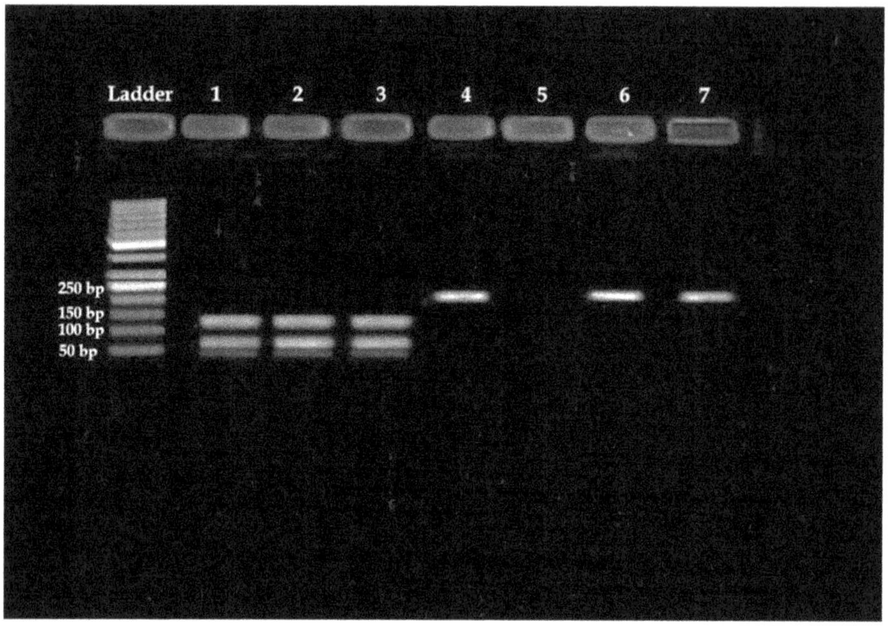

Fig. 1 Agarose gel electrophoresis (2.5%) of BstNI-digested PCR product for *IRS-1* G972R (rs 1801278). Ladder of 50-bp interval (50–1000 bp); lanes L1–3, AA; lanes 4, 6, and 7, amplified DNA before restriction; lane 5, negative control

High-density lipoprotein cholesterol (HDL-C) was significantly lower in patient groups (II, III, and IV) than in controls with $P < 0.001$ for all. And it was significantly higher in patients of group II than in patients of groups III and IV with $P < 0.001$.

Serum level of low-density lipoprotein cholesterol (LDL-C) was significantly higher in diabetes mellitus patient groups II and IV than in controls with $P < 0.001$. And it was significantly higher in patients of group II than in patients of group IV with $P = 0.012$. There was no significant difference between patients of group III and controls.

There was no significant difference between patients of group III and patients of group IV regarding HCV PCR level.

Fasting serum (FSG), postprandial serum glucose (PPSG), and glycosylated hemoglobin ($HbA_1C\%$) were significantly higher in DM patients (groups II and IV) than in controls ($P < 0.001$ for both) (Tables 2, 3, and 4).

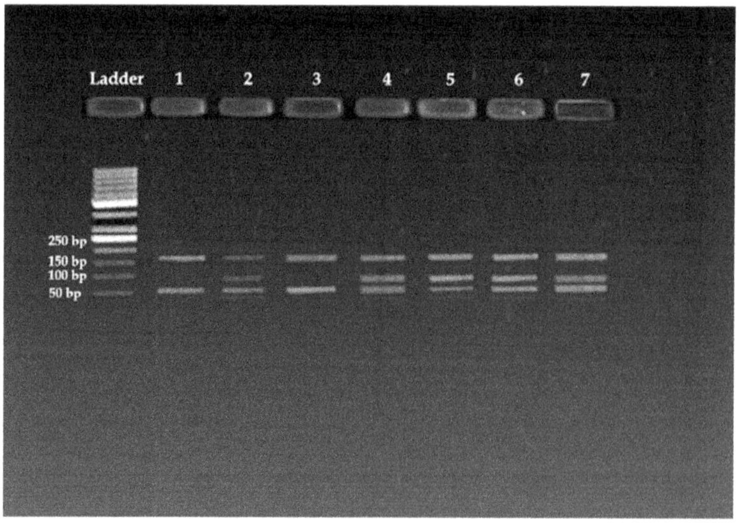

Fig. 2 Agarose gel electrophoresis (2.5%) of BstNI-digested PCR product for *IRS-1* G972R (rs 1801278). Ladder of 50-bp interval (50–1000 bp); lanes 1 and 3, GG; lanes 2 and 4–7, GA

Fasting insulin was significantly higher in the patient groups (groups II, III, and IV) than in controls ($P < 0.001$). It was significantly lower in group III than in groups II and IV ($P = 0.002$ and $P < 0.001$ respectively). It was significantly higher in group IV than in group II ($P < 0.001$) (Tables 2, 3, and 4).

HOMA-IR and QUICKI index was significantly different in the patient groups (groups II, III, and IV) than in controls ($P < 0.001$, $P = 0.019$, and $P < 0.001$ respectively) (Table 2).

Urea and creatinine and uric acid were significantly different in the patient groups (groups II, III, and IV) than in controls (Table 3).

There was no statistically significant difference between groups III and IV regarding severity of liver cirrhosis assessed by Child–Pugh classification ($P = 0.198$).

It was noticed that the observed frequencies of the different genotypes of IRS-1 G972R polymorphism were compared to the expected frequencies, according to the Hardy–Weinberg equilibrium, in the diseased group which showed $P > 0.05$ (after performing the chi-square test) indicating an agreement with the Hardy–Weinberg equilibrium.

The IRS-1 G972R polymorphism genotype distribution was significantly different between the four studied groups ($P = 0.034$). DM patients without HCV infection (group II), HCV patients without DM (group III), and HCV patients with DM (group IV) showed a significant decrease in GG genotypes and a significant increase in AA genotypes than the controls ($P = 0.017$, $P = 0.019$, and $P = 0.009$ respectively). There was no significant difference in genotype distribution between HCV-infected patients without DM (group III) and HCV-infected patients with DM (group IV) ($P = 0.880$). The highest frequency of wild genotype of IRS-1 polymorphism (GG) was in controls (70%), while the lowest one was in group IV (42%). The highest frequency of homozygous mutant genotype (AA) was in group II (8%), whereas the mutant genotype was absent in controls. HCV patients with DM (group IV) had the highest frequency of heterozygous genotype (GA) (54%) (Table 5, Fig. 3).

The allelic frequency was significantly different between the four studied groups ($P = 0.031$). There was a significant increase in minor allele (A) in groups II, III, and IV than in controls ($P = 0.007$, $P = 0.017$, and $P = 0.007$ respectively) (Table 5, Fig. 4).

Testing the dominant mode of inheritance, there was a statistically higher frequency of exposed genotypes "GA&AA" among the diabetics (group II) when compared to the control group (54% vs 30% respectively; $P = 0.016$) with a substantial increase in insulin resistance and DM risk among the exposed group (GA and AA) with a crude odds ratio of odds ratio (2.739) (95% confidence interval, 1.204–6.230) when compared to unexposed group (GG). After logistic regression analysis, the odds ratio was adjusted for BMI, age, and sex, to be 3.852 (95% confidence interval, 1.248–11.887) ($P = 0.019$).

Testing the recessive model was not applicable as the odds ratio cannot be estimated because of the absence of (AA) genotype among the control subjects.

Also, testing the dominant mode of inheritance, there was a statistically higher frequency of exposed genotypes "GA&AA" among HCV-infected patient group without diabetes (group III) than the control group (53.8 % vs 30% respectively; $P = 0.016$) with a substantial increase in insulin resistance and DM risk among the exposed group (GA and AA) with a crude odds ratio of OR (2.722) (95% confidence interval, 1.206–6.146) than the unexposed group (GG). After logistic regression analysis, the odds ratio was adjusted for BMI, age, and sex, to be insignificant 2.391 (95% confidence interval, 0.975–5.862) ($P = 0.057$).

Testing the recessive model was not applicable and the odds ratio cannot be estimated because of the absence of (AA) genotype among the control subjects.

Testing the dominant mode of inheritance, there was a statistically significant higher frequency of exposed genotypes "GA&AA" among group IV when compared to the control group (58% vs 30% respectively; $P = 0.005$) with apparently increased in insulin resistance and DM risk among the exposed group (GA and AA) with a crude odds ratio of odds ratio 3.2222 (95% confidence interval, 1.412–7.356) when compared to unexposed group (GG). After logistic regression analysis, the odds ratio was adjusted for BMI, age, and sex, to be insignificant 14.734 (95% confidence interval, 0.576–376.811) ($P = 0.104$), meaning that genotype exposure by itself was insignificant but with other confounders like BMI and the risk of IR and DM increased.

Testing the recessive model was not applicable and odds ratio cannot be estimated because of the absence of (AA) genotype among the control subjects.

There was a significant positive correlation between serum level of ALT and HOMA-IR with $r = 0.425$ and $P = 0.002$, and a significant negative correlation, inversely proportional, between serum level of ALT and QUICKI index in diabetic patients without chronic hepatitis C infection with $r = -0.408$ and $P = 0.003$.

There was a statistically significant difference regarding HOMA-IR and QUICKI index among different Child classes in groups III and IV, with HOMA-IR tending to increase and QUICK index tending to decrease with the increasing severity of liver cirrhosis, while there was no statistically significant difference regarding IRS-1 genotypes between different liver cirrhosis Child–Pugh classes in both groups (Tables 6 and 7).

Table 2 Statistical significance of fasting serum glucose level (FSG) (mg/dl), postprandial serum glucose (PPSG) (mg/dl), HbA_1C (%), fasting insulin (μIU/ml), and HOMA-IR and QUICKI index in the studied groups

	Group I (n = 50)	Group II (n = 50)	Group III (n = 52)	Group IV (n = 50)	Test of sig.	P
FSG (mg/dl)						
Min.–Max.	75.0–99.0	129.0–322.0	59.0–100.0	83.0–766.0	H = 143.378	< 0.001*
Mean ± SD.	86.3 ± 5.62	195.2 ± 51.82	82.31 ± 11.46	182.68 ± 106.6		
Median	87.0	189.0	80.0	168.50		
$P_{\text{Group I}}$		< 0.001*	0.239	< 0.001*		
Sig. bet. Grps		P_1 < 0.001*, P_2 = 0.132, P_3 < 0.001*				
PPSG (mg/dl)						
Min.–Max.	85.0–130.0	108.0–391.0	77.0–145.0	85.0–540.0	F = 72.836	< 0.001*
Mean ± SD.	102.3 ± 12.9	207.3 ± 70.44	101.6 ± 17.87	223.62 ± 81.85		
Median	99.0	201.0	95.0	210.0		
$P_{\text{Group I}}$		< 0.001*	1.000	< 0.001*		
Sig. bet. Grps		P_1 < 0.001*, P_2 = 0.447, P_3 < 0.001*				
HbA_1C (%)						
Min.–Max.	3.80–5.50	6.20–13.70	3.80–5.40	5.40–12.20	F = 145.963	< 0.001*
Mean ± SD.	4.68 ± 0.49	8.75 ± 2.01	4.58 ± 0.47	7.89 ± 1.42		
Median	4.80	8.10	4.50	7.75		
$P_{\text{Group I}}$		< 0.001*	0.974	< 0.001*		
Sig. bet. Grps		P_1 < 0.001*, P_2 = 0.005*, P_3 < 0.001*				
Fasting insulin (μIU/ml)						
Min.–Max.	1.20–10.10	5.40–77.0	2.40–25.30	10.0–514.2	H = 121.986	< 0.001*
Mean ± SD.	5.75 ± 2.65	17.09 ± 16.22	9.19 ± 3.65	40.68 ± 72.89		
Median	5.65	11.0	9.30	18.65		
$P_{\text{Group I}}$		< 0.001*	< 0.001*	< 0.001*		
Sig. bet. Grps		P_1 = 0.002*, P_2 < 0.001*, P_3 < 0.001*				
HOMA-IR						
Min.–Max.	0.30–2.20	2.70–49.0	0.50–5.30	4.60–65.10	H = 157.864	< 0.001*
Mean ± SD.	1.23 ± 0.55	9.14 ± 11.09	1.81 ± 0.73	12.76 ± 11.04		
Median	1.30	5.10	1.95	7.40		
$P_{\text{Group I}}$		< 0.001*	0.019*	< 0.001*		
Sig. bet. Grps		P_1 < 0.001*, P_2 = 0.055, P_3 < 0.001*				
QUICKI index						
Min.–Max.	0.34–0.49	0.23–0.33	0.30–0.43	0.21–0.31	F = 150.524	< 0.001*
Mean ± SD.	0.38 ± 0.04	0.30 ± 0.03	0.35 ± 0.02	0.28 ± 0.02		
Median	0.37	0.30	0.35	0.29		
$P_{\text{Group I}}$		< 0.001*	< 0.001*	< 0.001*		
Sig. bet. Grps		P_1 < 0.001*, P_2 = 0.009*, P_3 < 0.001*				

P_1 P value for comparing between group II and group III, P_2 P value for comparing between group II and group IV, P_3 P value for comparing between group III and group IV

Discussion

From the present study, it could be concluded that the minor allele "A" was associated with a statistically significant increased risk of developing insulin resistance and DM.

Although IRS-1 G972R polymorphism was studied in other Egyptian populations, the current study showed different genotype distributions. Shaker et al. [24] had studied the polymorphism on Egyptian patients, men and women, divided into three groups: DM lean, DM obese, and metabolic syndrome patients. The control group of healthy non-obese subjects. They found that most of the patient groups

Table 3 Statistical significance of serum urea, creatinine, and uric acid in the studied groups

Parameters	Group I (n = 50)	Group II (n = 50)	Group III (n = 52)	Group IV (n = 50)	Test of sig.	P
Urea (mg/dl)						
Min.–Max.	12.0–40.0	20.0–99.0	11.0–250.0	14.0–242.0	H = 41.355	< 0.001*
Mean ± SD.	26.32 ± 7.05	40.82 ± 20.38	47.58 ± 44.06	59.56 ± 43.55		
Median	26.0	34.0	35.0	45.0		
$P_{\text{Group I}}$		< 0.001*	< 0.001*	< 0.001*		
Sig. bet. Groups		P_1 = 0.829, P_2 = 0.028*, P_3 = 0.045*				
Creatinine (mg/dl)						
Min.–Max.	0.60–1.10	0.70–2.10	0.60–4.80	0.60–2.50	H = 50.629	< 0.001*
Mean ± SD.	0.81 ± .15	1.08 ± 0.38	1.25 ± 0.64	1.21 ± 0.42		
Median	0.80	0 .90	1.10	1.15		
$P_{\text{Group I}}$		< 0.001*	< 0.001*	< 0.001*		
Sig. bet. Groups		P_1 = 0.031*, P_2 = 0.031*, P_3 = 0.983				
Uric acid (mg/dl)						
Min.–Max.	2.90–5.80	3.80–10.0	2.10–6.70	3.50–9.30	F = 44.584	<0.001*
Mean ± SD.	4.33 ± .76	6.72 ± 1.74	4.17 ± 1.01	5.67 ± 1.40		
Median	4.30	6.50	4.10	5.30		
$P_{\text{Group I}}$		< 0.001*	0.916	< 0.001*		
Sig. bet. Groups		P_1 < 0.001*, P_2 < 0.001*, P_3 < 0.001*				

F, *F* for ANOVA test, pairwise comparison bet. each 2 groups was done using post hoc test (Tukey); *H*, *H* for Kruskal–Wallis test, pairwise comparison bet. each 2 groups was done using post hoc test (Dunn's for multiple comparisons test); *P*, *P* value for comparing between the different groups; $P_{\text{Group I}}$, *P* value for comparing between group I and each other groups; P_1, *P* value for comparing between group II and group III; P_2, *P* value for comparing between group II and group IV; P_3, *P* value for comparing between group III and group IV; *Sig. bet. Groups*, significance between groups
*Statistically significant at $P \leq 0.05$

were of GG genotype and the rest were of GA genotypes with no AA genotypes.

Elmougy et al. [23] studied IRS-1 G972R polymorphism on Egyptian subjects with PCOS in which patients and controls were divided into four categories based on their HOMA-IR results. They showed GA genotype only in HOMA-IR of > 6.4, suggesting the association of IRS-1 G972R polymorphism with higher insulin levels, as the study was conducted on females with PCOS categorized according to HOMA-IR illustrating the difference in genotype distribution between that study and the current study.

El-sisi et al. [25] also investigated the effect of IRS-1 G972R polymorphism on insulin secretion and how the polymorphism might predispose to sulfonylurea failure on 100 unrelated Egyptian patients with DM divided to two equal groups of those responsive to treatment and those resistant to sulfonylurea, 6% among controlled diabetic and 22% among uncontrolled were of GA genotype.

Recently, Yousef et al. [26] studied IRS-1 G972 R polymorphism on DM patients selected from the Department of Internal Medicine, Banha University. Patients who had a blood glucose level of > 250 mg/dL (severe hyperglycemia), aged over 30 years, and who used only insulin therapy during hospitalization were included. They found that genotype distribution was GG 70%, GA 26%, and AA 4%. They concluded that IRS-1 genetic factor may be a significant genetic determinant for IR in DM patients during severe/acute-phase hyperglycemia.

The discrepancy between the genotype distribution of previously mentioned studies and the current study might be due to different sub-classifications of the diabetic patients; inclusion or exclusion of different confounders of insulin resistance such as BMI, WHR, dyslipidemia, PCOS, metabolic syndrome (MS), intake of antidiabetic drugs, and HCV infection; and different sample size. Also, the existence of mutant allele in the control group in all previous studies may suggest that phenotype features of glucose intolerance might not be developed due to epigenetic elements or subjective factors.

Furthermore, in obese adults, the prevalence of the IRS-1 972 GA genotype among insulin-resistant PCOS

Table 4 Liver cirrhosis Child–Pugh class in groups III and IV

	Group III (n = 52)	Group IV (n = 50)	X^2	P
Child–Pugh class				
A	6	12	3.236	0.198
B	28	26		
C	18	12		

Table 5 Comparison between the four studied groups according to genotype distribution of IRS1 G972R (rs 1801278) polymorphism

Parameters	Group I (n = 50)		Group II (n = 50)		Group III (n = 52)		Group IV (n = 50)		χ^2	P
	N	%	N	%	N	%	N	%		
IRS1 G972R										
GG Homo wild	35	70.0	23	46.0	24	46.2	21	42.0	12.243*	$^{MC}P = 0.034^*$
GA Hetero	15	30.0	23	46.0	26	50.0	27	54.0		
AA Homo mutant	0	0.0	4	8.0	2	3.8	2	4.0		
Sig. bet. Grps	$^{MC}P_1 = 0.017^*$, $^{MC}P_2 = 0.019^*$, $^{MC}P_3 = 0.009^*$, $^{MC}P_4 = 0.700$, $^{MC}P_5 = 0.627$, $^{MC}P_6 = 0.880$									
G	85	85.0	69	69.0	72	69.2	74	74.0	8.861*	0.031*
A	15	15.0	31	31.0	32	30.8	26	26.0		
Sig. bet. Grps	$P_1 = 0.007^*$, $P_2 = 0.017^*$, $P_3 = 0.007$, $P_4 = 0.972$, $P_5 = 0.434$, $P_6 = 0.450$									

χ^2 chi-square test, *MC* Monte Carlo, *P P* value for comparing between the different groups, common letters are not significant (i.e., different letters are significant), P_1 *P* value for comparing between group I and group II, P_2 *P* value for comparing between group I and group III, P_3 *P* value for comparing between group I and group IV, P_4 *P* value for comparing between group II and group III, P_5 *P* value for comparing between group II and group IV, P_6 *P* value for comparing between group III and group IV, *Sig. bet. Grps* significance between groups
*Statistically significant at $P \leq 0.05$

patients in other studies ranged from 4.9 to 8% such as Sir-Petermann et al. [27], Sir-Petermann et al. [28], Villuendas et al. [29], and Dravecká et al. [30] found no heterozygous mutation. This was lower than in the current study. Still, the increased frequency of GA and AA in the present work might be due to the difference in racial and ethnic distribution and the lack of data concerning the prevalence of the polymorphism in DM specifically.

Assuming a dominant model of inheritance of IRS-1 G972R (rs1801278), the exposed group was considered as subjects with both (AA and GA) genotypes combined, while the unexposed group was considered as subjects with only (GG) genotype. Results of the present study revealed a statistically higher frequency of exposed genotypes (AA and GA) among DM patients without HCV (group II) than the control group, with a substantial increase in insulin resistance and DM risk among the exposed group (GA and AA).

This association between IRS-1 G972R (rs1801278), insulin resistance, and DM risk among DM patients without HCV infection (group II) remained after performing logistic regression analysis to adjust for some important insulin resistance confounding factors (BMI, age, and sex).

On the contrary, HCV-infected patients with DM (group IV) showed a statistically significant higher frequency of exposed genotypes (AA and GA) among group IV than the control group, with an apparent increase in insulin resistance and DM risk among the

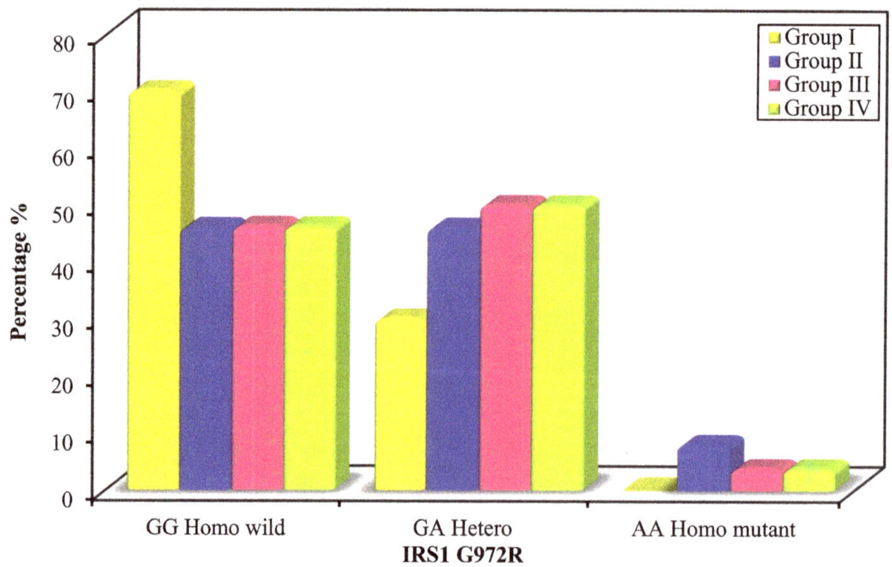

Fig. 3 Comparison between the four studied groups according to IRS1 G972R genotype distribution

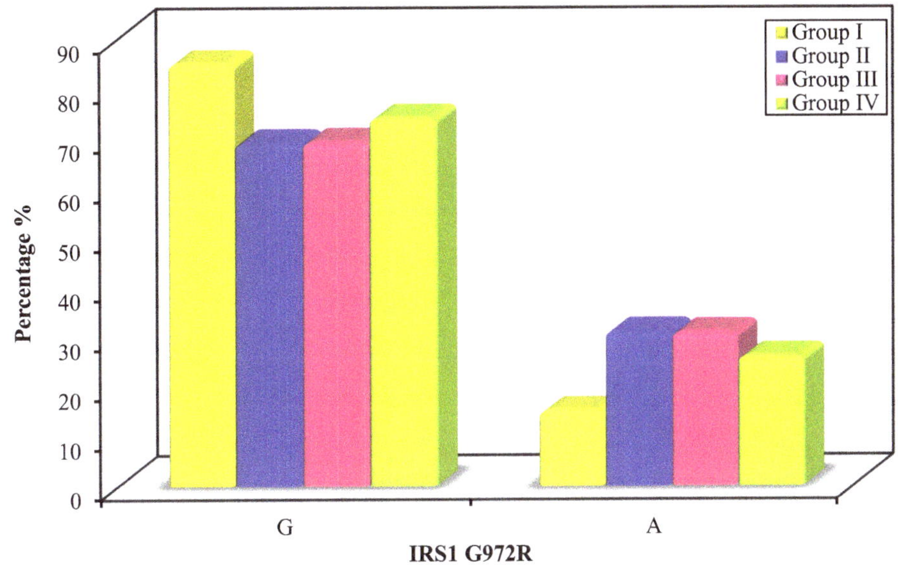

Fig. 4 Comparison between the four studied groups according to IRS1 G972R allele frequency

exposed group. After logistic regression analysis, the odds ratio was adjusted for BMI, age, and sex, to be insignificant, suggesting that genotype exposure by itself was insignificant but with other confounders like BMI, the risk of IR, and DM increased.

In agreement with the current study, IRS-1G972R polymorphism was shown to be associated with insulin resistance in many studies with different several populations and meta-analyses about DM. McGettrick et al. [31] determined the molecular mechanism by which this polymorphism was linked to insulin resistance. Burguete-Garcia et al. [32] in the Mexican population suggested the role of IRS-1G972R SNP in the genetic susceptibility to DM. Moreover, Huri et al. [33] in Malaysia using the polymerase chain reaction-restriction fragment length polymorphism method where a polymorphism in IRS-1 G972A showed a significant predictor of both insulin resistance and worsening of glycemic control.

However, the association between the IRS-1 G972R variant with DM has been controversial throughout the literature, and contrary to the current study, the lack of association has been also reported in other studies. Zeggini et al. [34] and Arikoglu et al. [12], in Turkish population; Bodhini et al. [35], in a South Indian; Elmougy et al. [23], in Egyptians; and Alsalman et al. [36], in Saudi Arabia population argued the lack of association between IRS-1 G972R and IR in their study due to multiple different genes and variants thought to be effective in the development of insulin resistance and DM.

These discrepancies in results might be due to insufficient statistical power and lack of adjustment for

Table 6 Insulin resistance (assessed by HOMA-IR and QUICKI index) and genotypes of IRS-1 SNP in relation to the degree of liver cirrhosis (assessed by Child–Pugh classification) in group III

	Child class A	Child class B	Child class C	Test of sig.	*P*
HOMA-IR					
Min.–Max.	0.80–5.30	0.50–2.40	0.90–2.40	$F = 3.324$	0.044
Mean ± SD.	2.267 ± 1.650	1.589 ± 0.501	1.994 ± 0.448		
QUICKI index					
Min.–Max.	0.30–0.40	0.33–0.43	0.33–0.39	$F = 3.444$	0.040
Mean ± SD.	0.352 ± 0.040	0.361 ± 0.022	0.342 ± 0.018		
Genotype					
GG	1	18	5	$X^2 = 8.934$	0.063
GA	5	9	12		
AA	0	1	1		

Table 7 Insulin resistance (assessed by HOMA-IR and QUICKI index) and genotypes of IRS-1 SNP in relation to the degree of liver cirrhosis (assessed by Child–Pugh classification) in group IV

	Child class A	Child class B	Child class C	Test of sig.	*P*
HOMA-IR					
Min.–Max.	4.60-29.60	5.10-27.50	5.00-65.10	$F = 8.689$	0.001
Mean ± SD.	8.867 ± 8.384	9.904 ± 5.418	22.833 ± 16.102		
QUICKI index					
Min.–Max.	0.25-0.31	0.21-0.30	0.23-0.30	$F = 6.668$	0.003
Mean ± SD.	0.291 ± 0.020	0.280 ± 0.022	0.260 ± 0.021		
Genotype					
GG	8	8	5	$X^2 = 5.173$	0.270
GA	4	17	6		
AA	0	1	1		

other potential insulin resistance confounding factors in some studies, recruitment procedures of the studied subjects, genetic heterogeneity, and differences in linkage disequilibrium between different populations as well as environmental backgrounds that might influence their phenotypes and may have an impact on the studied results.

In the current study, it was concluded that there was a statistically significant difference regarding HOMA-IR and QUICKI index among different Child classes in groups III and IV, with HOMA-IR tending to increase and QUICK index tending to decrease with the increasing severity of liver cirrhosis. In agreement with our results, Hideki Fujii et al. [37] concluded that HOMA-IR is an independent risk factor of advanced liver fibrosis in non-alcoholic and non-diabetic fatty liver disease. On the other hand, Dongiovanni et al. [38] had concluded that IRS-1 972Arg polymorphisms affecting insulin receptor activity predispose to liver damage and decrease hepatic insulin signaling in patients with NAFLD. This finding was in concordance with our conclusion of the lack of statistically significant difference regarding IRS-1 genotypes between different liver cirrhosis Child–Pugh classes in both liver patient groups (Tables 6 and 7). This disagreement can be attributed to different etiology of the liver cirrhosis between the current study, HCV infection, and Dongiovanni et al. study which was conducted on non-alcoholic liver disease patients.

Conclusions

From this study, it could be concluded that:

✓ IRS-1 G972R (rs 1801278) polymorphism might be contributing risk factors for the development of type 2 DM as established by the high frequency of minor allele (A) in type 2 diabetic patients without chronic hepatitis C infection.

✓ The increased frequency of mutant allele (A) than wild allele (G) of IRS-1 G972R polymorphism in type 2 diabetic patients with BMI < 25 kg/m^2 suggests the role of these SNPs as risk factors for type 2 diabetes mellitus even in subjects with normal body weight.

✓ The significant increase of body mass index in type 2 diabetics without HCV infection and HCV-infected patients with type 2 diabetes mellitus indicates its role as an independent risk factor for the development of type 2 diabetes mellitus.

✓ The study of other related gene polymorphisms that might contribute to the development of type 2 DM in chronic hepatitis C patients and additional studies on the association between IRS-1 G972R polymorphism and DM complications and its relation to the antidiabetic therapy response are recommended to be conducted on larger sample size; also, in the light of our study, it could be recommended that assessment of gene expression of IRS-1 in chronic hepatitis C-infected patients might be useful for early detection of type 2 diabetes in these patients.

Limitation of the study:

- Small size of subjects
- Lack of data about HCV genotype in the studied group

Acknowledgements

Not applicable.

Authors' contributions

SO analyzed and interpreted the patient data regarding the liver disease. EA performed the laboratory and molecular studies and was a major contributor in writing the manuscript. AW supervised the laboratory studies and subject selections. RB shared in research idea formulation and study design, and GM validated the data and managed and supervised the whole work. All authors read and approved the final manuscript.

Ethics approval and consent to participate
The study was conducted after approval of the Medical Research Institute, Alexandria University Ethical committee, no available reference number, and according to the Helsinki Declaration. The study was explained to all participating subjects, and written informed consents were taken from all of them.

Competing interests
The authors declare that they have no competing interests.

Author details
[1]Chemical Pathology Department, Medical Research Institute, Alexandria University, Alexandria, Egypt. [2]Experimental and Clinical Internal Medicine, Medical Research Institute, Alexandria University, Alexandria, Egypt.

References
1. Doss W, Shiha G, Hassany M, Soliman R, Fouad R et al (2015) Sofobuvir plus ribavirin for the treatment of Egyptian patients with hepatitis C genotype 4. J Hepatol 15:306–302
2. Mohamed R, Saeed R, Oun AR, Abdel-Halim K, Abdel-Aal M et al (2015) Hepatitis C virus vertical transmission in a sample of Egyptian pregnant women. J Am Sci 11:40–46
3. Negro F, Alaei M (2009) Hepatitis C virus and type 2 diabetes. World J Gastroenterol 15:1537–1547
4. Alvares da Silva MR, Wedemeyer H, Pinto HC, Souza CPM (2012) Hepatitis C and metabolic disorders: genetics, mechanism, and therapies (clinical and experimental). Int J Hepatol 2012:937202–937204
5. El Ray A, Asselah T, Moucari R, El Ghannam M, Taha AA et al (2013) Insulin resistance: a major factor associated with significant liver fibrosis in Egyptian patients with genotype 4 chronic hepatitis C. Eur J Gastroenterol Hepatol 25:421–427
6. Zakaria E, Fayad T, Rizk MN, Ghanem NS, Kamal M (2013) Association between insulin resistance, metabolic syndrome, and duration of hepatitis C in Egyptian patients. Egypt J Intern Med 25:213–217
7. Sesti G, Federici M, Hribal ML, Lauro D, Sbraccia P et al (2001) Defects of the insulin receptor substrate (IRS) system in human metabolic disorders. FASEB J 15:2099–2111
8. Rowland AF, Fazakerley DJ, James DE (2011) Mapping insulin/GLUT4 circuitry. Traffic 12:672–681
9. Menting JG, Whittaker J, Margetts MR, Whittaker L, Kong GKW, Smith BJ et al (2013) How insulin engages its primary binding site on the insulin receptor. Nature 493:241–245
10. Araki E, Sun XJ, Haag BL 3rd, Chuang LM, Zhang Y et al (1993) Human skeletal insulin receptor sustrate-1. Characterization of the cDNA, gene, and chromosomal localization. Diabetes 42:1041–1054
11. Alharbi KK, Khan IA, Abotalib Z, Al-Hakeem MM (2014) Insulin receptor substrate-1 (IRS-1) Gly927Arg: correlation with gestational diabetes mellitus in Saudi women. BioMed Res Int 2014:146495–146499
12. Arikoglu H, Hepdogru MA, Kaya DE, Asik A (2014) IRS1 gene polymorphisms Gly972Arg and Ala513Pro are not associated with insulin resistance and type 2 diabetes risk in non-obese Turkish population. Meta Gene 2:579–585
13. Banerjee S, Saito K, Goughoulte MA, Meyer K, Ray RB et al (2008) Hepatitis C virus core protein upregulates serine phosphorylation of insulin receptor substrate-1 and impairs the downstream Akt/Protein kinase B signaling pathway for insulin resistance. J Virol 82:2606–2612
14. Daud S, Javaid F (2012) Estimation of body mass index (BMI) in medical students. PJMHS 5:702–705
15. Wang C, Wang B, He H, Li X, Wei D, Zhang J et al (2012) Association between insulin receptor gene polymorphism and the metabolic syndrome in Han and Yi Chinese. Asia Pac J Clin Nutr 21:457–463
16. Verslype C, Rosmorduc O, Rougier P, Group EGW (2012) Hepatocellular carcinoma: ESMO-ESDO clinical practice guidelines for diagnosis, treatment and follow-up. Ann Oncol 23(Suppl 7):vii41–vii48
17. Burtis CA, Ashwood ER, Bruns DE (2012) Tietz textbook of clinical chemistry and molecular diagnostics, 5th edn. Elsevier Saunders Company, St Louis pp. 676-9 (albumin creatinine ratio), 718-22(glucose), 771-8 (lipid profile), 680-4(creatinine), 690 (uric acid), 143-6 (ALT, AST and GGT)
18. Guojun Z, Yanguo T, Ranxing Z, Yan Z, Tao K et al (2013) Analysis of current status of serum insulin determination by different chemiluminescence immunoassay systems. J Cap Med Univ 34:545–549
19. Matthews DR, Hosker JP, Rudenski AS, Naylor BA, Treacher DF, Turner RC (1985) Homeostasis model assessment: insulin resistance and beta-cell function from fasting plasma glucose and insulin concentrations in man. Diabetologia 28:412–419
20. Rabasa-Lhoret R, Bastard JP, Jan V (2003) Modified quantitative insulin sensitivity check index is better correlated to hyperinsulinemic glucose clamp than other fasting-based index of insulin sensitivity in different insulin-resistant states. J Clin Endocrinol Metab 88:4917–4923
21. Chakravarti A, Charhan MS, Dogra G, Banerjee S (2013) Hepatitis C virus core antigen assay: can we think beyond convention in resource limited settings? Braz J Infect Dis 17:369–374
22. Dufour R (2006) Hepatitis B surface antigen (HBs Ag) assays- are they good enough for their current uses? Clin Chem 52:1457–1459
23. Elmougy FA, Morgan MF, Elgayar DF, Mohey AM, Baz HN et al (2011) Allelic variants of insulin receptor substrate-1 gene in Egyptian women with polycystic ovary syndrome. Comp Clin Pathol 21:1689–1696
24. Shaker O, Abdel Hafez MA, Fayez S, Alsherif YM (2015) Phosphatidylinositol 3-kinase and insulin receptor substrate-1 gene polymorphism/ adipocytokines interaction in pathogenesis of insulin resistance among Egyptian patients: a pilot study. IJRSB 3(9):81–93
25. El-sisi AE, Hegazy SK, Metwally SS, Wafa AM, Dawood NA (2011) Effect of genetic polymorphisms on the development of secondary failure to sulfonylurea in Egyptian patients with type 2 diabetes. Adv Endocrinol Metab 2(4):155–164
26. Yousef AA, Behiry EG, Abd Allah WM, Hussien AM, Abdelmoneam AA, Imam MH et al (2018) IRS-1 genetic polymorphism (r.2963G>A) in type 2 diabetes mellitus patients associated with insulin resistance. Appl Clin Genet 11:99–106
27. Sir-Petermann T, Pérez-Bravo F, Angel B, Maliqueo M, Calvillan M, Palomino A (2001) G972R polymorphism of IRS-1 in women with polycystic ovary syndrome. Diabetologia 44(9):1200–1201
28. Sir-Petermann T, Angel B, Maliqueo M, Santos JL, Riesco MV, Toloza H et al (2004) Insulin secretion in women who have polycystic ovary syndrome and carry the Gly972Arg variant of insulin receptor substrate-1 in response to a high-glycemic or low-glycemic carbohydrate load. Nutrition 20(10):905–910
29. Villuendas G, Botella-Carretero JI, Roldán B, Sancho J, Escobar-Morreale HF, San Millán JL (2005) Polymorphisms in the insulin receptor substrate-1 (IRS 1) gene and the insulin receptor substrate-2 (IRS-2) gene influence glucose homeostasis and body mass index in women with polycystic ovary syndrome and non-hyperandrogenic controls. Hum Reprod 20(11):3184–3191
30. Dravecká I, Lazúrová I, Habalova V (2010) The prevalence of Gly972Arg and C825T polymorphisms in Slovak women with polycystic ovary syndrome and their relation to the metabolic syndrome. Gynecol Endocrinol 26(5):356–602
31. McGettrick AJ, Feener EP, Kahn CR (2005) Irs-1 Human insulin receptor substrate-1 (IRS-1) polymorphism G972R causes IRS-1 to associate with the insulin receptor and inhibit receptor autophosphorylation. J Biol Chem 280(8):6441–6446
32. Burguete-Garcia AI, Cruz-Lopez M, Madrid-Marina V, Lopez-Ridaura R, Hernandez-Avila M et al (2010) Association of Gly972Arg polymorphism of IRS1 gene with type 2 diabetes mellitus in lean participants of a national health survey in Mexico: a candidate gene study. Metabolism 59:38–45
33. Huri HZ, Makmor-Bakry M, Hashim R, Mustafa N, Wan Ngah WZ (2012) Optimisation of glycaemic control during episodes of severe/acute hyperglycaemia in patients with type 2 diabetes mellitus. Int J Clin Pharm 34:863–870
34. Zeggini E, Parkinson J, Halford S, Owen KR, Frayling TM et al (2004) Association studies of insulin receptor substrate 1 gene (IRS1) variants in type 2 diabetes samples enriched for family history and early age of onset. Diabetes 53:3319–3322
35. Bodhini D, Phil M, Radha V (2011) Association study of IRS1 gene polymorphisms with type 2 diabetes in South Indians. Diabetes Technol Ther 13(7):767–772

36. Alsalman HA, Kaabi YA (2015) Lack of association between the insulin receptor substrates-1 Gly972Arg polymorphism and type-2 diabetes mellitus among Saudis from Eastern Saudi Arabia. Saudi Med J 36(12):1420–1424
37. Fujii H, Imajo K, Yoneda M, Nakahara T, Hyogo H, Takahashi H et al (2019) HOMA-IR: An independent predictor of advanced liver fibrosis in nondiabetic non-alcoholic fatty liver disease. J Gastroenterol Hepatol 34(8): 1390–1395
38. Dongiovanni P, Valenti L, Rametta R, Daly AK, Nobili V, Mozzi E et al (2010) Genetic variants regulating insulin receptor signalling are associated with the severity of liver damage in patients with non-alcoholic fatty liver disease. Gut 59(2):267–273

3

Growth differentiation factor 15: an emerging diagnostic biomarker of liver fibrosis in chronic hepatitis C patients

Heba M. Adel Abou Zaghla[1*], Aziza Ahmed El Sebai[1], Ossama Ashraf Ahmed[2], Ayat Fawzy Ahmed[1] and Azza Abdel Rahman Saab[1]

Abstract

Background: Chronic liver disease and cirrhosis are of the major health concern worldwide. Assessment of liver fibrosis is necessary to determine disease severity and prognosis at the time of presentation to determine suitable treatment. Liver biopsy is considered as standard golden method in diagnosis of liver fibrosis. However, this procedure is invasive; thus, multiple laboratory and radiologic tests are used to help determination of the degree of fibrosis. Growth differentiation factor 15 (GDF-15) is a pleiotropic cytokine involved in regulating inflammatory and apoptotic pathways. It is suggested that GDF-15 plays an important role in pathogenesis of liver fibrosis. In this study, we aimed to evaluate efficiency of growth differentiation factor 15 in diagnosing liver fibrosis. The study was a case-control study conducted on 55 chronic HCV patients recruited from hepatitis C virus clinic at Faculty of Medicine Ain Shams Research Institute (MASRI), and 30 healthy subjects age- and sex-matched. The patients were classified into three subgroups according to the degree of liver fibrosis assessed by fibro-scan. Serum concentration of GDF-15 was determined by enzyme-linked immunosorbent assay.

Results: Our results revealed a highly significant statistical rise in GDF-15 levels among studied chronic HCV patients with liver fibrosis when compared to the control group ($p < 0.01$). Furthermore, there was a significant positive correlation between the degree of fibrosis assessed by fibro-scan and GDF-15 serum levels. Levels of GDF-15 were significantly higher in patients with mild degree of fibrosis (patients' subgroup I) when compared with the controls' group ($p < 0.01$) suggesting the role of this marker in early detection of liver fibrosis. A statistically significant increase in serum GDF-15 levels was noticed among patients with advanced fibrosis "subgroup III" compared to those with mild fibrosis "subgroup I" ($p < 0.05$). The diagnostic sensitivity and specificity of GDF-15 were 96.7%, 98.2%, respectively at a cut-off value of 150 ng/L for discrimination between patients' and controls' groups.

Conclusion: Growth differentiation factor 15 could be a potential marker of liver fibrosis especially in early detection as its levels were significantly higher in patients' group with liver fibrosis than controls' group and there was a significant positive correlation between the degree of liver fibrosis and GDF-15 serum levels.

Keywords: Liver fibrosis, Growth differentiation factor 15 (GDF-15)

* Correspondence: hebazaghla@hotmail.com
[1]Clinical Pathology, Ain Shams University, Cairo, Egypt
Full list of author information is available at the end of the article

Background

Liver fibrosis is a common pathological consequence of a variety of chronic stimuli including viral, autoimmune, drug induced, cholestatic, and metabolic diseases. Advanced liver fibrosis results in cirrhosis, portal hypertension, hepatocellular carcinoma, and liver cell failure [1].

Chronic liver disease has high global mortality rates. Egypt has a high hepatitis C virus (HCV) prevalence, where 11.5% of estimated populations are HCV positive [2]. Assessment of liver fibrosis helps clinicians to predict patient prognosis, to initiate treatment at early stage of fibrosis and to achieve high survival rate [3].

The degree of liver fibrosis is determined mainly by liver biopsy, but issues regarding its invasiveness and the small amount of liver tissue evaluated limit its applicability [4]. On the other hand, transient elastography (fibro-scan) is one of the most successful methods for assessment of liver fibrosis due to its noninvasive nature, reproducibility, and high diagnostic performance providing a quantifiable estimate of liver stiffness in unit known as kilopascals. Fibroscan measures liver stiffness in a volume of approximately a cylinder of 1-cm diameter and 5-cm long, which is roughly 100 times the volume of a percutaneous liver biopsy. In HCV fibroscan results ≤ 7 kPa account for F0–F1, results ≥ 7.1–8.6 kPa account for F1–F2, results ≥ 8.7–9.4 kPa account for F2, results ≥ 9.5–12.4 kPa accounts for F3, results ≥ 12.5–14.4 kPa account for F3–F4, results ≥ 14.5 kPa accounts for cirrhosis [5]. However, fibro-scan has some limitations in individuals with narrow intercostal spaces, morbid obesity, and increased liver stiffness for causes rather than fibrosis [6].

A series of serum markers of liver fibrosis had been developed. They are classified into direct and indirect markers. Direct markers refer to molecules involved in hepatic fibrogenesis and extracellular matrix turnover such as hyaluronic acid and Procollagen N-terminal peptide, while indirect markers involve molecules that reflect liver function such as ALT, AST, and GGT. Direct and indirect markers can be used alone or combined to form composite scores, e.g., AST-platelet ratio index (APRI), fibrosis-4 index (FIB-4 index), and hepascore. However, most of these markers are unable of accurate distinction of fibrosis stage especially early stages [7].

In the past few years, growth differentiation factor 15 (GDF-15) was the matter of research by many scientists. It is a transforming growth factor β (TGF-β) protein related to infection, fibrosis, and apoptosis pathways in case of tissue damage or disease. Its mRNA is known to be found particularly in the liver. In the presence of hypoxia, anoxia, inflammation, radiation exposure, and tissue injuries, the GDF-15 gene is expressed by activated macrophages which increase synthesis of GDF-15 protein [8]. Immediate induction of GDF-15 is an initial response to liver injury which can happen via TNF and p53 dependent and independent processes. Direct liver injury can induce GDF-15 expression in hepatocytes in the absence of other cell types such as inflammatory cells. GDF-15 has been put forward as a predictive biomarker of liver fibrosis and severity in patients with chronic liver disease. As a result of chronic damage to hepatocytes, prolonged stimulation of hepatic stellate cells results in the release of profibrogenic abundant factors such as GDF-15, leading to the development of liver cirrhosis. GDF-15 was found to not only stimulate transforming growth factor beta 1 (TGF-β1) expression, but it also induces fibrosis by directly increasing phosphorylation of SMAD2 and SMAD3, which play a crucial role in HSC activation and fibrogenesis. GDF-15 leads to increase expression of fibrosis markers, such as α-SMA and collagen I. Also, it leads to ECM accumulation by inhibition of tissue collagenases expression as well as increasing synthesis of tissue inhibitors of metalloproteinases [9].

Aim of the work

The aim of this work was to investigate the clinical utility of GDF-15 serum level as a predictor of the degree of liver fibrosis in patients with chronic HCV infection and correlation of its serum level with the fibro-scan value.

Methods

This case-control study was conducted from January 2019 to February 2020 on 55 HCV-positive patients who underwent fibro-scan for assessment of liver fibrosis. They were recruited from hepatitis C virus Clinic at Faculty of Medicine Ain Shams Research Institute (MARSI). In addition, 30 age- and sex- matched apparently healthy subjects served as healthy controls. The study was in accordance with the Declaration of Helsinki (2013). All participants gave their written consent to enter the study. The study has been approved by the ethical committee of Faculty of Medicine, Ain Shams University.

Subjects were classified into the following groups

Patient group (n = 55)

This group included 55 patients undergoing fibro-scan for assessment of liver fibrosis caused by chronic HCV infection. They were 35 males and 20 females. Their ages ranged from 27 to 75 years. They were further divided into the following subgroups according to the degree of fibrosis.

Subgroup I "F0 and F1" (*n* = 18) This group included 18 patients with fibrosis stage of F0 and F1 with liver stiffness measure (LSM) less than or equal 7 kPa. Their ages range from 26 to 67 years.

Subgroup II "F2" (n = 13) This group included 13 patients with fibrosis stage of F2 with LSM (7.1–9.4 kPa). Their ages range from 28 to 74 years

Subgroup III "F3–F4" (n = 24) This group included 24 patients with fibrosis stag of F3 with LSM (9.5–12.4 kPa) and F4 with LSM (≥ 12.5 kPa). Their ages range from 38 to 75 years.

Control group (n = 30)

This group included thirty age- and sex-matched subjects. Their HCV antibody test was negative, and their pelvi-abdominal U/S showed no abnormality. They were 19 males and 11 females. Their ages range from 25 to 70 years.

Subjects with any of the following conditions were excluded from the study; HCV, alcohol abuse, evidence of autoimmune liver disease, BMI of more than 35 kg/m^2, hepatocellular carcinoma or any extrahepatic malignancy and intake of any medication known to have injurious effect on the liver.

All individuals in this study were subjected to the following

- Full history taking: focusing on chronic liver disease and its complications, smoking, alcohol, drugs, and any immunological disease.
- Thorough clinical examination with special emphasis on abdominal examination, presence of jaundice, edema, or ascites.
  Radiological investigations including transient elastography (for patients only) and pelvi-abdominal ultrasound.
- Laboratory investigations including:
  - Routine laboratory investigations; including complete blood count, fasting blood sugar, liver profile (total and conjugated bilirubin, serum ALT, AST, INR, total protein, and albumin), and alfa fetoprotein.
  - HCV Ab testing and polymerase chain reaction for HCV.
  - Assay of serum concentration of GDF-15 by enzyme-linked immunosorbent assay (ELISA).

Analytical method of GDF-15

Growth differentiation factor-15 concentration was measured using a commercially available ELISA kit supplied by Shanghai Korain Biotech Co.., Ltd. The level of GDF-15 in samples was determined using a double-antibody sandwich ELISA. In this technique, GDF-15 is captured between two antibodies. The first is GDF-15 monoclonal antibody that was fixed to the inner wall of ELISA wells plate and the second is labeled with biotin to which Streptavidin-horse radish peroxidase (HRP) is combined forming immune complex. Addition of substrate results in color development that is stopped by acidic stopping solution. Absorbance of the developed color is measured spectrophotometrically at a wavelength of 450 nm. The concentration of GDF-15 is proportional to the intensity of the color of test sample. A standard curve is constructed from which the concentrations of GDF-15 in the samples are determined.

Results

Statistical analysis

IBM SPSS statistics (V. 26.0, IBM Corp., USA, 2019) was used for data analysis. p value > 0.05 will be considered statistically significant.

The results obtained in the present study are shown in Tables 1, 2, 3, 4, and 5 and Figs. 1, 2, 3, 4, 5, 6, and 7.

Table 1 demonstrates the descriptive statistics of the different studied parameters in the control group.

Table 2 demonstrates the descriptive and comparative statistics of the various studied parameters between the three patients' subgroups included in this study using Kruskal-Wallis test. Significant difference was revealed between the three subgroups regarding different studied parameters (age, AST, ALT, total and direct bilirubin, albumin, platelets count, INR, and AFP) (p < 0.05). Nine results of AFP were only available with subgroup I patients among 18 patients in this retrospective study (as they may be considered as low-risk patients for cancer liver). Borderline significant difference was revealed as regards GDF-15 (p value 0.075) among the three patients' subgroups using Kruskal-Wallis test but by doing post hook test using Wilcoxon rank sum test between each two groups, levels of GDF-15 were significantly higher in subgroup III patients when compared with subgroup I patients. No significant difference was

Table 1 Descriptive statistics of the different studied parameters in the control group

Parameter	Median (n = 30)	Q1–Q3 (n = 30)
Age (years)	31	27–46.25
Weight (kg)	76	69–87.25
AST (IU/L)	18	8–20
ALT (IU/L)	17	7–19
T. bilirubin (mg/dl)	0.7	0.5–0.8
D. bilirubin (mg/dl)	0.2	0.1–0.2
Albumin (g/L)	4.3	4–4.5
Platelets (10^3/ul)	240	190.25–260
INR	1	0.987–1.025
AFP (IU/ml)	2	1–4.25
GDF-15 (ng/L)	110	100–120

Table 2 Descriptive and comparative statistics of the different studied parameters in the different patient subgroups

Parameter	Liver fibrosis patient group (n = 55)									Kruskal-Wallis test	
	Subgroup I F0-F1			Subgroup II F2			Subgroup III F3–F4			H	p value
	n.	Median	Q1–Q3	*n.*	Median	Q1–Q3	*n.*	Median	Q1–Q3		
Age (years)	16	32	28–47.25	12	37.5	32–47.5	22	52.5	43.75–57.5	12.522	0.002
Weight (kg)	18	73.5	68–78.25	13	75	67.5–86.5	24	70	66.5–84.5	0.273	0.873
AST (IU/L)	18	28	21–36.25	13	25	19–43	24	50.5	8.75–72.5	20.873	0
ALT (IU/L)	18	27	20.25–43.5	13	35	21.5–48	24	47	35.5–64.25	9.367	0.009
T. bilirubin (mg/dl)	18	0.65	0.475–0.8	13	0.6	0.35–0.8	24	1	0.8–1.75	16.122	0
D. bilirubin (mg/dl)	18	0.2	0.1–0.2	13	0.2	0.1–0.3	24	0.3	0.2–0.7	13.276	0.001
Albumin (g/L)	17	4.1	3.95–4.45	13	4.2	4–4.5	24	3.55	3.2–4.1	14.857	0.001
Platelets (10^3/ul)	18	232	188.25–256	13	256	219–295.5	24	135	91–223.75	15.835	0
INR	18	1	0.987–1.025	13	1	1–1.1	23	1.1	1–1.3	10.895	0.004
AFP (IU/ml)	9	2.5	1.2–5.45	11	2.9	1.9–4.5	23	9.2	2.9–13.6	9.89	0.007
GDF-15 (ng/L)	18	340	220–500	13	500	405–510	24	415	335–587.5	5.185	0.075

Q1–Q3* = interquartile range (25th–75th percentiles); p value > 0.05 is non-significant; p value < 0.01 is highly significant

revealed among the three patients' subgroups using Kruskal-Wallis test as regards weight (p value 0.8).

The statistical comparison of different studied parameters was done between each two patients' subgroup using Wilcoxon rank sum test. A high significant difference was revealed between subgroups II and III patients, and between subgroups I and III patients regarding different studied parameters (age, AST, ALT, total and direct bilirubin, albumin, platelets count, INR, and AFP), p value < 0.01. While no significant difference was revealed between subgroups I and II patients regarding all studied parameters (p > 0.05). Also, no significant difference was revealed between each two patients' subgroup regarding weight as p value > 0.05.

Table 3 demonstrates comparative statistics of GDF-15 level between different groups using Wilcoxon rank sum test. Levels of GDF-15 were significantly higher in all patients' group when compared with the controls' group (p value = 0). Also, levels of GDF-15 were significantly higher in subgroup I patients when compared with the controls' group (p value = 0). Levels of GDF-15 were higher but not significantly in subgroup II patients

Table 3 Comparative statistics of GDF-15 between control group and whole patients' group and between each two patients' subgroups using Wilcoxon's rank sum test

Group	**Control (n = 30)**		**Patient group (n = 55)**		**Wilcoxon rank sum test**	
Parameter	**Median**	**Q1–Q3**	**Median**	**Q1–Q3**	***Z***	***p* value**
GDF-15 (ng/L)	110	100–120	410	300–530	− 7.442	0
Group	**Control (n = 30)**		**Patient subgroup I (n = 18)**		**Wilcoxon rank sum test**	
Parameter	**Median**	**Q1–Q3**	**Median**	**Q1–Q3**	***Z***	***p* value**
GDF-15 (ng/L)	110	100–120	340	220–500	− 5.753	0
Group	**Subgroup I F0–F1 (n = 18)**		**Subgroup II F2 (n = 13)**		**Wilcoxon rank sum test**	
Parameter	**Median**	**Q1–Q3**	**Median**	**Q1–Q3**	***Z***	***p* value**
GDF-15 (ng/L)	340	220–500	500	405–510	− 1.834	0.067
Group	**Subgroup I F0–F1 (n = 18)**		**Subgroup III F3–F4 (n = 24)**		**Wilcoxon rank sum test**	
Parameter	**Median**	**Q1–Q3**	**Median**	**Q1–Q3**	***Z***	***p* value**
GDF-15 (ng/L)	340	220–500	415	335–587.5	− 2.065	0.039
Group	**Subgroup II F2 (n = 13)**		**Subgroup III F3–F4 (n = 24)**		**Wilcoxon rank sum test**	
Parameter	**Median**	**Q1–Q3**	**Median**	**Q1–Q3**	***Z***	***p* value**
GDF-15 (ng/L)	500	405–510	415	335–587.5	− 0.08	0.936

Q1–Q3* = Interquartile range (25th–75th percentiles) p value > 0.05 is non-significant, p value < 0.01 is highly significant

Table 4 Three models of logistic multi regression analysis used to predict the most sensitive predictors of liver fibrosis

Module	Module 1				Module 2				Module 3			
Item	Reg. Coef.	*t*	*p*	Sig.	Reg. Coef.	*t*	*p*	Sig.	Reg. Coef.	*t*	*p*	Sig.
Platelets (10^3/ul)	− 0.003	− 1.605	0.126	NS	− 0.003	− 2.55	0.01	S	− 0.002	− 1.66	0.014	S
GDF-15 (ng/L)	0	− 0.463	0.649	NS	0.001	2.112	0.04	S	0.001	2.002	0.05	S
Weight (kg)	− 0.023	− 2.201	0.041	S	0.006	0.828	0.41	NS				
Prothrombin time (s)	0.21	1.609	0.125	NS	0.065	0.705	0.48	NS				
INR	− 2.712	− 1.917	0.071	NS	0.474	0.43	0.67	NS				
Age (years)	− 0.002	− 0.204	0.841	NS								
Height (cm)	0.016	0.885	0.388	NS								
AST (IU/L)	0.006	0.862	0.4	NS								
ALT (IU/L)	0.003	0.468	0.645	NS								
Bilirubin (mg/dl)	0.2	0.041	0.968	NS								
Direct bilirubin (mg/dl)	0.238	0.049	0.962	NS								
Indirect bilirubin (mg/dl)	0.431	0.089	0.93	NS								
Albumin (g/L)	− 0.017	− 0.065	0.949	NS								
Creatinine (mg/dl)	0.01	0.101	0.921	NS								
Fasting blood sugar (mg/dl)	− 0.003	− 0.818	0.424	NS								
Alfa fetoprotein (IU/ml)	0.016	0.803	0.433	NS								
F ratio	2.16				2.984				6.003			
p	0.059				0.02				0.005			
Sig.	Not significant				Significant				Highly significant			

$p > 0.05$ is non-significant; $p < 0.05$: significant; $p < 0.001$ highly significant

when compared with subgroup I patients, and levels of GDF-15 were significantly higher in subgroup III patients when compared with subgroup I patients. Levels of GDF-15 were higher but not significantly in subgroup III patients when compared with subgroup II patients.

Spearman's rank correlation analysis was done between different stages of fibrosis classified according to fibro-scan and measured in kilopascal (kPa) and the studied parameters in patients' group and also, Spearman's rank correlation analysis was done between GDF-15 serum levels and the studied parameters in patients' group. As seen in Fig 1, a significant positive correlation was found between the degree of fibrosis and GDF-15 serum levels in all patients' group ($r = 0.286$ and p value = 0.034), but no significant correlation was found between the degree of fibrosis and GDF-15 serum levels in different patients' subgroups (Figs. 2, 3, and 4). Spearman's rank correlation analysis also revealed a highly significant positive correlation between fibrosis degree and age, AST, ALT, and INR with p value < 0.01 and a highly significant negative correlation between fibrosis degree and both albumin and platelets count p value <

Table 5 Diagnostic performance of GDF-15 as a marker of liver fibrosis for discriminating different groups

	Cut-off	Sensitivity (%)	Specificity (%)	NPV (%)	PPV (%)	EFF (%)	AUC
GDF-15(ng/L) for discriminating HCV patients' group from the control group	150	96.7	98.2	96.7	98.2	97.6	0.99
GDF-15(ng/L) for discriminating subgroup I patients from control group	150	100	96.7	100	94.7	97.9	0.798
GDF-15(ng/L) for discriminating subgroup I (F0–F1) patients from subgroup II (F2)	400	66.7	76.9	80.8	62.5	71.0	0.694
GDF-15(ng/L) for discriminating subgroup I (F0–F1) patients from subgroup III (F3–4)	220	27.8	95.8	83.3	63.9	66.7	0.687
GDF-15(ng/L) for discriminating subgroup II (F2) patients from subgroup III (F3–F4).	420	54.2	69.2	76.5	45.0	59.5	0.508

AUC area under the curve, *NPV* negative predictive value, *PPV* positive predictive value, *EFF* efficiency

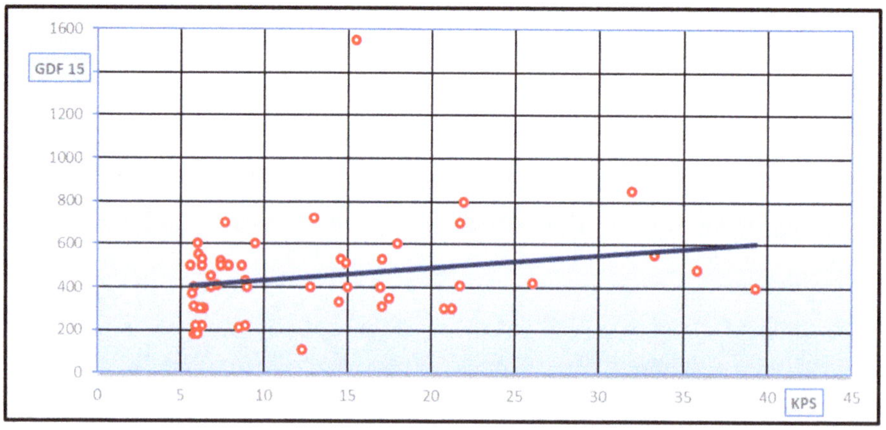

Fig. 1 Correlation study between GDF-15 and fibroscan in KPS in all patients group [$r = 0.086$ and $p = 0.034$ (significant)]

0.01. It was found a significant negative correlation between GDF-15 serum levels and the weight ($r = -0.314$ and p value = 0.019).

Logistic regression was used as shown in Table 4 to estimate the association between the degree of liver fibrosis and different independent variables. It showed that the most sensitive independent variables to predict liver fibrosis were GDF-15 (p value 0.05) and platelets (p value 0.01).

Receiver operating characteristic (ROC) curve analysis was also applied to assess the diagnostic performance GDF-15 (ng/L) in diagnosis of liver fibrosis. The best-balanced cut-off level of GDF-15 that discriminates between chronic HCV patient with liver fibrosis and controls was 150 ng/L, at which sensitivity was 96.7%, specificity 98.2%, positive predictive value (PPV) 98.2%, negative predictive value (NPV) 96.7%, and the diagnostic efficiency was 97.6%, with an area under the curve (AUC) of 0.99 as shown in Fig. 5 and Table 5.

Receiver operating characteristic (ROC) curve analysis was applied to assess the diagnostic performance GDF-15 (ng/L) in diagnosis of liver fibrosis. The best-balanced cut-off level of GDF-15 that discriminates between subgroup I patients and controls was 150 ng/L, at which sensitivity was 100%, specificity 96.7%, positive predictive value (PPV) 94.7%, negative predictive value (NPV) 100%, and the diagnostic efficiency was 97.9%, with an area under the curve 0.798 as shown in Fig. 6 and Table 5.

Another ROC curve analysis was applied to assess the diagnostic performance GDF-15 for discriminating between subgroups I and Ц patients. The best diagnostic cut-off for GDF-15 was 400 ng/L, which had a diagnostic specificity of 76.9%, sensitivity 66%, NPV 80%, PPV 62.5%, and efficacy 71%. AUC was 0.694 as shown in Fig. 7 and Table 5. The combined use of GDF-15 and platelets count at cut-off 400 ng/L and 320,000/ul, respectively, achieved an increase in sensitivity (100%),

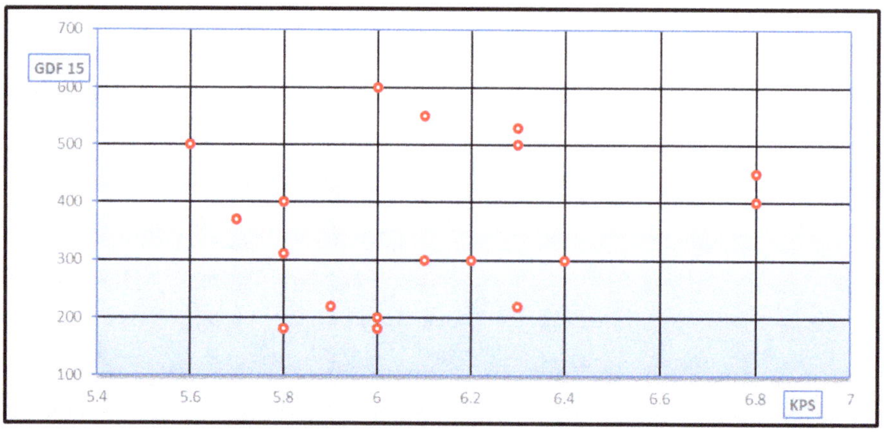

Fig. 2 Correlation study between GDF-15 and fibroscan in KPS in group I patients [$r = 0.15$ and $p = 0.553$ (non-significant)]

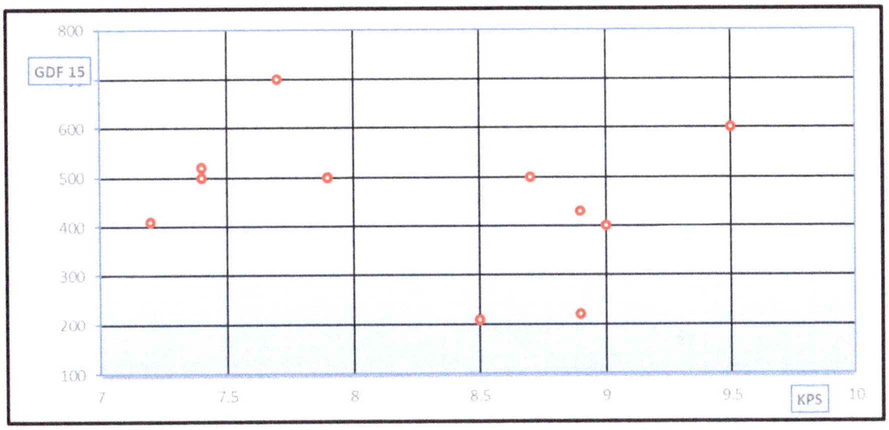

Fig. 3 Correlation study between GDF-15 and fibroscan in KPS in group II patients [$r = -0.251$ and $p = 0.409$ (non-significant)]

specificity (84.6%), NPV 90%, PPV 100%, and efficacy 93.5% by multi-ROC analysis with AUC = 0. 897.

Also, another ROC curve analysis was applied to assess the diagnostic performance GDF-15 for discriminating between subgroups I and III patients. The best diagnostic cut-off for GDF-15 was 220 ng/L, with a diagnostic specificity of 95.8%, sensitivity 27.8%, NPV 83.3%, PPV 63.9%, efficacy 66.7%, and AUC 0.687 as shown in Fig. 7 and Table 5. An increase in sensitivity (100%), specificity (95.8%), NPV 94.7%, PPV 100%, and efficacy 97.6% was achieved after adding PLTs at cut-off of 330,000/ul by the multi-ROC analysis with AUC = 0.93.

The last ROC curve analysis was applied to assess the diagnostic performance of GDF-15 for discriminating between subgroups II and III patients. The best diagnostic cut-off for GDF-15 was 420 ng/L, with a diagnostic specificity of 69.2%, sensitivity 54.2%, NPV 76.5%, PPV 45%, efficacy 59.5%, and AUC 0.508 as shown in Fig. 7 and Table 5. Also, an increase in sensitivity (100%), specificity (92.3%), NPV (96%), PPV (100%), and efficacy (97.3%) was observed after adding PLTs at cut-off 254, 000/ul by Multi-ROC analysis with AUC = 0.914.

Discussion

Growth differentiation factor 15 (GDF-15), a distant member of the transforming growth factor β (TGF-β) superfamily, has been identified as a pleiotropic protein that plays key roles in fetal development, inflammation, regulation of cellular responses to stress signals, and in tissue repair [10].

Serum GDF-15 levels were significantly increased in patients with liver cirrhosis and hepatocellular carcinoma [11]. Furthermore, high serum GDF-15 level is associated with a risk of advanced fibrosis among NAFLD subjects [12].

Growth differentiation factor 15 leads to the extracellular matrix (ECM) accumulation directly by increasing the synthesis of ECM components as procollagen 1a and indirectly by inhibition of tissue collagenases expression and increasing synthesis of ECM-degrading enzyme

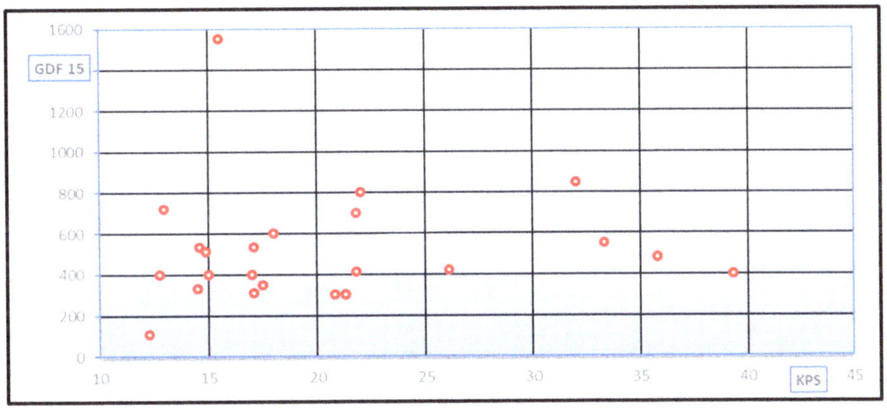

Fig. 4 Correlation study between GDF-15 and fibroscan in KPS in group III patients [$r = 0.203$ and $p = 0.342$ (non-significant)]

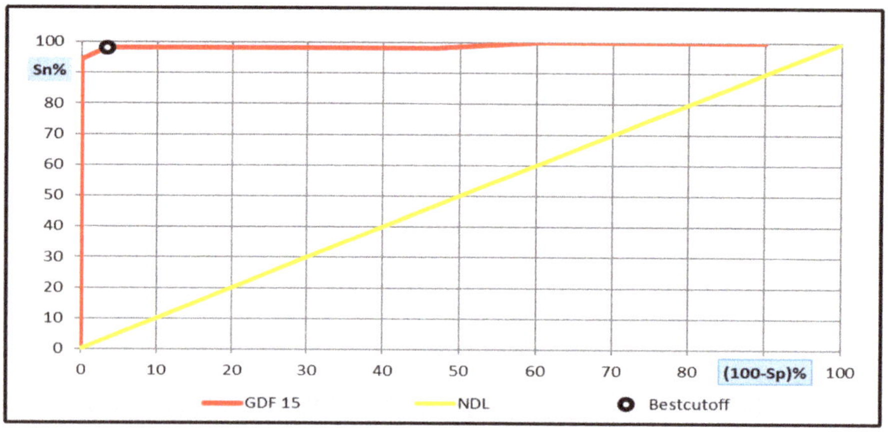

Fig. 5 Receiver operating characteristic curve (ROC) analysis showing the diagnostic performance of GDF-15 for discriminating HCV patients with liver fibrosis from those control with area under the curve (AUC) = 0.99

inhibitors (as plasminogen activator inhibitor type 1 and tissue inhibitors of metalloproteinases) [8]. Thus GDF-15 has been put forward as a predictive biomarker of liver fibrosis and severity in patients with chronic liver disease [13].

The aim of this work was to study the clinical utility of GDF-15 serum level in prediction of the degree of liver fibrosis in patients with chronic HCV infection through correlation of its levels with fibrosis degree assessed by fibro-scan.

Results of our study revealed a highly significant statistical rise in GDF-15 levels among studied chronic HCV patients when compared to the control group. Similar results were obtained by Cheng et al. [11] who measured serum GDF-15 levels in 54 patients with chronic HCV. They reported that GDF-15 was associated with the pathogenesis of hepatitis C virus as a host response to viral proteins, infection-induced cell stress or both. Also, Abdulla et al. [14] reported that GDF-15 levels were increased in the serum of patients with cirrhosis and/or hepatocellular carcinoma compared with controls.

Subgroup I patients with mild degree of liver fibrosis showed significantly higher GDF-15 levels than control group (p value = 0), suggesting the role of this marker in early detection of liver fibrosis. A statistically significant increase in serum GDF-15 levels was noticed among patients with advanced fibrosis (subgroup III) compared to those with mild fibrosis (subgroup I), while there was no significant difference in the GDF-15 level among patient subgroups I and II and between patient subgroups II and III. Krawczyk et al. [15] assessed degree of liver fibrosis in 229 patients by both liver biopsy and fibro-scan and in 605 patients by fibro-scan only. They reported that GDF-15 could not discriminate between significant

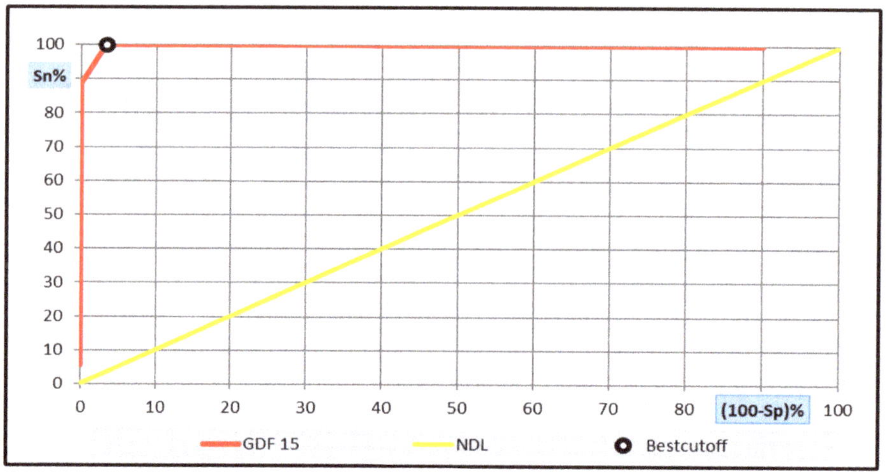

Fig. 6 Receiver operating characteristic curve (ROC) analysis showing the diagnostic performance of GDF-15 for discriminating patients with subgroup-1 (F0–1) from those control with area under the curve (AUC) = 0.798

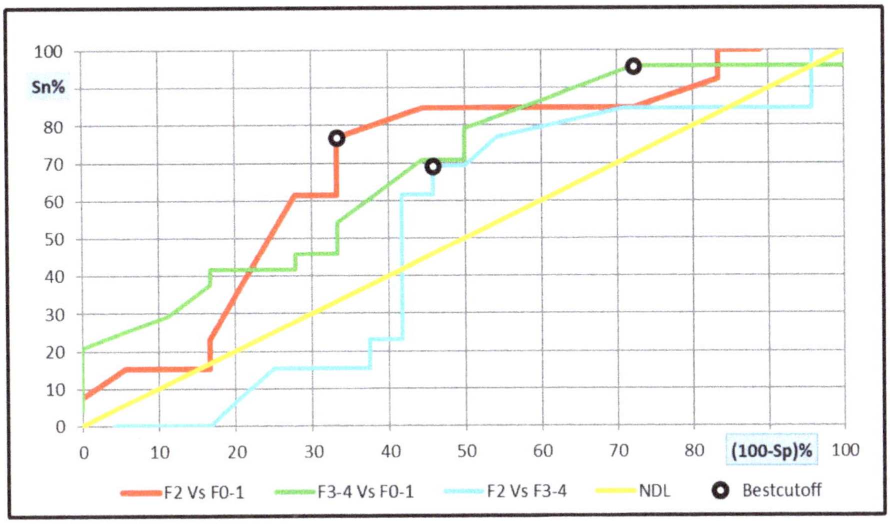

Fig. 7 ROC curve analysis showing the diagnostic performance of GDF-15 for discriminating patients of different patients'groups

fibrosis (≥F2) and cirrhosis (≥F4) in patients staged with fibro-scan only.

The present study revealed a significant positive correlation between the degree of fibrosis assessed by transient elastography and GDF-15 serum levels in all patients' group, but no significant correlation was found between transient elastography and GDF-15 in the three patients' groups separately. These results are in contrast with those of Krawczyk et al. [15] who proved that there is a highly significant correlation between GDF-15 level and histological stages of fibrosis; this might be due to small sample size in each patients' subgroup in our study. In addition, Kim et al. [8] found that patients with more severe chronic liver diseases had proportionately higher GDF-15 values. Furthermore, they stated that the increase in GDF-15 is caused by fibrosis rather than the hepatocellular damage by the infections in chronic liver diseases.

Also, our study showed a highly significant positive correlation between the degree of fibrosis and AST, ALT, total bilirubin, direct bilirubin and prothrombin time and a highly significant negative correlation between the degree of fibrosis and both albumin and PLTs count. Our study showed a significant negative correlation between GDF-15 levels and the weight. However, there was no significant correlation between GDF-15 and the other studied parameters.

In our study, a cut-off of 150 ng/L was found to discriminate both liver fibrosis degree of F0–1 from control and chronic HCV patients with liver fibrosis from controls. However, Kim et al. [8] who studied 246 Asian subjects, reported a cut-off of 574 ng/L for discriminating chronic hepatitis patients from controls. This discrepancy may be attributed to different performance of the used kits, our relatively small sample size, and difference between ethnic groups.

Also, ROC curve analysis was applied to assess the diagnostic performance of GDF-15 in detecting early fibrosis, and also discriminating between early and advanced fibrosis. The best diagnostic cut-off early detection of fibrosis for GDF-15 was 150 ng/L, which had a diagnostic specificity of 96.7%, sensitivity 100%, NPV 100%, PPV 94.7%, and efficacy 97.9%. The best diagnostic cut-off for discriminating between early and advanced fibrosis for GDF-15 was 220 ng/L, which had a diagnostic specificity of 95.8%, sensitivity 27.8%, NPV 83.3%, PPV 63.9%, and efficacy 66.7%. AUC was 0.687. Fortunately, the combined use of GDF-15 and platelets count at cut-off 220 ng/L and 330,000/ul respectively achieved in an increase in sensitivity (100%), specificity (95.8%), NPV (94.7%), PPV (100%), and efficacy (97.6%) by multi-ROC analysis with AUC = 0.930.

It is noteworthy that the platelet count is a convenient marker of liver fibrosis in several hepatic diseases, such as nonalcoholic fatty liver disease, hepatitis B and C; nevertheless, there are studies reporting conflicting results as thrombocytopenia is valuable marker of advanced liver disease and combined assessment of the AST/ALT ratio and platelet had a high diagnostic value for cirrhosis [16].

Conclusion

Serum GDF-15 levels can significantly differentiate between chronic HCV patients with liver fibrosis and healthy controls, and also can discriminate between early and advanced liver fibrosis. Therefore, GDF-15 can be used as an early predictor of liver fibrosis assisting physicians initiating treatment earlier hence achieving higher survival rate.

Abbreviations

AFP: Alpha fetoprotein; ALT: Alanine transaminase; APRI: AST-platelet ratio index; AST: Aspartate transaminase; AUC: Area under curve; BMI: Body mass index; ECM: Extracellular matrix; ELISA: Enzyme-linked immunosorbent assay; FIB-4 index: Fibrosis-4 index; GDF-15: Growth differentiation factor 15; GGT: Gamma glutamyl transferase; HCV: Hepatitis C virus; HRP: Streptavidin-horse radish peroxidase; INR: International normalized ratio; MARSI: Medicine Ain Shams Research Institute; NAFLD: Nonalcoholic fatty liver disease; NPV: Negative predictive value; PPV: Positive predictive value; ROC: Receiver operating characteristic; TGF-β: Transforming growth factor beta

Acknowledgements

To our institute and our families.

Authors' contributions

HAZ and AAS supervised, reviewed, and validated the final manuscript and were responsible for conceptualization. AAR contributed to the writing and editing of the manuscript and contributed to setting the research methodology, while OAA contributed to the manuscript review and sample collection. Finally, AFA was responsible for original draft preparation and writing, sample funding collection, and research methodology. All authors read, revised, and approved the final manuscript.

Ethics approval and consent to participate

The study was in accordance with the Declaration of Helsinki. All participants gave their written consent to enter the study. The study has been approved by the ethical committee of Faculty of Medicine, Ain Shams University. The reference number is not applicable. Ethical issues (including plagiarism, data fabrication, double publication) have been completely observed by the authors.

Competing interests

The authors declare that they have no competing interests.

Author details

[1]Clinical Pathology, Ain Shams University, Cairo, Egypt. [2]Internal Medicine, Faculty of Medicine, Ain Shams University, Cairo, Egypt.

References

1. Elpek GÖ (2014) Cellular and molecular mechanisms in the pathogenesis of liver fibrosis: an update. World J Gastroenterol 20(23):7260–7276
2. Abu-Raddad LJ, Kouyoumjian SP, Chemaitelly H (2018) Characterizing hepatitis C virus epidemiology in Egypt: systematic reviews, meta-analyses, and meta-regressions. Sci Rep 8:1661
3. Milani S, Stasi C (2016) Non-invasive assessment of liver fibrosis: between prediction/prevention of outcomes and cost-effectiveness. World J Gastroenterol 22(4):1711–1720
4. Alves V, Ragazzo T, Paranagua-Vezozzo D, Lima F, Mazo D, Pessoa M, Oliveira C, Carrilho F (2017) Accuracy of transient elastography-fibroscan, acoustic radiation force impulse (ARFI) imaging, the enhanced liver fibrosis (ELF) test, APRI, and the FIB-4 index compared with liver biopsy in patients with chronic hepatitis C. Clinics 72(9):516–525
5. de Lédinghen V, Vergniol J (2008) Transient elastography (FibroScan). Gastroenterol Clin Biol 32(6):58–67
6. Cequera A, García de León Méndez MC (2014) Biomarkers for liver fibrosis; advances, advantages and disadvantages. Rev Gastroenterol Mex 79(3):187–199
7. Khalili K, Sharma S, Nguyen GC (2014) Non-invasive diagnosis of advanced fibrosis and cirrhosis. World J Gastroenterol 20(45):16820–16830
8. Kim HJ, Lee ES, Kim SH, Kim KH, Lee BS, Ku BJ (2017) Growth differentiation factor 15 predicts chronic liver disease severity. Gut Liver 11(2):276–282
9. Koo BK, Um SH, Seo DS, Joo SK, Bae JM, Park JH, Chang MS, Kim W et al (2018) Growth differentiation factor 15 predicts advanced fibrosis in biopsy-proven non-alcoholic fatty liver disease. Liver Int 38(4):695–705
10. Delanghe JR, Desmedt S, Desmedt V, De Vos L, Speeckaert R, Speeckaert MM (2019) Growth differentiation factor 15: a novel biomarker with high clinical potential. Crit Rev Clin Lab Sci 56(5):333–350
11. Cheng M, Liu X, Chi X, Gong Q, Gao L, Niu Y, Chi X, Si Y, Wang M, Zhong J, Niu J, Yang W (2015) Association of serum level of growth differentiation factor 15 with liver cirrhosis and hepatocellular carcinoma. PLoS One 10(5): e0127518
12. Bae JM, Koo BK, Um SH, Seo DS, Joo SK, Park JH, Chang MS, Kim JH, Lee J, Jeong W, Kim W (2018) Growth differentiation factor 15 predicts advanced fibrosis in biopsy-proven non-alcoholic fatty liver disease. Liver Int 38(4): 695–705
13. Cheng M, Si Y, Liu X, Wang M, Gong Q, Yang Y, Wang T, Yang W (2011) Growth differentiation factor 15 is induced by hepatitis C virus infection and regulates hepatocellular carcinoma-related genes. PLoS One 6(5):e19967
14. Abdulla NA, Halim MH, Kamel A, Abdel El Maksoud N, Ragab HM (2017) Significance of growth differentiation factor 15 in chronic HCV patients. J Genet Eng Biotechnol 15(2):403–407
15. Krawczyk M, Zimmermann S, Hess G, Holz R, Dauer M et al (2017) Correlation: panel of three novel serum markers predicts liver stiffness and fibrosis stages in patients with chronic liver disease. PLoS ONE 12(6): e0179205
16. Shao L-N, Zhang S-T, Wang N, Yu W-J, Chen M, Xiao N et al (2020) Platelet indices significantly correlate with liver fibrosis in HCV-infected patients. PLoS ONE 15(1):e0227544

4

Effectiveness and safety of ombitasvir/paritaprevir/ritonavir in treatment of chronic hepatitis C Egyptian hemodialysis patients, case-control study

Nahla Mohamed Teama[1*], Waleed Anwar Abdel-Mohsen[1], Ossama Ashraf Ahmed[2], Sarah Mohamed El Sayed[1] and Ahmed Mohamed ElGhandour[2]

Abstract

Background: Prevalence of hepatitis C virus infection in patients with renal diseases is higher compared to the general population. FDA has approved ombitasvir/paritaprevir/ ritonavir for the treatment of patients with severe renal disease. This study aimed to evaluate the efficacy and safety of *ombitasvir/paritaprevir/ritonavir* with or without ribavirin in treatment of chronic hepatitis C Egyptian hemodialysis patients to compare it with the same treatment result in chronic hepatitis C Egyptian patients with normal renal functions. This case-control study was conducted on one hundred patients with confirmed diagnosis of HCV-positive infection at the Center of National Committee for Control of Viral Hepatitis [NCCVH] at Ain Shams University Hospital. Patients were divided into two groups: group I (control group) with 50 chronic hepatitis C virus patients with normal renal functions and group II (Case Group) with 50 chronic hepatitis C virus hemodialysis patients.

Results: 95.1% of prevalent hemodialysis patients achieved sustained virological response (SVR), while 100% of patients with normal kidney functions achieved sustained virological response. Most common side effects were hemoglobin drop, gastrointestinal disturbance, severe fatigue, and itching.

Conclusion: Ombitasvir, paritaprevir, and ritonavir are considered a safe and effective in treatment in HCV infection in patients on regular hemodialysis as in chronic hepatitis C virus infection patients with normal kidney functions.

Keywords: Ombitasvir, Paritaprevir, Ritonavir, Ribavirin chronic hepatitis C, Hemodialysis

Background

Hepatitis C virus infection is a major global health problem. Over 80 million are estimated to be chronically infected throughout the world, with 3–4 million new infections and 350,000 deaths occurring due to HCV-related complications such as cirrhosis and hepatocellular carcinoma annually [1]. Egypt's prevalence of infection with hepatitis C virus (HCV) is the highest in the globe. The high prevalence is mainly due to the parenteral antischistosomal therapy campaigns that were conducted between the 1950s and the 1980s in which more than 6 million individuals received 36 million injections, almost all with shared unsterilized syringes and needles. This is the greatest iatrogenic spread of blood-borne infection ever to occur [2]. Direct-acting antivirals (DAAs) transformed HCV management into a curable disease. The use of standard interferon-based therapies was correlated with low efficacy and elevated toxicity in patients with elevated renal functions. Recent advancement of DAAs has dramatically altered the treatment of chronic hepatitis C and interferon-free regimens have become the preferred therapy in clinical practice [3].

* Correspondence: nahlateama@med.asu.edu.eg
[1]Department of Internal Medicine and Nephrology, Faculty of Medicine, Ain Shams University, Ramsis 38 Street, Abassia, Cairo 11211, Egypt
Full list of author information is available at the end of the article

Three direct-acting antiviral (3D) regimen is an all-oral interferon-free combination of the protease inhibitor paritaprevir co-formulated with ritonavir as a systemic PK enhancer and the nonstructural protein 5A (NS5A) inhibitor ombitasvir [4].

Recently, the FDA has endorsed ombitasvir/paritaprevir/ ritonavir (OBV/PTV/ RITONA) for treatment of patients with severe renal disease. Metabolism of these compounds is mediated mainly by the liver. Treatment with OBV/PTV/RITONA ± RBV is currently approved for patients infected with HCV, based on the results of several clinical trials in which sustained virological response (SVR) rates at week 12 (SVR12) reached 95–100% [5].

The aim of this study was to evaluate the efficacy and safety of *ombitasvir/paritaprevir/ritonavir* with or without ribavirin in treatment of chronic hepatitis C Egyptian hemodialysis patients and compare it with the same treatment result in chronic hepatitis C Egyptian patients with normal renal functions.

Methods

This study was performed in accordance with the ethical standards of Ain Shams University Research Committee and with the 1964 Helsinki Declaration and its later amendments or comparable ethical standards. Ethics committee's reference number is 00017585.

Written informed consent was obtained from all individual participants included in the study. Informed consent to publish patient's data was signed by all participants prior to the beginning of the research.

Patient selection

One hundred patients were enrolled in this study and were selected from the Center of National Committee for Control of Viral Hepatitis [NCCVH] in Ain Shams University Hospital. All patients with chronic hepatitis C were treated with ombitasvir/paritaprevir/ritonavir with or without ribavirin during the period between May 2018 and December 2018.

Study design

The patients were assigned into 2 groups:

Group I (control group): Fifty chronic hepatitis C virus patients with normal renal functions as assessed by serum creatinine and by calculation of GFR. All patients in this group received ombitasvir/paritaprevir/ritonavir with ribavirin [1000/1200 mg on the basis of bodyweight ≤ 75/> 75 kg].

Group II (case group): Fifty chronic hepatitis C virus infection prevalent hemodialysis patients for more than 6 months; these patients received conventional hemodialysis 3 sessions per week each 4 h long using standard dialysate containing bicarbonate and biocompatible hemodialysis (HD) membrane and heparin as an anticoagulant; they received ombitasvir/paritaprevir/ritonavir with ribavirin at a dose of 200 mg three times/week, 4 h before session of hemodialysis. Ribavirin was stopped when hemoglobin level less than 8.5 gm/dl.

All patients in the drug and control groups were subjected to the following: full history, full clinical examination, and laboratory investigations before treatment including liver function tests (alanine transaminase (ALT), aspartate transaminase (AST), total bilirubin, serum albumin, hepatitis B surface antigen (HBsAg), Alpha Fetoprotein (AFP), HCV PCR quantitative), serum creatinine, hemoglobin A1c (HbA1c), complete blood picture (CBC), and pelvi-abdominal ultrasound. Laboratory investigations during treatment included AST, ALT, total bilirubin, serum albumin, serum creatinine, international normalized ratio (INR), and CBC. Laboratory investigations after treatment were HCV PCR quantitative at week 16 and 24 from start of treatment.

All patients were subjected to regular follow-up monthly visits at NCCVH at Ain Shams University Hospitals and side effects were detect during these visits and in between monthly visits by telephone or extra visits if needed.

Patients with ages less than 18, chronic hepatitis B, decompensated liver cirrhosis [child C], severe anemia (hemoglobin level less than 10 gm), known HCC or other malignancy or known cardiac or neuropsychiatric disease were excluded from the study.

Statistical analysis

Data were collected, revised, coded, and entered to the Statistical Package for Social Science (IBM SPSS) version 23. The quantitative data were presented as mean, standard deviations, and ranges when their distribution was found to be parametric and median with interquartile range (IQR) when their distribution was found to be non-parametric. Also, qualitative variables were presented as number and percentages. The comparison between groups regarding qualitative data was done using *Chi-square test.* The comparison between two independent groups with quantitative data and parametric distribution were done using *Independent t test* while data with non-parametric distribution were done using *Mann-Whitney test.* The comparison between more than two paired groups with quantitative data and parametric distribution were done using *repeated measure ANOVA test,* while comparison between more than two paired groups with quantitative data and non-parametric distribution was done using *Friedman test.* The confidence interval was set to 95% and the margin of error accepted was set to 5%.

So, *p* value was considered significant as the following: *p* value < 0.05, significant (S)

Results

This study included 100 patients divided into two groups. Group I included 50 patients; 35 males and 15 females with mean age 47 years. Five patients had hypertension and eight patients had diabetes mellitus. Group II included 50 patients, 30 males and 20 females with mean age 51 years. Twenty-five patients had hypertension and 14 patients had diabetes. All patients were naïve to antiviral treatment.

Of 100 participants, 91 patients completed the course of treatment, six patients stopped treatment due to adverse effects, two patients died during the course of treatment, and one patient died after the course of treatment but before performing HCV PCR quantitative at week sixteen of treatment.

95.1% of prevalent hemodialysis patients achieved cure which means they achieved sustained virological response (SVR), while 100% of patients with normal kidney functions achieved sustained virological response. The most common side effects were hemoglobin drop, gastrointestinal disturbance, severe fatigue, and itching.

Table 1 shows that 95.1 % of hemodialysis patients and 100% of control group achieved end of treatment response and sustained virologic response. There was no statistically significant difference between two groups regarding the cure rate.

There was highly statistically significant differences between the two groups regarding presence of gastrointestinal (GIT) symptoms which includes nausea, vomiting, and GIT upset with *p* value of 0.006 and statistically significant difference between two groups regarding patients that stopped treatment during course due to severe anemia and sever fatigue with *p* value of 0.012 (Table 2). There was statistically significant difference between two groups regarding patients needed blood transfusion during treatment with *p* value of 0.022 and no statistical difference between two groups regarding itching and sever fatigue; no statically significant difference between the two groups regarding death rate. Three patients died during the course of treatment, 2 patients had sudden death, and 1 patient died due to cerebral hemorrhage despite normal platelet level and normal INR.

Table 1 Comparison between group I (control group) and group II (case group) regarding cure rate after treatment

Cure	Group I No. = 50	Group II No. = 41	Test value*	*p* value
Complete	50 (100.0%)	39 (95.1%)	2.494	0.114
Relapse	0 (0.0%)	2 (4.9%)		

*Chi-square test

Table 2 Comparison between group I (control group) and group II (case group) regarding complications occurred during the course of treatment

	Group I		Group II		Test value[a]	*p* value
	No.	%	No.	%		
Patient stopped treatment	0	0.0	6	12.0	6.383	0.012
Death	0	0.0	3	6.0	3.093	0.079
Blood transfusion	0	0.0	5	10.0	5.263	0.022
Itching	0	0.0	2	4.0	2.041	0.153
Sever fatigue	0	0.0	3	6.0	3.093	0.079
Gastrointestinal symptoms	0	0.0	7	14.0	7.527	0.006

[a]Chi-square test

There is a difference in hemoglobin, albumin, and creatinine levels between dialysis and normal group with high statistically significant difference (*p* value, 0.001), but there is no significant change in AST, ALT, total bilirubin, INR, and platelet levels.

There is a difference in hemoglobin, total bilirubin, and creatinine levels between dialysis and normal group with high statistically significant difference (*p* value 0.001); there is statistical difference in albumin and platelet levels with *p* value of 0.028, but there is no significant change in AST, ALT, and INR.

There is a difference in hemoglobin, total bilirubin, and creatinine levels between dialysis and normal group with high statistically significant difference (*p* value, 0.001); there is statistical difference in albumin level with *p* value of 0.030.

There is a difference in hemoglobin, albumin, and creatinine levels between the dialysis and normal group with high statistically significant difference (*p* value, 0.001); there is statistically difference in total bilirubin level with *p* value of 0.047, but there is no significant change in AST, ALT, INR, and platelet levels.

From Tables 3, 4, 5, and 6, there is a decrease in hemoglobin level along the treatment course with high statistically significant difference (*p* value, 0.001), a decrease in AST and ALT levels along the course of treatment with high statistically significant difference (*p* value, 0.001) and there is increase at total bilirubin level with high statistically significant difference (*p* value, 0.001), but there is no significant change in albumin, INR, platelet, and creatinine levels during the course of treatment.

Also, from the Tables 3, 4, 5, and 6, there is a decrease in hemoglobin level along the treatment course in the case group with high statistically significant difference (*p* value, 0.001), a decrease in AST and ALT level along the course of treatment with high statistically significant difference (*p* value, 0.001), and an increase at total bilirubin level and INR with

Table 3 Comparison between group I (control group) and group II (case group) regarding levels of hemoglobin, AST, ALT, albumin, total bilirubin, INR, platelets, and creatinine before start of treatment

		Group I	Group II	Test value	*p* value
Hemoglobin (gm/dl)	Mean ± SD	14.56 ± 1.72	12.09 ± 1.75	7.111	0.001
	Range	10.8–17.6	10–16.4		
AST (U/L)	Normal	31 (62.0%)	37 (74%)	1.654	0.198
	High	19 (38.0%)	13 (26%)		
ALT (U/L)	Normal	31 (62%)	35 (70%)	0.407	0.523
	High	19 (38%)	15 (30%)		
Albumin (gm/dl)	Mean ± SD	4.28 ± 0.41	4.03 ± 0.37	3.253	0.002
	Range	2.6–5	3.1–5.1		
Bilirubin (mg/dl)	Mean ± SD	0.65 ± 0.24	0.58 ± 0.19	1.610	0.111
	Range	0.2–1.4	0.19–1		
INR	Mean ± SD	1.09 ± 0.09	1.12 ± 0.11	− 1.675	0.097
	Range	0.9–1.3	0.89–1.4		
Platelets (10^3/mm^3)	Mean ± SD	233.88 ± 67.28	215.18 ± 67.56	1.387	0.169
	Range	94–400	108–372		
Creatinine (mg/dl)	Median (IQR)	0.85 (0.8–0.91)	7.3 (6.1–9.49)	− 8.631	0.001
	Range	0.5–1.3	3.6–12.75		

statistically significant difference (*p* value, 0.034, and *p* value, 0.017, respectively) but there is no significant change in albumin, total bilirubin, platelet, and creatinine levels during the course of treatment.

Discussion

Egypt used to be on the top of the countries with heavy HCV burden. Treatment of HCV in Egypt has become one of the top national priorities since 2007. Egypt started a national treatment program intending to provide cure for Egyptian HCV-infected patients. Mass HCV treatment program had started using pegylated interferon and ribavirin between 2007 and 2014. Yet, with the development of highly effective direct-acting antivirals (DAAs) for HCV, elimination of viral hepatitis has become a real possibility. Egypt adopted a strategy

Table 4 Comparison between group I (control group) and group II (case group) regarding levels of hemoglobin, AST, ALT, albumin, total bilirubin, INR, platelets, and creatinine 4 weeks after treatment

		Group I	Group II	Test value	*p* value
Hemoglobin (gm/dl)	Mean ± SD	12.63 ± 1.59	10.27 ± 1.97	6.581	0.001
	Range	8.8–16	7.1–15.1		
AST (U/L)	Normal	49 (98.0%)	47 (94%)	1.042	0.307
	High	1 (2%)	3 (6%)		
ALT (U/L)	Normal	45 (90%)	47 (94%)	0.543	0.461
	High	5(10%)	3(6%)		
Albumin (gm/dl)	Mean ± SD	4.26 ± 0.40	4.03 ± 0.57	2.261	0.026
	Range	3.2–5.4	2.7–5.3		
Bilirubin (mg/dl)	Mean ± SD	0.99 ± 0.43	0.73 ± 0.33	3.324	0.001
	Range	0.2–2	0.2–2		
INR	Mean ± SD	1.08 ± 0.13	1.05 ± 0.08	1.197	0.234
	Range	1–1.65	0.9–1.21		
Platelets (10^3/mm^3)	Mean ± SD	250.27 ± 92.85	213.56 ± 69.12	2.234	0.028
	Range	132–663	92–430		
Creatinine (mg/dl)	Median (IQR)	0.88 (0.7–0.95)	7.38 (5.6–9)	− 8.634	0.001
	Range	0.3–1.2	3–16.8		

Table 5 Comparison between group I (control group) and group II (case group) regarding levels of hemoglobin, AST, ALT, albumin, total bilirubin, INR, platelets, and creatinine 8 weeks after treatment

		Group I	Group II	Test value	*p* value
Hemoglobin (gm/dl)	Mean ± SD	12.53 ± 1.35	9.43 ± 1.75	9.763	0.001
	Range	9.8–15.5	6.4–13		
AST (U/L)	Normal	50 (100%)	46 (100%)	0.930	0.335
	High	0 (0%)	0 (0%)		
ALT (U/L)	Normal	49 (98%)	46 (100%)	0.930	0.335
	High	1(2%)	0(0%)		
Albumin (gm/dl)	Mean ± SD	4.18 ± 0.39	3.97 ± 0.54	2.202	0.030
	Range	2.6–5.1	2–5.4		
Bilirubin (mg/dl)	Mean ± SD	0.90 ± 0.42	0.62 ± 0.24	3.848	0.001
	Range	0.3–2.08	0.1–1.39		
INR	Mean ± SD	1.11 ± 0.16	1.10 ± 0.13	0.618	0.538
	Range	0.95–2	0.67–1.4		
Platelets (10^3/mm^3)	Mean ± SD	234.44 ± 65.96	225.95 ± 68.82	0.610	0.543
	Range	135–439	105–400		
Creatinine (mg/dl)	Median (IQR)	0.9 (0.8–1)	7 (5.9–9.1)	− 8.310	0.001
	Range	0.6–1.2	3.5 –13.8		

that represents a model of care that could help other countries with high HCV prevalence rate in their battle against HCV Omran et al. [6].

The results of our study revealed that 95.1% of prevalent hemodialysis patients achieved SVR12 to the combination of ombitasvir/paritaprevir/ritonavir but treatment failure was observed in 4% of patients. Most of patients tolerated treatment; only 6 patients (12%) discontinued treatment due to side effects including severe anemia, fatigue, and GIT intolerance. In our study, three patients died during the treatment course. The most common side effects were anemia in 5 (10%) patients, requiring blood transfusion; gastrointestinal disturbance including nausea and

Table 6 Comparison between group I (control group) and group II (case group) regarding levels of hemoglobin, AST, ALT, albumin, total bilirubin, INR, platelets, and creatinine 12 weeks after treatment

		Group I	Group II	Test value	*p* value
Hemoglobin	Mean ± SD	12.36 ± 1.62	8.92 ± 1.63	10.021	0.001
	Range	8.8–15.7	4.2–12.4		
AST (U/L)	Normal	50 (100%)	40 (95.2%)	2.434	0.119
	High	0 (0%)	2 (4.8%)		
ALT (U/L)	Normal	50 (100%)	40 (95.2%)	2.434	0.119
	High	0 (0%)	2 (4.8%)		
Albumin (gm/dl)	Mean ± SD	4.25 ± 0.35	3.89 ± 0.41	4.682	0.001
	Range	3.5–5.1	2.9–4.8		
Bilirubin (mg/dl)	Mean ± SD	0.87 ± 0.43	0.70 ± 0.33	2.019	0.047
	Range	0.3–2.6	0.1–1.9		
INR	Mean ± SD	1.09 ± 0.08	1.08 ± 0.11	0.592	0.555
	Range	1–1.26	0.88–1.36		
Platelets (10^3/mm^3)	Mean ± SD	242.57 ± 69.99	233.35 ± 91.59	0.538	0.592
	Range	155–501	114–570		
Creatinine (mg/dl)	Median(IQR)	0.9 (0.8–1)	7 (5.87–8.9)	− 8.051	0.001
	Range	0.6–1.2	3.6–12.8		

vomiting in 7 patients (14%); severe fatigue in 3 (6%) patients; and itching in 2 (4%) patients.

The three patients that died during the course of treatment 2 patients had sudden death and 1 patient died due to cerebral hemorrhage despite normal platelet level and normal INR.

During the course of treatment, our study showed that patient had hemoglobin level drop, AST and ALT level improvement, increase at bilirubin level, and no change at albumin level, platelet level, total leukocyte count, and creatinine level.

Similar to our study, Liu et al. [7] investigated paritaprevir/ritonavir/ombitasvir for East-Asian non-cirrhotic hepatitis C virus patients receiving hemodialysis. Their study sample included 46 patients. The primary efficacy endpoint was sustained virologic response 12 weeks off-therapy (SVR_{12}). The SVR_{12} rate was 100% (46 of 46 patients) like our study common side effects were hemoglobin drop (23%), pruritus (19.6%), and fatigue (15.2%). Their study results were different from the results of the present study as our study listed 6 patients that stopped treatment due to adverse effects but the other study reported that all patients tolerated treatment well.

In agreement with the present study, Lawitz et al. [8] investigated the efficacy and safety of ombitasvir/paritaprevir/ritonavir in patients with hepatitis C virus genotype 4 infection and advanced kidney disease. They selected 65 patients including 50 (76%) on dialysis and 15 (23%) had compensated cirrhosis. They reported that SVR12 rate was 95% (63/66); 3 patients discontinued treatment due to adverse events. Seventy-three percent (27/37) of patients receiving RBV had adverse events leading to RBV dose modification.

Another study, the results of which came similar to ours, is the study in which Mekky et al. [9] investigated the efficacy of ombitasvir/paritaprevir/ritonavir with ribavirin in the management of HCV genotype 4 and end-stage kidney disease study which enrolled 110 patients. As regards SVR12, it was 96% in HD and 91.4% in non-HD patients. Treatment failure was observed in 6 patients. There were no reported serious adverse events. Anemia was observed in 66.6% in HD group and in 31.4% in non-HD group.

The study by El Kassas et al. [10] observed high rates for the use of ombitasvir/paritaprevir/ritonavir containing regimens study which included 325 patients (age, 47.63 ± 12.63 years); SVR12 was attained by 100% of patients who received OBV/rPTV/RBV as assessed by modified intention to treat analysis. In concordance with the present study, they found that there was a significant improvement of baseline alanine aminotransferase and aspartate aminotransferase. The most common reported adverse effects were anemia, fatigue, and elevated indirect bilirubin four patients stopped treatment at week 4.

In contrast to our study, Said et al. [11] investigated ritonavir-boosted paritaprevir and ombitasvir plus ribavirin and 171 patients were included. All included patients reached the end of treatment with no treatment discontinuations. The overall end of treatment response was 100%; 16 patients required blood transfusions.

The study by Yaraş et al. [12] was different from the results of the present study as they reported that all 25 patients well tolerated the treatment regimen. Serious side effects causing treatment interruption were not observed. But their study agreed with the present study as they reported that the most frequent side effects were fatigue and itching. In accordance with the present results of the current study, a significant decrease in the level of serum alanine transaminase from 16.6 to 8.7 U/l after treatment was observed. This study enrolled 25 hemodialysis-dependent patients; they found that there was no difference in serum albumin levels. The mean serum bilirubin levels increased from 0.49 to 0.56 mg/dL after treatment.

To study the efficacy of paritaprevir/ritonavir/ombitasvir plus dasabuvir regimen in the treatment of chronic hepatitis C infection in patients with severe renal impairment and end-stage renal disease. Sperl et al. [13] enrolled 23 patients; SVR12 rate was 100%. Unlike our study, none of the patients presented with a significant decrease in hemoglobin level during the treatment period. The most frequent adverse events were nausea, hypotension, and diarrhea. Four patients presented with a serious adverse event unrelated to the antiviral drugs (salmonellosis, non-functional kidney graft rejection, early gastric cancer, renal cyst infection). Concomitant medication had to be modified with the treatment initiation in 10 out of 23 (43.5%) patients (calcium channel blockers, ACE inhibitors, statins, diuretics); four patients required further adjustment of antihypertensive drugs. Our study listed that no patients required dose adjustment of their medications.

In concordance with the present study, Atsukawa et al. [14] investigated the efficacy and safety of ombitasvir/paritaprevir/ritonavir and ribavirin for chronic hepatitis patients in 94 patients. In agreement with the current study, they found that SVR were 97.9%. Only two patients failed to achieve SVR. The median ALT levels decreased significantly after treatment. The hemoglobin levels decreased significantly during the treatment period, the most frequent adverse event was anemia (20.2%; 19/94 patients) and pruritus.

In agreement to our study, Liu et al. [15] assessed effectiveness and safety of paritaprevir/ritonavir/ombitasvir. One hundred and three patients were enrolled in the study. One patient prematurely discontinued treatment due to hepatic decompensation, 23 patients complained of fatigue, 23 patients had nausea, 14 had pruritus, and 9 patients had dropped hemoglobin level.

Abad et al. [16] observed sustained viral response to the combination of ombitasvir/paritaprevir/ritonavir. Thirty-five patients with genotypes 1 and 4 were treated with that DAA regimen. Sustained viral response was achieved in 100% of patients. Adverse effects were negligible, and no patient had to discontinue treatment. The most significant side effect was anemia, which led to a significant increase in the dose of erythropoiesis-stimulating agents. Anemia was more marked in patients receiving ribavirin. No patients required transfusions.

Atsukawa et al. [17] studied efficacy and safety of ombitasvir/paritaprevir/ritonavir in dialysis patients with chronic hepatitis C. The study enrolled 31 patients and end-of-treatment response SVR12 were 93.5%, while our study reported that SVR12 at hemodialysis group was 96.0% and at normal group was 100%. The incidence of adverse events was 35.5%. One discontinued the treatment. The most common adverse effect was pruritus (6.5%), while our study reported that 12% of patients stopped treatment and the most common adverse effect was hemoglobin drop.

Another study, the results of which came similar to ours, is the study in which Pockros et al. [18] studied the efficacy of direct-acting antiviral combination for patients with hepatitis C. Study sample included 20 patients completed 12 weeks of treatment. Eighteen of the 20 patients achieved SVR, one patient died after the end of the treatment (unrelated to the treatment) and 1 relapse accounted. Adverse events were primarily mild or moderate, and no patient discontinued treatment due to an adverse effect. Four patients experienced serious adverse effects all were considered unrelated to treatment. Ribavirin therapy was interrupted in 9 patients due to anemia. No blood transfusions were needed in contrast to our study in which patients needed blood transfusion. Most patients experienced side effects, the majority of which were mild or moderate in severity. No patient discontinued DAAs due to adverse effects. In agreement to our study, the most common side effects were anemia (45%), fatigue (35%), diarrhea (25%), and nausea (25%).

Arai et al. [19] studied efficacy and safety of ombitasvir/paritaprevir/ritonavir combination therapy for genotype 1b chronic hepatitis C patients complicated with chronic kidney disease; their study included 54 patients with impaired renal functions and 181 patients with normal renal functions. They concluded that only one patient among normal renal function group had increased in his serum creatinine level. This comes in agreement with our study that found that there is no effect of ombitasvir/paritaprevir/ritonavir on serum creatinine level during the course of treatment.

Conclusion

From the result of the present study, we concluded that ombitasvir, paritaprevir, and ritonavir are considered a safe and effective in treatment of HCV infection in patients on regular hemodialysis.

Abbreviations

FDA: Food and Drug Administration; HCV: Hepatitis C virus; NCCVH: National Committee for Control of Viral Hepatitis; SVR: Sustained virological response; DAAs: Direct-acting antivirals; PK: Pharmacokinetic; NS5A: Nonstructural protein 5A; RBV: Ribavirin; HD: Hemodialysis; ALT: Alanine aminotransferase; AST: Aspartate aminotrasferase; HBsAg: Hepatitis B surface antigen; AFP: Alpha fetoprotein; HCV PCR: Hepatitis C virus polymerase chain reaction; HbA1c: Glycosylated hemoglobin; CBC: Complete blood count; INR: International normalized ratio; IQR: Interquartile range; ANOVA: Analysis of variance; ACE: Angiotensin converting enzyme

Acknowledgements

Not applicable.

Authors' contributions

NMT and WAA selected the patients from hemodialysis units at Ain Shams University Hospitals and made the design for the study. AME and OAA contributed to follow-up of the patients at the Center of National Committee for Control of Viral Hepatitis [NCCVH] at Ain Shams University Hospital and analysis and interpretation of data. SME contributed to data collection. All authors provided critical feedback and helped shape the research, analysis, and manuscript. All authors have read and approved the manuscript.

Ethics approval and consent to participate

This study was performed in accordance with the ethical standards of Ain Shams University Research Committee and with the 1964 Helsinki Declaration and its later amendments or comparable ethical standards. Ethics committees reference number, 00017585.

A written informed consent was obtained from all individual participants included in the study.

Competing interests

The authors declare that they have no competing interests.

Author details

Department of Internal Medicine and Nephrology, Faculty of Medicine, Ain Shams University, Ramsis 38 Street, Abassia, Cairo 11211, Egypt. [2]Department of Internal Medicine and Gastroenterology, Faculty of Medicine, Ain Shams University, Cairo, Egypt.

References

1. Gower E, Estes C, Blach S et al (2014) Global epidemiology and genotype distribution of the hepatitis C virus infection. Journal of Hepatology 61(1): S45–S57. https://doi.org/10.1016/j.jhep.2014.07.027
2. Gomaa A, Allam N, Elsharkway A et al (2017) Hepatitis C infection in Egypt: prevalence, impact and management strategies. Hepatic Medicine: Evidence and Research 9:17. https://doi.org/10.2147/HMER.S113681
3. McConachie SM, Wilhelm SM, Kale-Pradhan PB (2016) New direct-acting antivirals in hepatitis C therapy: a review of sofosbuvir, ledipasvir, daclatasvir, simeprevir, paritaprevir, ombitasvir and dasabuvir. Expert Rev Clin Pharmacol 9(2):287–302
4. Feld JJ, Kowdley KV, Coakley E et al (2014) Treatment of HCV with ABT-450/r–ombitasvir and dasabuvir with ribavirin. N Engl J Med 370(17):1594–1603. https://doi.org/10.1056/NEJMoa1315722
5. American Association for the study of Liver Disease/Infectious Disease Society of America/ International Antiviral Society (2016) Recommendations for testing, managing, and treating hepatitis C virus.
6. Omran D, Alboraie M, Zayed RA et al (2018) Towards hepatitis C virus elimination: Egyptian experience, achievements and limitations. World J Gastroenterol 24(38):4330 4340. https://doi.org/10.3748/wjg.v24.i38.4330

7. Liu CH, Shih YL, Yang SS et al (2019) Paritaprevir/ritonavir, ombitasvir plus dasabuvir for East-Asian non-cirrhotic hepatitis C virus genotype 1b patients receiving hemodialysis. Journal of Gastroenterology and Hepatology 34(11): 1977–1983. https://doi.org/10.1111/jgh.14672
8. Lawitz E, Makara M, Akarca US et al (2019) Efficacy and safety of ombitasvir, paritaprevir, and ritonavir in an open-label study of patients with genotype 1b chronic hepatitis C virus infection with and without cirrhosis. Gastroenterology 149(4):971–980
9. Mekky MA, Abdel-Malek MO, Osman HA et al (2019) Efficacy of ombitasvir/ paritaprevir/ritonavir/ribavirin in management of HCV genotype 4 and end-stage kidney disease. Clinics and research in hepatology and gastroenterology 43(1):82–87. https://doi.org/10.1016/j.clinre.2018.08.003
10. El Kassas M, Alboraie M, Omar H et al (2019) High success rates for the use of ombitasvir/paritaprevir/ritonavir containing regimens in treatment of naive and experienced chronic hepatitis C genotype 4: real world results. J Med Virol. https://doi.org/10.1002/jmv.25478
11. Said M, Omar H, Soliman Z et al (2019) Ritonavir-boosted paritaprevir, ombitasvir plus ribavirin could improve eGFR in patients with renal impairment and HCV: an Egyptian cohort. Expert Review of Gastroenterology & Hepatology 13(1):89–93. https://doi.org/10.1080/ 17474124.2019.1544070
12. Yaraş S, Üçbilek E, Özdoğan O et al (2019) Real-life results of treatment with ombitasvir, paritaprevir, dasabuvir, and ritonavir combination in patients with chronic renal failure infected with HCV in Turkey. Turk J Gastroenterol 30(4):331
13. Sperl J, Kreidlova M, Merta D et al (2018) Paritaprevir/ritonavir/ombitasvir plus dasabuvir regimen in the treatment of genotype 1 chronic hepatitis C infection in patients with severe renal impairment and end-stage renal disease: a real-life cohort. Kidney Blood Press Res 43(2):594–605. https://doi.org/10.1159/000488965
14. Atsukawa M, Tsubota A, Koushima Y et al (2018) Efficacy and safety of ombitasvir/paritaprevir/ritonavir and ribavirin for chronic hepatitis patients infected with genotype 2a in Japan. Hepatolo Res. 2(3):55–61. https://doi.org/10.1111/hepr.13292
15. Liu CH, Liu CJ, Su TH et al (2018) Real-world effectiveness and safety of paritaprevir/ritonavir, ombitasvir, and dasabuvir with or without ribavirin for patients with chronic hepatitis C virus genotype 1b infection in Taiwan. J Gastroenterol Hepatol. 33(3):710–717. https://doi.org/10.1111/jgh.13912
16. Abad S, Vega A, Hernández E et al (2017) Universal sustained viral response to the combination of ombitasvir/paritaprevir/ritonavir and dasabuvir with/ without ribavirin in patients on hemodialysis infected with hepatitis C virus genotypes 1 and 4. Am J Nephrol 45(3):267–272. https://doi.org/10.1159/ 000454819
17. Atsukawa M, Tsubota A, Koushima Y et al (2017) Efficacy and safety of ombitasvir/paritaprevir/ritonavir in dialysis patients with genotype 1b chronic hepatitis C. Hepatology Research 47(13):1429–1437. https://doi.org/ 10.1111/hepr.12910
18. Pockros PJ, Reddy KR, Mantry PS et al (2016) Efficacy of direct-acting antiviral combination for patients with hepatitis C virus genotype 1 infection and severe renal impairment or end-stage renal disease. Gastroenterology 150(7):1590–1598. https://doi.org/10.1053/j.gastro.2016.02. 078
19. Arai T, Atsukawa M, Tsubota A et al (2018) Efficacy and safety of ombitasvir/ paritaprevir/ritonavir combination therapy for genotype 1b chronic hepatitis C patients complicated with chronic kidney disease. Hepatol Res 48(7):549–555. https://doi.org/10.1111/hepr.13058

5

The role of IL-4 gene polymorphism in HCV-related hepatocellular carcinoma in Egyptian patients

Mohy-Eldin Abd-Elfattah[1*], Mary Naguib[2], Mohammed Elkheer[1], Eman Abdelsameea[3] and Ali Nada[3]

Abstract

Background: Interleukin-4 (IL-4), a pleiotropic anti-inflammatory cytokine, is produced mainly by activated T helper 2 (Th2). Hepatocellular carcinoma (HCC) is a typical inflammation-related cancer. Alterations influencing IL-4 expression may disturb immune response and may be associated with HCC risk. We aimed to verify role of IL4 gene polymorphism (*IL-4-589C/T (rs2243250)*) in HCV-related hepatocellular carcinoma in Egyptian patients. *IL-4-589C/T (rs2243250)* polymorphism was examined in 50 patients with HCC on top of HCV, 40 patients with HCV-induced liver cirrhosis, and 30 healthy controls using the polymerase chain reaction- restriction fragment length polymorphism method.

Results: Overall IL-4 gene polymorphism (*IL-4-589C/T (rs2243250)*) showed significant difference between hepatocellular carcinoma group versus liver cirrhosis and healthy control groups. *TT* homozygous genotype was more prevalent in HCC group (24%) versus (5%) in liver cirrhosis and (3.3%) in control. *TT* homozygous genotype had 10 times more risk of hepatocellular carcinoma versus healthy control group and 6.33 times more risk versus cirrhotic patients group (p value = 0.018 and 0.016 respectively).

Conclusion: *IL-4-589C/T (rs2243250)* polymorphism, *TT* homozygous genetic model, may be a risk factor in HCV-related HCC in Egyptian patients.

Keywords: Interleukin-4 (IL-4), Hepatocellular carcinoma (HCC), Hepatitis C virus (HCV)

Background

Hepatocellular carcinoma (HCC) is one of the main causes of cancer-related mortality. In Egypt, it is considered a major health problem being the fourth common malignancy [1]. The increased incidence of HCC cases in Egypt is related to the high prevalence of hepatitis C virus (HCV) infection [2].

HCC is diagnosed at late stages in most cases. This limits the treatment options especially it is refractory to the available chemotherapeutic drugs. So, current available therapies are effective only to small group of patients [3].

HCC is considered an inflammation-related cancer initiated by different etiological factors such as hepatitis virus, alcohol, and non-alcoholic steatohepatitis [4]. Chronic inflammatory state is characterized by the continued expression of cytokines and recruitment of immune cells to the liver which appears to be necessary for the initiation and development of liver cancer [5].

IL-4 is a short four α-helix bundle glycoprotein secreted mainly by activated T helper 2 (Th2) cells. In addition, it is secreted from other immune cells within the lymphoid lineage compartment as type 2 innate lymphoid cells (ILC2s) and myeloid lineage compartment as basophils and mast cells. In its turn IL-4 delineates, Th2 phenotype [6]. It was reported that Th2 dominance might provoke carcinogenesis in chronic HCV patients [7].

Together with IL-13, which have 25% sequence similarity with IL-4 and encoded by adjacent genes that share several *cis*-acting regulatory regions, receptor subunits, and signaling molecules, they are classic inducers of M2,

* Correspondence: mohy_abdelfattah@yahoo.com
[1]Bioorganic Chemistry Department, Faculty of Science, Suez Canal University, Sheikh Zayed City, Ismailia 42524, Egypt
Full list of author information is available at the end of the article

an alternatively activated macrophage [8, 9] which was reported to promote HCC development [10, 11].

Therefore, in this study we aimed to study the contribution of promoter polymorphism of *IL-4-589C/T (rs2243250)* to the susceptibility of HCV-related HCC.

Methods

Study participants

A total of 90 Egyptian chronic HCV-infected patients were recruited in the current study from the Hepatology and Gastroenterology Department, National Liver Institute, Menoufia University. After history taking, clinical evaluation, laboratory, and radiological investigations, patients were classified into 2 groups; (cirrhosis group 40 cirrhotic patients) with no radiological evidence of hepatocellular carcinoma and (HCC group 50 HCC patients) (arterial enhancement and washout in venous or delayed phase). In addition, 30 healthy age and sex matched individuals (control group) were enrolled as control group.

Patients with other coexistent morbidity such as HBV infection, autoimmune hepatitis, non-alcoholic steatohepatitis, and genetic metabolic diseases were excluded from the study. The protocol was approved by the local ethical committee of National Liver Institute and informed consent was taken before the study.

Routine investigations

Sera were subjected to routine laboratory study including liver and renal function tests performed on Micro lab 300 auto analyzer (vital scientific, Netherlands) using Diamond Kits (Germany) for measuring urea, total, and direct bilirubin; Human Kits (Germany) for measuring Aspartate Aminotransferase (AST), Alanine Aminotransferase (ALT) and creatinine and spinreact kits (Spain) for measuring albumin according to manufacturer's instructions. Hepatitis B surface antigen (HBsAg), anti-hepatitis B core antibody (HBcAb), anti-hepatitis C antibodies (HCV Abs), and serum alpha fetoprotein were detected by Cobas e411 immunoassay analyzer (Roche diagnostics-Mannhein, Germany). Complete blood count was measured using Sysmex XT-1800i (Sysmex Corporation, Kobe, Japan) and HCV RNA level which was assessed by COBAS AmpliPrep/COBAS TaqMan (Roche Diagnostics Ltd., Germany) with detection limit of 15 IU/ml.

Study of *IL-4 rs2243250 C/T* polymorphism by PCR-RFLP

Genomic DNA was extracted from EDTA treated blood samples using Quick-gDNA™MiniPrep Genomic DNA Purification Kit (Zymo Research, USA). PCR amplification of the 195 base pair (bp) stretch within the promoter region of IL-4 gene was performed followed by Ava II restriction enzyme digestion (Biolabs, Inc., England) as was previously described [12]. The primers used were 5′-TAAACTTGGGAGAACATGGT-3′forward and 5′-TGGGGAAAGATAGAGTAATA-3′ reverse. PCR reaction mixture consisted of 1 μl of each of primers, 12.5 μl of MyTaq Red PCR master mix (Bioline USA Inc., USA), 5.5 μl of nuclease-free water and 5 μl of extracted DNA.

Amplification was performed in Perkin Elmer Gene Amp PCR System 2400 Thermal Cycler in the following conditions; 95 °C for 5 min, followed by 35 cycles, of 95 °C for 45 s, annealing at 50 °C for 45 s, 72 °C for 45 s and final extension at 72 °C for 10 min.

The genotyping analysis of the 195 bp amplicon was performed through digestion with Ava II restriction enzyme at 37 °C for 20 min. Detection of the digested products was carried out by 3% agarose gel electrophoresis. PCR products with *C* at the polymorphic site were digested showing two fragments 177 and 18 bp, while those with *T* were not. Samples yielding 177 and 18 bp fragments were scored as *CC* genotypes, those with single 195 bp fragment as *TT* genotype and 195, 177, 18 bp fragments as *CT* genotype (Fig. 1).

Statistical methods

Results were statistically analyzed by using statistical package of social sciences (SPSS 22.0, IBM/SPSS Inc., Chicago, IL, USA). Descriptive statistics were applied for summarizing clinical and demographical data as mean (X), standard deviation (SD), median (Med), and range or interquartile range (IQR) for quantitative data, and frequency with percentage (%) for qualitative data. Inferential statistics were conducted to test significant difference among the studied groups. For comparing continuous variables, ANOVA or Student's t test were used when normality and homogeneity assumptions were met, instead, their non-parametric equivalents Kruskal-Wallis or Mann-Whitney test were applied upon violation. Dunn-Sidak used as a post hoc test for multiple pairwise comparisons after significant Kruskal-Wallis test. Chi-square (χ^2) test was used to compare allele frequency and genotype distribution of IL-4 gene polymorphism and to estimate the disease risk via odds ratio (OR) also Fisher's exact test was used when Chi-square assumptions were violated. Binary logistic regression analysis was applied to calculate the adjusted odds ratios (ORs) and 95% confidence intervals (CIs) after controlling for after age and gender status to exclude potential confounding effect. The p values indicating the significance level was set at level < 0.05.

Result

Characteristics of the study participants

Table 1 summarizes characteristics of the study population. There was no statistical difference concerning age and gender between different studied groups (p value > 0.05); however, male gender in HCC group (64%) was

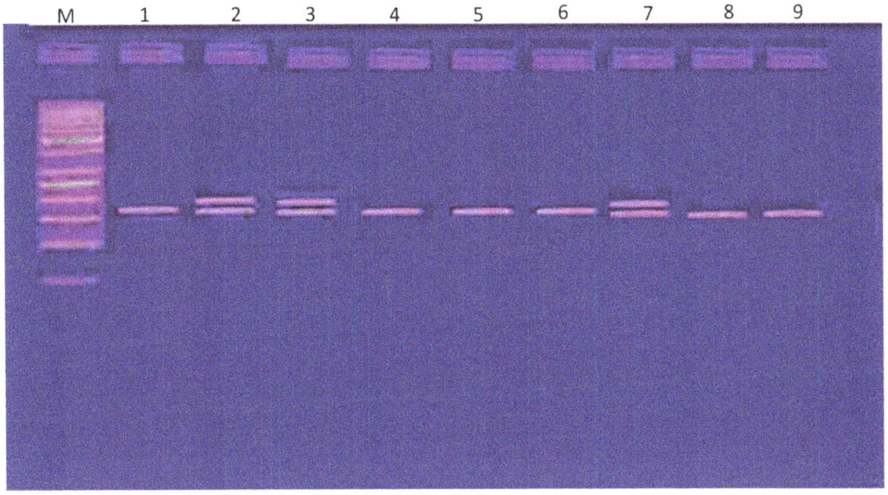

Fig. 1 Genotyping analysis of IL-4-589C/T polymorphism using PCR-RFLP technique. PCR-RFLP assay for analyzing IL-4-589C/T polymorphism. PCR product was digested by AVA II restriction enzyme and visualized on 3% agarose gel. M: marker (50 bp ladder). Lanes 1, 4, 5, 6, 8, and 9 show CC homozygous (177 bp band, 18 bp is not seen); lanes 2, 3, and 7 show CT heterozygous (195 and 177 bp bands)

more prevalent than female gender (36%). On the other hand, comparing liver and renal function tests between studied groups showed highly statistical significance difference between studied groups. HCC group had statistically significant elevated alanine aminotransferase (ALT), aspartate aminotransferase (AST), total and direct bilirubin, urea, and creatinine and significant decreased albumin level compared to control group ($p <$ 0.001). On the other hand, there was no statistical significance between HCC and cirrhotic patients.

Genotype polymorphism and risk of hepatocellular carcinoma

Studying genotype distribution and allele frequency of IL-4 promotor polymorphism *(-589C/T)* among different groups showed that there was increase of *TT* genotype

Table 1 Studying demographic data, liver, and renal profile among studied groups

	Control (n = 30)	Cirrhosis (n = 40)	HCC (n = 50)	p value
Age (years) Median (range)	50.00 (40.00–59.00)	52.5 (43.00–66.00)	52.5 (42.00–67.00)	**0.066**
Gender				**0.562**
Male (n, %)	16 (53.3)	22 (55.0)	32 (64.0)	
Female (n, %)	14 (46.7)	18 (45.0)	18 (36.0)	
ALT (U/L) Median (range)	17.00 (9.0–36.0)	48.50 (16.0–146.0)	55.50 (20.0–102.0)	**< 0.001** [a,b]
AST (U/L) Median (range)	19.00 (9.0–36.0)	60.50 (16.0–146.0)	62.50 (20.0–102.0)	**< 0.001** [a,b]
Total bilirubin (mg/dL) Median (range)	0.50 (0.10–0.80)	1.19 (0.45–4.18)	1.50 (0.73–3.63)	**< 0.001** [a,b]
Direct bilirubin (mg/dL) Median (range)	0.10 (0.07–0.23)	0.38 (0.09–3.08)	0.62 (0.18–2.53)	**< 0.001** [a,b]
Albumin (g/dL) Median (range)	4.40 (3.50–5.10)	3.68 (2.20–4.90)	3.32 (2.20–4.52)	**< 0.001** [a,b]
Urea (mg/dL) Median (range)	27.50 (17.0–41.0)	37.50 (22.0–56.0)	38.00 (22.0–67.0)	**< 0.001** [a,b]
Creatinine (mg/dL) Median (range)	0.80 (0.50–1.20)	0.87 (0.58–1.50)	1.00 (0.50–1.50)	**0.001** [a,b]

ALT alanine aminotransferase, *AST* aspartate aminotransferase
Data are median and range in parenthesis, otherwise are n (%)
Significant p value < 0.05
[a]On comparing a control and cirrhotic patients
[b]Control and HCC patients
[c]Cirrhotic and HCC patients

(24%) in HCC group compared to cirrhotic patients group (5%) and control group (3.3%) with *T* allele predominance in HCC group (44%) compared to cirrhotic group (28.8%) and control group (26.7%).

The study revealed that *CC* genotype was more prevalent (50%) in healthy control and (47.5%) in cirrhotic patients than hepatocellular carcinoma group (36%). *CT* genotype frequency was increased in control, cirrhotic patients groups (46.7%, 47.5% respectively) compared to HCC group (40%) as shown in Table 2.

TT homozygous genotype was significantly increased in HCC group with OR (95% CI) 10 times more risk compared to control (p value = 0.018). *T* allele was associated with a significant increase of hepatocellular carcinoma with OR (95% CI) 2.16 more times risk (p value = 0.028). The *T* allele variant showed significant association with HCC risk in the recessive genetic model *(CC + CT* vs *TT)* (p = 0.025) not the dominant genetic model *(CC* vs *CT + TT)* (p = 0.218) as shown in Table 2.

Also, the homozygous *TT* genotype was more prevalent in HCC group compared to cirrhotic patients group with OR (95% CI) 6.33 times risk of hepatocellular carcinoma (p value = 0.016). Additionally, the *T* allele showed significant prevalence in HCC group with OR (95% CI) 1.95 more risk (p = 0.035). The *T* allele variant showed significant association with HCC risk in the recessive genetic model *(CC + CT* vs *TT)* (p = 0.013) not the dominant genetic model *(CC* vs *CT + TT)* (p = 0.271) as shown in Table 2.

On studying foci size and numbers in HCC group regarding the recessive genetic model of *-589C/T* SNP *(CC + CT* vs *TT)* (Table 3), we could not detect statistical significance difference between 2 groups.

Discussion

Chronic hepatitis C virus infection is considered a major risk factor for HCC development [13]. As an RNA virus, HCV does not integrate into the host genome, so pathogenesis of HCV-related HCC is proposed to involve generation of oxidative stress and increased expression of inflammatory cytokines associated with chronic hepatitis [14], in addition to the direct effect of HCV viral products [15].

Interleukin-4 (IL-4), a pleiotropic anti-inflammatory cytokine, is involved in humoral and cell-mediated immunity [16]. It suppresses a number of pro-inflammatory cytokines and expands anti-inflammatory effect [17]; thus, it is suggested that any alterations that influence IL-4 expression or function may disturb immune responses increasing the liability to infections.

In addition, IL-4, together with other Th2 cytokines, induces M2 macrophage polarization. Traditionally, macrophages are classified into classically activated M1 phenotype and the alternatively activated M2 macrophages according to their responses to different microenvironmental stimuli [18].

M2-polarized macrophages are main components of tumor-infiltrating stromal cells. They are key factors participating in tumor progression. M2-polarized macrophages were also related to promote tumor growth, invasion, and metastasis by secreting certain chemokines growth factors, cytokines, and matrix metalloproteases [19].

IL-4 gene is located on chromosome 5q31 [17]. In the current study, we aimed to study the contribution of promoter polymorphism of *IL-4 -589C/T (rs2243250)* to the susceptibility of HCV-related HCC. It had been

Table 2 Genotypes distribution and allele frequencies of polymorphism *-589 C/T (rs2243250)* in control, cirrhotic, and HCC groups

polymorphism *-589 C/T (rs2243250)*	Control *n* = 30(%)	LC *n* = 40 (%)	HCC *n* = 50 (%)	*p* value	LC vs control		HCC vs. control		HCC vs. LC	
					OR (95% CI)	*P* value	OR (95% CI)	*P* value	OR (95% CI)	*p* value
Genotypes				**0.044**						
CC	15 (50.0)	19 (47.5)	18 (36.0)		Ref	–	Ref	–	Ref	–
CT	14 (46.7)	19 (47.5)	20 (40.0)		1.07 (0.41–2.82)	0.889	1.19 (0.45–3.13)	0.724	1.11 (0.45–2.73)	0.818
TT	1 (3.3)	2 (5.0)	12 (24.0)		1.58 (0.13–19.12)	1.000	**10.0 (1.16–86.02)**	**0.018**	**6.33 (1.24–32.32)**	**0.016**
Dominant model				**0.391**						
CC	15 (50.0)	19 (47.5)	18 (36.0)		Ref	–	Ref	–	Ref	–
CT+TT	15 (50.0)	21 (52.5)	32 (64.0)		1.11 (0.43–2.85)	0.836	1.78 (0.71–4.46)	0.218	1.61 (0.69 – 3.76)	0.271
Recessive model				**0.008**						
CC+CT	29 (96.7)	38 (96.0)	38 (76.0)		Ref	–	Ref	–	Ref	–
TT	1 (3.3)	2 (5.0)	12 (24.0)		1.53 (0.13–17.66)	1.000	**9.16 (1.13–74.52)**	**0.025**	**6.00 (1.26–28.64)**	**0.013**
Alleles				**0.034**						
C	44 (73.3)	57 (71.3)	56 (56.0)		Ref	–	Ref	–	Ref	–
T	16 (26.7)	23 (28.8)	44 (44.0)		1.11 (0.52–2.35)	0.786	**2.16 (1.08–4.33)**	**0.028**	**1.95 (1.04–3.64)**	**0.035**

Data are *n* (%), *CI* confidence interval, significant p value < 0.05

Table 3 Studying Data are *n* (%). Significant *p* value < 0.05 size and number of foci in HCC group regarding recessive genetic model of *-589 C/T SNP ((CC + CT vs TT)*

Parameters	Genetic model for *-589 C/T* SNP (*CC + CT vs TT*)		*p* value
	CT + CC (*n* = 38)	*TT* (*n* = 12)	
	Number of foci [*n* (%)]		
Single	19 (50)	7 (58.3)	0.614
Multiple	19 (50)	5 (41.7)	
	Size of foci [*n* (%)]		
Small (≤ 2 cm)	10 (26.3)	2 (16.7)	0.834
Moderate (> 2–5 cm)	18 (47.4)	6 (50.0)	
Large (> 5 cm)	10 (26.3)	4 (33.3)	

Data are *n* (%). Significant *p* value < 0.05

stated the *T* allele of *IL-4 (-589C/T)* polymorphism is associated with an increased IL-4expression [20].

Our study showed that *TT* genotype was more prevalent in HCC group (24%) compared to control group (3.3%) and cirrhotic patient group (5%). *TT* homozygous genotype had 10 times more risk of hepatocellular carcinoma versus healthy control group and 6.33 times more risk versus cirrhotic patients group (*p* value = 0.018 and 0.016, respectively). The *T* allele frequency was increased in HCC group (44%) versus (26.7% and 28.8%, OR (95% CI) = 2.16 and 1.95) in control and cirrhotic patients group, respectively.

This was consistent with the study led by Khalil et al. among HCV-infected Egyptian patients, they reported that *IL-4-589 TT* genotype was significantly increased in HCV-infected patients (*p* = 0.001) with strong reduction in the control group (3.3%), the patients samples revealed only *CT* (82%) and *TT* (18%) genotypes [21].

Also, there was a study conducted by Yousif et al. among HBV-infected patients in Sudan. They noted that *CT* and *TT* genotypes were 73.2% and 19.6%, respectively among infected patients [22].

In addition, the meta-analysis study directed by Zheng et al. who reported significant association between the *IL4-589T* polymorphism and increased risk of liver diseases in Caucasian populations; however, this was not detected in Asian populations [23].

It is worth noting that in our study, the significant association of *IL4-589C/T* polymorphism among HCC patient group was related to *TT* genotype which was contrary to the *CC* genotype detected in chronic HBV-infected Chinese male patients in the study conducted by Lu et al. in 2014 [24].

It is proposed that there are differences in the IL-4 genetic background among different ethnic groups. As on studying genotype distribution and allele frequency in control group of our study, the *IL4–589 C* allele frequencies were (73.3%), which were similar to healthy Egyptian (61.7%) and healthy Caucasians results (86.3%) in the studies conducted by Khalil et al. in 2017 [21] and Zheng et al. in 2013 [23] respectively but higher than frequencies among healthy Chinese (17.4%) in the study conducted by Lu et al. [24], while the *T* allele frequencies accounted for (26.7%), which was similar to healthy Egyptian (38.3%) [21] and healthy Caucasians frequency results (13.7%) [23] but was lower than that of healthy Chinese (82.6%) [24]. Thus, the *T* allele may be the variant responsible for various diseases in Egyptian population, while the opposite is true for Chinese population. This suggests that distinct allele frequencies in the same polymorphism site may play different roles in the same disease. A larger-scale multicenter study is recommended to confirm this suggestion.

On the other hand, we studied size and number of foci lesions in HCC group in relation to recessive genetic model of *-589C/T* SNP (*CC + CT* vs *TT*), we did not find statistical significance between 2 groups.

Conclusion

Our study revealed that there was statistically significant association between the *IL-4-589C/T (rs2243250)* polymorphism (*TT* genotype) and HCV-related HCC. The *T* allele may be a variant responsible for the disease production among Egyptian population.

Abbreviations

IL-4: Interleukin-4; HCC: Hepatocellular carcinoma; HCV: Hepatitis C virus; HBV: Hepatitis B virus; LC: Liver cirrhosis; HCC: Hepatocellular carcinoma; Th2: T helper 2; ILC2s : Type 2 innate lymphoid cells; HBsAg: Hepatitis B surface antigen; AST : Aspartate aminotransferase; ALT: Alanine aminotransferase; HBsAg: Hepatitis B surface antigen; HCV Abs : Hepatitis C virus antibodies; CIs: Confidence intervals

Acknowledgements

All authors are greatly indebted to members of National Liver Institute, Menoufia University, Egypt. Also, many thanks to all members of Bioorganic Chemistry Department, Faculty of Science, Suez Canal University.

Authors' contributions

M-E A initiated the project, designed and implemented the study for application. MN analyzed the data, drafted and revised the paper. ME contributed to the data collection, analyzed the data, and revised the paper. EA analyzed the data, drafted and revised the paper. AN analyzed the data, drafted and revised the paper. All authors have read and approved the manuscript.

Ethics approval and consent to participate

The study was conformed to the ethical guidelines of the 1975 Declaration of Helsinki and was approved by the institutional review board of National Liver Institute (NLI), Menoufia University, Egypt (approval no. 00198/2020). Written consents were filled and signed by all participants.

Competing interests

The authors declare that they have no competing interests.

Author details

[1]Bioorganic Chemistry Department, Faculty of Science, Suez Canal University, Sheikh Zayed City, Ismailia 42524, Egypt. [2]Clinical Pathology Department, National Liver Institute, Menoufia University, Shibin El Kom, Egypt. [3]Hepatology and Gastroenterology Department, National Liver Institute, Menoufia University, Shibin El Kom, Egypt.

References

1. Rashed WM, Kandeil MAM, Mahmoud MO, Ezzat S (2020) Hepatocellular carcinoma (HCC) in Egypt: a comprehensive overview. J Egypt Natl Canc Inst. 32(1):5
2. Abdelmoez FA, Imam HM, Nk I, Wahid LA, Abbas WA, Ali Abozaid MA, Abdelwahab HM (2019) The role of hepatitis C virus and possible risk factors in development of hepatocellular carcinoma: 400 patients based study. Egypt J Intern Med 31:64–72
3. Kumari R, Sahu MK, Tripathy A, Uthansingh K, Behera M. Hepatocellular carcinoma treatment: hurdles, advances and prospects. Hepat Oncol. 2018; 5(2):HEP08. Published 2018 Sep 28. doi:10.2217/hep-2018-0002
4. Tu T, Buhler S, Bartenschlager R (2017) Chronic viral hepatitis and its association with liver cancer. Biol Chem. 398(8):817–837. https://doi.org/10.1515/hsz-2017-0118
5. Porta C, Riboldi E, Sica A (2011) Mechanisms linking pathogens-associated inflammation and cancer. Cancer Letters. 305(2):250–262
6. Zhu J (2015) T helper 2 (Th2) cell differentiation, type 2 innate lymphoid cell (ILC2) development and regulation of interleukin-4 (IL-4) and IL-13 production. Cytokine. 75(1):14–24. https://doi.org/10.1016/j.cyto.2015.05.010
7. Kogame M, Nagai H, Shinohara M, Igarashi Y, Sumino Y, Ishii K. Th2 dominance might induce carcinogenesis in patients with HCV-related liver cirrhosis. Anticancer Res. 2016;36(9):4529–4536. doi:10.21873/anticanres.11000
8. LaPorte SL, Juo ZS, Vaclavikova J et al (2008) Molecular and structural basis of cytokine receptor pleiotropy in the interleukin-4/13 system. Cell 132:259–272
9. McCormick SM, Heller NM (2015) Commentary: IL-4 and IL-13 receptors and signaling. Cytokine. 75(1):38–50. https://doi.org/10.1016/j.cyto.2015.05.023
10. Capece D, Fischietti M, Verzella D, Gaggiano A, Cicciarelli G, Tessitore A et al (2013) The inflammatory microenvironment in hepatocellular carcinoma: a pivotal role for tumor-associated macrophages. Biomed Res Int. 2013: 187204. https://doi.org/10.1155/2013/187204
11. Yeung OW, Lo CM, Ling CC et al (2015) Alternatively activated (M2) macrophages promote tumour growth and invasiveness in hepatocellular carcinoma. J Hepatol. 62(3):607–616. https://doi.org/10.1016/j.jhep.2014.10.029
12. Micheal S, Minhas K, Ishaque M, Ahmed F, Ahmed A (2013) IL-4 gene polymorphisms and their association with atopic asthma and allergic rhinitis in Pakistani patients. J Investig Allergol Clin Immunol 23(2):107–111
13. Goossens and Hoshida Hepatitis C virus-induced hepatocellular carcinoma Clin Mol Hepatol. 2015 Jun; 21(2): 105–114.
14. Yu LX, Ling Y, Wang HY. Role of nonresolving inflammation in hepatocellular carcinoma development and progression. NPJ Precis Oncol. 2018;2(1):6. Published 2018 Feb 23. doi:10.1038/s41698-018-0048-z
15. El-Nady GM, Ling R, Harrison TJ (2003) Gene expression in HCV-associated hepatocellular carcinoma--upregulation of a gene encoding a protein related to the ubiquitin- conjugating enzyme. Liver Int 23:329–337
16. Luzina IG, Keegan AD, Heller NM et al (2012) Regulation of inflammation by interleukin-4: a review of "alternatives". J LeukocBiol 92:753–764
17. Park HK, Kim SK, Kweon HY, Lee KG, Arasu MV, Kim YO (2017) Promoter polymorphism (-590, T/C) of interleukin 4 (IL4) gene is associated with Rheumatoid arthritis: An updated meta-analysis. Saudi J Biol Sci. 24(2):444–449
18. Martinez FO, Gordon S. The M1 and M2 paradigm of macrophage activation: time for reassessment. F1000Prime Rep. 2014;6:13. Published 2014 Mar 3. doi:10.12703/P6-13
19. Yao RR, Li JH, Zhang R, Chen RX, Wang YH. M2-polarized tumor-associated macrophages facilitated migration and epithelial-mesenchymal transition of HCC cells via the TLR4/STAT3 signaling pathway. World J Surg Oncol. 2018; 16(1):9. Published 2018 Jan 16. doi:10.1186/s12957-018-1312-y
20. Saxana MK and Kaur M.Th1/Th2 cytokines and their genotypes as predictors of hepatitis B virus related hepatocellularcarcinoma, World J Hepatol. 2015 Jun 18;7(11):1572-80. doi: 10.4254/wjh.v7.i11.1572.
21. Khalil H, Arfa M, El-Masrey S, El-Sherbini SM, Abd-Elaziz AA.(2017) Single nucleotide polymorphisms of interleukins associated with hepatitis C virus infection in Egypt. J Infect Dev Ctries. 31;11(3):261-268
22. Yousif N, Khair O, El Hussein ARM, Elkhidir IM, Enan KA (2017) The polymorphism of interleukin 4 in chronic hepatitis B virus infection in hemodialysis patients at Khartoum State. Sudan Arch Microbiol Immunology 1(1):33–40
23. Zheng Z, Li X, Li Z, Ma XC (2013) IL-4 -590C/T polymorphism and susceptibility to liver disease: a meta-analysis and meta-regression. DNA Cell Biol 32:443–450
24. Lu Y, Wu Z, Peng Q et al (2014) Role of IL-4 Gene Polymorphisms in HBV-Related Hepatocellular Carcinoma in a Chinese Population. PLoS One. 9(10): e110061

6

Safety and efficacy of directly acting antivirals (sofosbuvir and daclatasvir) in treatment of chronic HCV in HIV-HCV co-infected Egyptian patients

Inas E L-Khedr Mohamed[1], Kadry Mohamed EL-Saeed[1], Mahmoud Hassan Al-Sadik[2] and Christina Alphonse Anwar[1*]

Abstract

Background: Cure of chronic hepatitis C (HCV) in HIV/HCV co-infected patients is a priority due to their increased risk of complications. Daclatasvir and sofosbuvir treatment regimens with or without ribavirin are considered an important chance for better HCV treatment in patients with HIV/HCV co-infection. This study aimed at the assessment of safety and efficacy of sofosbuvir-daclatasvir treatment regimens in HIV/HCV co-infected Egyptian patients.

Results: Thirty HIV/HCV co-infected adult patients were included. All patients completed the study duration without major problems or drug interactions, HCV PCR was negative for all patients at the end of treatment, yet 12 weeks after ending treatment, only one patient (3.33%) had HCV relapse.

Liver enzymes showed a significant decrease by the end of treatment and 12 weeks after end of treatment in comparison with their values before treatment (*P*-value = 0.0001). CD4 counts as well showed significant increase. There was non-significant change in serum albumin, total bilirubin, alfa fetoprotein, complete blood count (CBC), coagulation profile, random blood sugar, or serum creatinine. Ultrasonographic findings did not show significant difference.

Conclusion: Combination of daclatasvir and sofosbuvir have showed 96.67% sustained virologic response at 12 weeks after treatment (SVR 12) among HIV/HCV co-infected patients, with a good safety profile. Moreover, the treated patients showed a significant increase in CD4 lymphocytic count.

Keywords: Sofosbuvir, Daclatasvir, HCV, HIV, SVR

Background

Five million people are HIV/HCV co-infected [1] those are at a higher risk of cirrhosis, hepatocellular carcinoma, hepatic decompensation and death than HCV mono-infected patients [2]. The widespread use of antiretroviral therapy made HIV as a chronic disease, with significant improvement in acquired immune deficiency syndrome (AIDS) related mortality; however the effect of HIV co-infection on the course of HCV disease, although reduced, but still not eliminated by antiretroviral therapy. Moreover, liver-related mortality is the most common cause of death in HIV/HCV co-infected individuals. Therefore, treatment of HCV infection in HIV/HCV co infected individuals is a priority [2].

Treatment of HCV with interferon-based regimens in HIV/HCV co-infected patients was associated with low rates of sustained virologic response, high rates of treatment-related cytopenias, and complex interactions with concomitant antiretroviral drugs [3].

Daclatasvir and sofosbuvir co-administration has pangenotypic anti HCV effect through inhibition of both NS5A, NS5B proteins, and are safe and effective for

* Correspondence: christinalfons7@gmail.com
[1]Gastro-enterology and Hepatology Faculty of Medicine, Ain Shams University, Cairo, Egypt
Full list of author information is available at the end of the article

treatment of chronic hepatitis C genotype 4 infected patients with minimal adverse events [4]. According to literature, 93% of HCV infected patients in Egypt are infected with genotype 4 [5].

Daclatasvir and sofosbuvir have limited pharmacokinetic interactions with antiretroviral drugs, and dose adjustments for daclatasvir in patients receiving moderate inducers or strong inhibitors of cytochrome P-450 3A4 are straightforward. Thus, this combination may be valuable for treating patients with HIV/HCV co-infection [6].

To our knowledge, safety and efficacy of DAA on Egyptian HIV/HCV co infected patients receiving antiretroviral treatment is not well studied. So we conducted this study aiming at assessing safety and efficacy of daclatasvir plus sofosbuvir regimens in treatment of chronic HCV in HIV/HCV co-infected Egyptian patients.

Methods

A prospective cohort study has been performed on 30 HIV/HCV co-infected adult Egyptian patients receiving treatment at Abbasia Fever Hospital in the period from July 2019 to February 2020.

Included patients were adults (age > 18), HCV infected patients (fulfilling NCCVH criteria for DAA treatment protocols) and were already on anti-retroviral drugs for HIV.

The following patients were excluded from the study according to NCCVH protocol: hepatocellular carcinoma, Child C, thrombocytopenic (platelets< 50000), HBsAg positive, Advanced HIV (CD4< 200), pregnant, uncontrolled diabetic (HbA1c > 9%), end stage renal disease (Glomerular filtration rate< 30) patients.

Subjected patients were already receiving highly active antiretroviral therapy (HAART), According to Al-Abbassia Fever Hospital protocol and Egyptian national guidelines for antiretroviral therapy, December 2017: efavirenz 600 mg one tablet daily + truvada (tenofovir 300 mg + emtricitabine 200 mg) one tablet daily.

Concerning directly acting anti-viral drug regimen; 25 patients (83.30%) were easy to treat according to NCCV H criteria and received sofosbuvir (400 mg/day) + daclatasvir (90 mg/day) for 12 weeks while only 5 patients were considered to be difficult to treat (due to thrombocytopenia, PLT: 50,000–149,000) and received sofosbuvir (400 mg/day) + daclatasvir (90 mg/day) + ribavirin (800 mg/day) for 12 weeks.

All participants were subjected to full history taking, clinical examination, laboratory investigations (including complete blood count (CBC), alanine aminotransferase (ALT), aspartate aminotransferase (AST), serum bilirubin, serum albumin, prothrombin time (PT), international normalized ratio (INR), alfa feto protein (AFP), serum creatinine, random blood sugar, quantitative PCR for HCV and HIV, CD4 T-lymphocyte count) and abdominal ultrasonography .

Patients were under regular follow-up during the study period (before the start of treatment, at the end of treatment and after12 weeks) by clinical examination and laboratory assessment.

Statistical analysis was conducted by using statistical SPSS Package program version 24 for Windows (SPSS, Inc., Chicago, IL) including the mean and standard deviation for all quantitative variables, number and percentage for all qualitative variables, normality test of data using Shapiro-Wilk test was used, Levene's test for testing the homogeneity of variance. Chi-square test ($\chi2$ test) , Independent t-test to compare two groups for all quantitative variables, one-way analysis of variance (ANOVA-test). Quantitative data was screened, normality test of data using Shapiro-Wilk test was used, Levene's test for testing the homogeneity of variance. All statistical analysis was significant at 0.05 level of probability ($P \leq 0.05$). Quantitative data was screened, normality test of data using Shapiro-Wilk test was used, Levene's test for testing the homogeneity of variance.

Ethics approval and consent to participate

This study had been performed in accordance with the ethical standards. Faculty of Medicine, Ain Shams University Ethical Committee approval was taken before starting the study, and the study protocol conforms to the ethical guidelines of the 1975 Declaration of Helsinki. A written consent was obtained from each participant.

Results

Thirty HIV/HCV co-infected patients, their ages ranged between 21 and 46 years, 80% of them were males, almost half of the patients were married and 86 % were unemployed. 50% of them were smokers and IV addicts. All enrolled patients were Child A, all of them completed the study duration without any major problems, quantitative HCV PCR was negative for all patients at the end of treatment, yet 12 weeks after ending treatment only one patient (3.33%) had HCV relapse.

With regard to route of HIV infection, the commonest was through intravenous drug abuse in 53.3%, different sexual routes in 20%, blood transfusion in 10%, and the rest was not identified.

As regard laboratory data before, after, and 12 weeks of end of treatment, there was no statistically significant differences on comparing values for CBC, coagulation profile, random blood sugar, or serum creatinine.

In addition, Ultrasonographic findings did not show any statistically significant difference throughout the study duration (liver parenchyma, portal vein diameter, spleen, ascites, hepatic focal lesions).

On pair-wise comparison, there was a significant decrease in ALT and AST levels by the end of treatment and 12 weeks after treatment in comparison with ALT and AST levels before treatment (*P*-value: 0.0001). Yet there was non-significant change in serum albumin, total bilirubin, alfa fetoprotein (Table 1).

Difference between CD4 lymphocytic counts before, at the end and 3 months after end of treatment was highly significant (*p* value = 0.0001).

With respect to adverse effects of both drug regimens, fatigue (73.33%), headache (46.67%), insomnia (33.33%), diarrhea (23.33%), nausea (20.00%), and pruritus (13.33%) were the most commonly documented adverse effects, yet there was no reported severe adverse effects requiring drug discontinuation or hospitalization.

Discussion

Although effect of HIV co-infection on the course of HCV disease is reduced but yet not eliminated by antiretroviral therapy and liver-related mortality is still considered the most common cause of death in HIV/HCV co-infected individuals [2].

Poor adherence of patients with HIV/HCV coinfection receiving HCV antiviral therapy owing to lots of ongoing challenges was reported by Grebely et al. (2012) [7].

HIV coinfection negatively impacts both sustained virological response and viral kinetics during treatment with pegylated interferon plus ribavirine in subjects infected with HCV genotype 1 or 4. Yet directly acting antivirals has narrowed the gap in SVR between HIV/HCV co-infected and HCV mono-infected persons for most of the used directly acting antiviral drug combinations [8].

Accordingly, treatment of HCV infection in HIV/HCV coinfected individuals is a priority.

In the current study, thirty HIV–HCV coinfected patients with mean age 33.8 years received 12 weeks of daclatasvir plus sofosbuvir with or without ribavirin. 96.67% of them had a sustained virologic response at week 12 post treatment (SVR 12). This matches with Wyles et al. (2015) [9] study that revealed SVR rate of 97% when the same combinations of DAAs were evaluated in patients co-infected with HIV and HCV. Yet our results are higher than the results of Milazzo and his colleges (2017) [10] and Hezode et al. (2016) [11] in their real life studies showing that the SVR 12 in HIV/HCV co-infected patients receiving antivirals was about 91% SVR. This difference may be due to genotypic variance or patient compliance.

In the current study, all patients were receiving antiretroviral combination of truvada (tenofovir+emtricitabine) and efavirenz. As regards drug-drug interactions, there were no drug interactions between DAAs and ARVs. No patient discontinued treatment because of drug-drug interactions. No modifications in HIV therapy were needed with the receipt of daclatasvir or sofosbuvir during treatment in our study and we administered a 90 mg dose of daclatasvir with efavirenz according to Garimella et al. (2016) [12]. This agrees with Panel et al. (2015) [13] who found that both daclatasvir and sofosbuvir have limited pharmacokinetic interactions with other antiretroviral drugs.

As regards achieving SVR on CD4 count, in our study, there was a significant increase in CD4 count in treated patients; Dazley et al. (2015) [14] agreed with our study. This matches with Sarah et al. [15], who documented that the use of DAA therapy in HIV-HCV co-infected patients resulted in a significant increase in CD4 count in patients with pre-DAA CD4 < 350 cells/mm^3. This can be explained by the persistent immune activation and CD4 T cell apoptosis involved with HCV infection in the co-infected patients [16], this activation decreases in response to the success of the HCV treatment (Table 2).

As regards efficacy, a significant decrease in ALT and AST over time in the studied patients 12 weeks after the end of treatment, this agrees with Elsharkawy et al. (2017) [17, 18]. This came in accordance with one previous study by Mehta et al. in 201 7[19] who studied safety and efficacy of the same regimen in B-Thalassemia major patients with chronic HCV, where responders showed significant improvement in AST and ALT values

Table 1 Comparison of liver function tests findings before, after, and 12 weeks after end of treatment

Items	Liver function tests findings (mean ± SD)				
	Alanine amino transferase	Aspartate amino transferase	Serum albumin	Total bilirubin	αfetoprotein
Before treatment	54.80±39.10	52.20±39.93	4.13±0.38	0.86±0.25	7.13±5.02
End of treatment	30.90±11.91	32.20±10.31	4.06±0.29 0	0.88±0.27	6.76±3.42
SVR at 12 weeks	28.23±10.49	30.28±10.46	4.14±0.24	0.76±0.22	6.75±3.83
F-value	10.815	7.319	0.588	1.175	0.081
P-value	0.0001	0.001	0.557	0.180	0.923
Significance	S	S	NS	NS	NS

SD standard deviation, *P-value* probability, *S* significant

Table 2 CD4 lymphocytic level changes before and after treatment

Items	CD4 lymphocytic count (mean ± SD)
Before treatment	310.60 ±89.9
End of treatment	385.90 ±108.71
SVR at 12 weeks	445.13 ±125.44
F-value	11.482
P-value	0.0001
Significance	S

SD standard deviation, *P-value* probability, *S* significant

compared to pretreatment values after 12 weeks of treatment which indicates Sof/Dac role in improving necroinflammation in patients with chronic HCV [19].

Daclatasvir plus sofosbuvir combination regimen was well tolerated with no reported serious adverse events and no discontinuations, The majority of events observed were categorized as mild or moderate as (fatigue 73.33%, headache 46.67%, nausea 20% and GI upset by 23.33%). This was similar to what was reported by Sulkowski et al. (2014) [20–22] about safety of DAAs in HIV/HCV co-infected patients and what was reported by Wyles et al. (2015) [9] about the safety of daclatasvir plus sofosbuvir combination in co-infected patients.

Limitation

Our study is limited by the small sample size, short observation period, and that all cases were studied in a single center.

Conclusion

Combination of daclatasvir and sofosbuvir have showed 96.67% sustained virologic response at 12 weeks after treatment (SVR 12) among HIV/HCV co-infected patients, with a very good safety profile. Moreover, the treated patients showed a significant increase in CD4 count. Accordingly, HIV/HCV co-infected patients should be treated with sofosbuvir and daclatesvir containing regimens.

Abbreviations

HIV: Human immune deficiency virus; HCV: Hepatitis C virus; ALT: Alanine amino tranaminase; AST: Aspartate amino tranaminase; SVR: Sustained virological response; PCR: Polymerase chain reaction; CBC: Complete blood count; CD4: Cluster of differentiation; NS: Non-structural protein; DAA: Directly acting antiviral drugs; NCCVH: National Committee for the Control of Viral Hepatitis; HBsAg: Hepatitis B surface antigen

Acknowledgements

Thanks should be applied to Fever hospital staff due to their help in facilitating data collection.

Authors' contributions

KE: Final approval of the version to be published. IE: Critical revision of the article. MH: Data collection, data analysis, and interpretation. CA: Conception or design of the work and drafting the article. All authors have read and approved the manuscript.

Declarations

Ethics approval and consent to participate

This study had been performed in accordance with the ethical standards. Faculty of Medicine, Ain Shams University Ethical Committee approval was taken before starting the study, and the study protocol conforms to the ethical guidelines of the 1975 Declaration of Helsinki. A written consent was obtained from each participant.

Competing interests

The authors declare that they have no competing interests.

Author details

[1]Gastro-enterology and Hepatology Faculty of Medicine, Ain Shams University, Cairo, Egypt. [2]Abbassia Fever Hospital, Cairo, Egypt.

References

1. UNAIDS (2014): Report on the Global AID Epidemic. Retrieved from: http://www.data.unaids.org/pub/ GlobalReport/2014.
2. Smith CJ, Ryom L, Weber R, Morlat P, Pradier C, Reiss P, Kowalska JD, de Wit S, Law M, el Sadr W, Kirk O, Friis-Moller N, Monforte A'A, Phillips AN, Sabin CA, Lundgren JD (2014) Trends in underlying causes of death in people with HIV from 1999 to 2011 (D: A: D): a multicohort collaboration. The Lancet 384(9939):241–248. https://doi.org/10.1016/S0140-6736(14)60604-8
3. Sulkowski MS, Thomas DL (2003) Hepatitis C in the HIV-infected person. Annals of internal medicine 138(3):197–207. https://doi.org/10.7326/0003-4819-138-3-200302040-00012
4. Ossama Ashraf Ahmed, Eslam Safwat, Mohamed Omar Khalifa et al., Sofosbuvir Plus Daclatasvir in Treatment of Chronic Hepatitis C Genotype 4 Infection in a Cohort of Egyptian Patients: An Experiment the Size of Egyptian Village. Int J Hepatol. 2018;2018:9616234. doi: 10.1155/2018/9616234.
5. Gower E, Estes C, Blach S et al (2014) Global Epidemiology and genotype distribution of the hepatitis C virus infection. J Hepatol 61(1)
6. Bifano M, Hwang C, Oosterhuis B et al (2013) Assessment of pharmacokinetic interactions of the HCV NS5A replication complex inhibitor daclatasvir with antiretroviral agents: ritonavir-boosted atazanavir, efavirenz and tenofovir. Antivir Ther 18(7):931–940
7. Grebely J, Hellard M, Applegate T et al (2012) Virological responses during treatment for recent hepatitis C virus: potential benefit for ribavirin use in HCV/HIV co-infection. AIDS (London, England) 26(13):1653
8. Monje-Agudo A, Castro-Iglesias A, Rivero-Juárez et al (2015) Impact of HIV infection on sustained virological response to treatment against hepatitis C virus with pegylated interferon plus ribavirin. Eurobian J Clin Microbiol Infect Dis:1929–1936
9. Wyles DL, Ruane PJ, Sulkowski MS, Dieterich D, Luetkemeyer A, Morgan TR, Sherman KE, Dretler R, Fishbein D, Gathe JC Jr, Henn S, Hinestrosa F, Huynh C, McDonald C, Mills A, Overton ET, Ramgopal M, Rashbaum B, Ray G, Scarsella A, Yozviak J, McPhee F, Liu Z, Hughes E, Yin PD, Noviello S, Ackerman P (2015) Daclatasvir plus sofosbuvir for HCV in patients coinfected with HIV-1. New England J Med 373(8):714–725. https://doi.org/10.1056/NEJMoa1503153
10. Milazzo L, Lai A, Calvi E, Ronzi P, Micheli V, Binda F, Ridolfo AL, Gervasoni C, Galli M, Antinori S, Sollima S (2017) Direct-acting antivirals in hepatitis C virus (HCV)-infected and HCV/HIV-coinfected patients: real-life safety and efficacy. HIV Med 18(4):284–291. https://doi.org/10.1111/hiv.12429
11. Hézode C, Abergel A, Chas J, Conti F, Cotte L, Tateo M, Alric L, Vergniol J, Tomei C, Bernard PH, Loustaud-Ratti V, Arpurt JP, Blaisoṅ D, Larrey D, Fedchuk L, Bennai Y, Filipovics A, Fontaine H, Pageaux GP (2016) Sustained virologic response to daclatasvir and sofosbuvir, with or without ribavirin, among patients in the French daclatasvir ATU programme infected with HCV genotypes 4, 5 and 6. J Hepatol 64(2):S755. https://doi.org/10.1016/S0168-8278(16)01471-9

12. Garimella T, You X, Wang R, Huang SP, Kandoussi H, Bifano M, Bertz R, Eley T (2016) A review of daclatasvir drug–drug interactions. Adv Ther 33(11): 1867–1884. https://doi.org/10.1007/s12325-016-0407-5
13. Panel Chung RT, Davis GL, Jensen DM et al (2015) Hepatitis C guidance: AASLD-IDSA recommendations for testing, managing, and treating adults infected with hepatitis C virus. Hepatology 62(3):932–954
14. Dazley J, Sison R, Slim J (2015) Long-Term Consequences of Hepatitis C Viral Clearance on the CD4. AIDS Res Treat 2015:1–4. https://doi.org/10.1155/2015/687629
15. Sarah M Michienzi, Jiaqi Cai, Cydnee Harris, et al., HIV-HCV Coinfection: An Investigation of CD4 T-Cell Reconstitution after HCV Direct-Acting Antiviral Treatment. Open Forum Infect Dis. 2019; 6(Suppl 2): S187.Published online 2019 Oct 23. doi: https://doi.org/10.1093/ofid/ofz360.429
16. Braitstein P, Zala C, Yip B, Brinkhof MWG, Moore D, Hogg RS, Montaner JSG (2006) Immunologic response to antiretroviral therapy in hepatitis C virus–coinfected adults in a population-based HIV/AIDS treatment program. J Infect Dis 193(2):259–268. https://doi.org/10.1086/498908
17. Elsharkawy A, Alem SA, Fouad R, el Raziky M, el Akel W, Abdo M, Tantawi O, AbdAllah M, Bourliere M, Esmat G (2017) Changes in liver stiffness measurements and fibrosis scores following sofosbuvir based treatment regimens without interferon. J Gastroenterol Hepatol 32(9):1624–1630. https://doi.org/10.1111/jgh.13758
18. Bachofner JA, Valli PV, Kröger A, Bergamin I, Künzler P, Baserga A, Braun D, Seifert B, Moncsek A, Fehr J, Semela D, Magenta L, Müllhaupt B, Terziroli Beretta-Piccoli B, Mertens JC (2017) Direct antiviral agent treatment of chronic hepatitis C results in rapid regression of transient elastography and fibrosis markers fibrosis-4 score and aspartate aminotransferase platelet ratio index. Liver Int 37(3):369–376. https://doi.org/10.1111/liv.13256
19. Mehta R, Kabrawala M, Nandwani S et al (2017) Safety and efficacy of sofosbuvir and daclatasvir for hepatitis C virus infection in patients with β-thalassemia major. J Clin Exper Hepatol
20. Sulkowski MS, Gardiner DF, Rodriguez-Torres M, Reddy KR, Hassanein T, Jacobson I, Lawitz E, Lok AS, Hinestrosa F, Thuluvath PJ, Schwartz H, Nelson DR, Everson GT, Eley T, Wind-Rotolo M, Huang SP, Gao M, Hernandez D, McPhee F, Sherman D, Hindes R, Symonds W, Pasquinelli C, Grasela DM (2014) Daclatasvir plus sofosbuvir for previously treated or untreated chronic HCV infection. New England J Med 370(3):211–221. https://doi.org/10.1056/NEJMoa1306218
21. Molina J, Chloe O, David MI et al (2015) Sofosbuvir plus ribavirin for treatment of hepatitis C virus in patients coinfected with HIV (PHOTON-2): a multicentre, open-label, non-randomised, phase 3 study. The Lancet 385(9973):1098–1106. https://doi.org/10.1016/S0140-6736(14)62483-1
22. Naggie S, Cooper C, Saag M, Workowski K, Ruane P, Towner WJ, Marks K, Luetkemeyer A, Baden RP, Sax PE, Gane E, Santana-Bagur J, Stamm LM, Yang JC, German P, Dvory-Sobol H, Ni L, Pang PS, McHutchison J, Stedman CA, Morales-Ramirez JO, Bräu N, Jayaweera D, Colson AE, Tebas P, Wong DK, Dieterich D, Sulkowski M, ION-4 Investigators (2015) Ledipasvir and sofosbuvir for HCV in patients coinfected with HIV1. New England J Med 373(8):705–713. https://doi.org/10.1056/NEJMoa1501315

7

Hepatitis C core antigen: a simple predictive marker for treatment response to the new direct-acting antiviral drugs in chronic HCV Egyptian patients

Asmaa M. Elbrolosy[1*], Moamena S. Elhamouly[2], Emad M. Eed[1], Gamalat A. El Gedawy[3], Mai Abozeid[4] and Naglaa S. Elabd[2]

Abstract

Background: Successful eradication of hepatitis C virus (HCV) has great impact on the prognosis of HCV-related complications and the associated mortality. The development of the new direct-acting antiviral drugs (DAAs) has revolutionized the treatment of HCV infection. HCV core antigen (HCVcAg) is a recently developed marker that displayed a good correlation with HCV RNA assays. Our main objectives were to correlate between serum levels of HCVcAg and HCV RNA loads in chronic HCV patients as well as to explore the potential value of HCVcAg assay in predicting treatment response to the new DAAs. The study enrolled a total of 280 chronic HCV-infected patients scheduled to start the new regimen for treatment of chronic HCV by all-oral, interferon-free DAAs. According to the viral load, the studied individuals were arranged into three groups corresponding to mild, moderate, and sever viremia. Serum level of HCVcAg was determined by ELISA technique and HCV RNA viral loads were quantified using the real-time PCR system. The assays were performed three times for all participants: prior to initiation of treatment, at the end of treatment (week 12), and 3 months post-treatment cessation (week 24).

Results: A statistically significant difference between HCV RNA and HCVcAg baseline levels among different viremia groups was detected ($P < 0.001$). There was a significant positive correlation between HCV RNA and HCVcAg baseline values among all the studied cases ($P < 0.05$) with a correlation coefficient of 0.752, 0.976, and 1.00 respectively for mild, moderate, and severe viremia groups. 92.9% (260/280) of the studied patients achieved sustained virologic response, 3.6% (10/280) were non-responders, and 3.6% (10/280) had recurrent viremia/relapse as regards RT-PCR results.

Conclusion: HCVcAg is a promising alternative to HCV RNA assay. The ELISAs for HCVcAg proved excellent correlations with HCV RNA levels. Moreover, HCVcAg can be introduced as a simple and highly specific tool for monitoring the new DAA regimens particularly in low-resource settings.

Keywords: HCV core antigen, HCV RNA assay, New direct-acting antiviral drugs

* Correspondence: asmaaelbrolosy@yahoo.com
[1]Department of Medical Microbiology and Immunology, Faculty of Medicine, Menoufia University, Shibin El Kom, Egypt
Full list of author information is available at the end of the article

Background

The prevalence of HCV infection varies significantly all over the world. Treatment and monitoring of HCV infection are of great concern, especially in developing countries [1]. The highest prevalence of HCV in the world occurs in Egypt with estimates higher than 10% among the general population. There are approximately 3.7 million persons in Egypt that have chronic HCV infection in 2015 [2].

In clinical practice, serological detection of anti-HCV antibodies is usually used for diagnosis of HCV infection. However, most assays are not able to distinguish patients with an ongoing active infection from those who have spontaneously cleared the virus [3]. Sometimes, there is a long seronegative interval throughout the course of HCV infection during which anti-HCV antibodies are undetectable. Immunosuppression may result in an insufficient antibody response as well. Therefore, anti-HCV assays still need additional confirmation [4].

Nucleic acid-based techniques for HCV RNA are currently used to confirm the diagnosis of HCV infection and to monitor the antiviral therapy because of their high specificity and sensitivity. However, the complexity and cost of such molecular diagnostics can constrain their use in low-resourced settings [5]. Likewise, cheaper and simple diagnostic tools and follow-up algorithms are in urgent need to enhance the global efforts for HCV eradication by the year 2030 particularly in low- and middle-income countries [6].

The HCV core antigen (HCVcAg) is a 21-kDa structural phosphoprotein of the HCV capsid and comprising the first 191 amino acids of the viral polyprotein. Hepatitis C virus core antigen is highly conserved across HCV genotypes. It exists in both complete virions and RNA-free core protein structures [5]. During viral assembly, HCVcAg is released into the plasma/serum and can be detected earlier than antibodies during the course of HCV infection. Recently, less-expensive and time-consuming immunoassay techniques for detecting HCVcAg have become available [7].

Viral kinetics of HCV no longer predict treatment duration or outcome; consequently, there is no longer value for repeated measurement of HCV RNA load. There is however great evidence that the amount of HCVcAg in the blood correlates well with the HCV RNA level. Thus, HCVcAg can identify patients with active HCV infection and is a surrogate marker for viral replication. Furthermore, HCVcAg assay may be superior to the current two-step diagnostic approach in terms of time and cost-saving benefits. The novel approach has also established its clinical utility in the screening of active HCV infections for anti-HCV antibody-positive individuals [8].

During the last decade, great interest has been focused on the development of direct-acting antiviral drugs (DAAs). These agents have the ability to block essential enzymes regulating HCV replication. Several new oral, interferon-free antiviral drugs were approved, representing an additional bonus of extension into pan-genotypic activity [9].

The proximate target of anti-HCV therapy is to achieve sustained virologic response (SVR)/virologic cure meaning that HCV RNA is undetectable for at least 12 weeks after cessation of therapy. In the year 2011, the FDA accepted SVR-12 as endpoint for future trials because HCV relapse usually occurs within the first 12 weeks after the end of treatment [10].

In the era of DAAs, many studies reported that HCVcAg could be employed as a simple marker to establish active infection, to initiate the requirement for treatment and then to evaluate viremia after completion of DAAs therapy as well [11]. The main objectives were to verify the utility HCVcAg assay in predicting treatment response to the new oral, interferon-free DAA regimen by comparing it with the established methods for quantification of HCV RNA.

Methods

This prospective study was carried out at the Department of Medical Microbiology and Immunology, in collaboration with Tropical Medicine Department, Faculty of Medicine, Menoufia University, and Department of Hepatology and Gastroenterology, National Liver Institute, Menoufia University, during the period from December 2018 to April 2020. The study involved 280 patients (100 females and 180 males). All patients were over 18 years of age, had compensated liver disease, and were diagnosed to have chronic HCV infection by enzyme-linked immunosorbent serum anti-HCV assay and confirmed by real-time PCR. All the recruited cases were scheduled to receive the new DAAs therapy for treatment of HCV infection as recommended by the Egyptian National Committee for Control of Viral Hepatitis (NCCVH).

The included patients were prescribed sofosbuvir (SOF)/daclatasvir (DCV) (easy to treat) or SOF/DCV/ribavirin (RVN) (difficult to treat) according to the NCCV H as follows:

- *Easy to treat group*: Comprises treatment-naïve patients, total bilirubin < 1.2 mg/dl, serum albumin > 3.5 g/dl, INR < 1.2, and platelet count > 150,000/mm^3
- *Difficult to treat group*: Comprises IFN-experienced patients, total bilirubin ≥ 1.2 mg/dl, serum albumin (2.8–3.5 g/dl), INR (1.2–1.7), and platelet count of 50,000–150,000/mm^3

Table 1 Baseline routine and specific laboratory investigations of the studied groups

Lab investigations	Total cases (No. = 280)			Test of significance	P value
	Group I (No. = 140)	Group II (No. = 80)	Group III (No. = 60)		
	Mean ± SD	Mean ± SD	Mean ± SD		
ALT (IU/ml)	58.6 ± 7.8	75.0 ± 20.6	122.0 ± 66.4	**Kruskal-Wallis test** = 17.6	< 0.001**
AST(IU/ml)	44.1 ± 13.3	65.0 ± 23.3	114.2 ± 67.6	**Kruskal-Wallis test** = 17.14	< 0.001**
ALP (IU/ml)	29.8 ± 14.8	75.1 ± 24.4	134.8 ± 68.8	**Kruskal-Wallis test** = 21.24	< 0.001**
GGT (IU/ml)	12.7 ± 7.5	30.1 ± 10.8	63.3 ± 12.1	**Kruskal-Wallis test** = 20.14	< 0.001**
Total bilirubin (mg/dl)	1.1 ± 0.27	1.2 ± 0.84	1.8 ± 1.2	**Kruskal-Wallis test** = 0.73	0.69
Albumin (g/dl)	3.8 ± 0.54	3.7 ± 0.39	3.4 ± 0.37	**ANOVA test** = 0.85	0.44
PT (s)	14.5 ± 2.1	14.5 ± 1.6	14.9 ± 2.2	**ANOVA test** = 0.08	0.92
PT concentration (%)	86.3 ± 19.5	86.8 ± 9.5	84.9 ± 13.9	**ANOVA test** = 0.05	0.95
INR	1.2 ± 0.17	1.2 ± 0.15	1.2 ± 0.18	**ANOVA test** = 0.09	0.91
Hb (gm/dl)	13.6 ± 1.7	13.6 ± 1.3	12.8 ± 2.8	**ANOVA test** = 0.41	0.67
PLT ($X10^3$/mm)	186.2 ± 48.3	189.9 ± 57.4	157.0 ± 62.6	**Kruskal-Wallis test** = 1.60	0.45
Glucose (mg/dl)	92.9 ± 30.5	90.1 ± 25.6	98.2 ± 36.9	**Kruskal-Wallis test** = 0.16	0.92
Creatinine(mg/dl)	0.81 ± 0.12	0.81 ± 0.09	0.83 ± 0.13	**ANOVA test** = 0.88	0.92
Urea (mg/dl)	35.0 ± 10.9	44.5 ± 9.1	39.5 ± 11.3	**ANOVA test** = 2.08	0.15

Exclusion criteria were determined as per the Supreme Council and National treatment programme of Hepatitis C updated Treatment Protocol December 2019 [12]. These included Child's C cirrhotic patients, platelet count less than 50,000/mm^3, serum albumin < 2.8 g/dl, total serum bilirubin > 3 mg/dl, INR > 1.7, patients co-infected with HIV, hepatocellular carcinoma (HCC) except 6 months after intervention aiming at cure with no evidence of activity by dynamic imaging (CT or MRI), extra-hepatic malignancy except after 2 years of disease-free interval, pregnancy or inability to use effective contraception, and inadequately controlled diabetes mellitus.

All patients had given informed consent about the study and ethical approval was provided by the Ethics Committee of Menoufia University which came in accordance with the ethical guidelines of the 2013 "Helsinki Declaration".

According to the HCV viral load, the studied patients were arranged into three groups: group I involved 140 patients with mild viremia (< 200,000 IU/ml), group II involved 80 patients with moderate viremia (200,000:2, 000,000 IU/ml), and group III involved 60 patients with severe viremia (> 2,000,000 IU/ml) [13].

All patients were subjected to proper history taking and clinical examination. Laboratory investigations regarding complete blood picture, liver profile (including ALT, AST, ALP, GGT, serum albumin, total bilirubin, direct bilirubin, and INR), kidney function tests, and viral hepatitis markers for HbsAg and HCV antibodies were collected from each patient's file.

Blood samples were collected from all participants and then sera were stored at − 20 °C until assayed for quantitative estimation of HCV RNA and HCVcAg levels.

Quantitative estimation of HCV RNA level by real-time reverse transcription-polymerase chain reaction (RT-PCR)

The assay was done 3 times for each patient as follows: PCR-1, prior to initiation of treatment to ensure the diagnosis of HCV infection and to determine the

Table 2 Mean values of baseline levels for both HCV RNA (IU/ml) and HCVcAg (Peiu/ml) assays among the studied groups

Studied groups	Baseline levels					
	HCV RNA serum level (IU/ml) Mean ± SD	Kruskal-Wallis test P value	Post hoc test	HCVcAg serum level (Peiu/ml) Mean ± SD	ANOVA test and P value	Post hoc test
Group I (*n* = 140)	95648.1 ± 50814.0	Test = 22.76 *P* < 0.001**	P1 < 0.001** P2 = 0.001** P3 = 0.002*	1.4 ± 0.35	Test = 69.69 *P* < 0.001**	P1 = 0.002* P2 < 0.001** P3 < 0.001**
Group II (*n* = 80)	1082313.0 ± 558186.7			2.6 ± 0.68		
Group III (*n* = 60)	4812067.8 ± 1837006.9			5.9 ± 1.5		

*Significant
**Highly significant

baseline viral load; PCR-2, at the end of treatment (week 12) to assess end of treatment response (ETR) [14]; and PCR-3, 3 months post-treatment cessation (week 24) as a follow-up step to assess sustained virologic response (SVR-12) [14].

Procedure

The procedure involved three main steps: HCV RNA extraction, conversion of HCV RNA to complementary DNA (Cdna), and amplification and detection of the amplified products. HCV RNA extraction was performed by using artus® HCV RG RT-PCR kit (Qiagen GmbH, Germany, Cat No. 4518263) according to the manufacturer's instructions. HCV levels were determined using the Rotor-Gene Q MDx (Rotor-Gene Q MDx, Qiagen, Germany) Light Cycler Real-Time PCR System using Rotor-Gene-3000 software version 6.0.23. An internal quality control serum was included during RT-PCR [15].

HCVcAg assay

HCV core antigen serum levels were measured by enzyme-linked immunosorbant assay according to the manufacturer's instructions (Sinogeneclon Co., Ltd, China). The concentration of HCVcAg in the samples was then determined by comparing the optical density (O.D.) of the samples to the standard curve. The assay was done at the same intervals of the PCR assay.

Statistical analysis

Statistical analysis was done using SPSS version 20. Continuous/numerical data were presented as mean ± standard deviation (SD) and were compared by Kruskal-Wallis test and ANOVA test. Categorical variables were shown as numbers (percentages) and were compared by Chi-square (χ^2) test. Linear regression analysis was applied to evaluate the association between HCVcAg and HCV RNA levels. The diagnostic performance of HCVcAg and HCV RNA in the prediction of SVR-12 was expressed as sensitivity, specificity, positive predictive value (PPV), negative predictive value (NPV), and area under the receiver operating characteristic (AUROC) curve. Statistical significance was set at P value < 0.05.

Results

Baseline routine and specific laboratory investigations of the studied groups are shown in Table 1. A highly significant statistical difference was recorded regarding serum ALT, AST, ALP, and GGT levels among the three studied viremia groups ($P < 0.001$). Other parameters revealed no significant difference ($P > 0.05$).

Baseline levels of both HCV RNA and HCVcAg assays were represented in Table 2 and Figs. 1 and 2. The

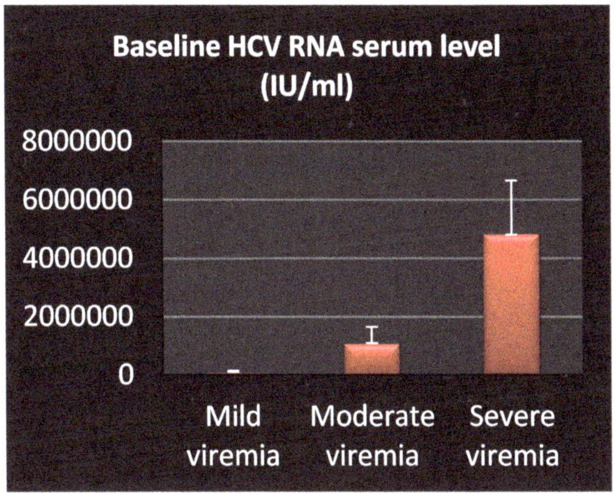

Fig. 1 Baseline HCV RNA levels (IU/mL)

recorded data denoted a statistically significant difference between the mean values of both HCV RNA and HCVcAg baseline levels among different viremia groups ($P < 0.001$). The level of HCVcAg was significantly higher in moderate viremia if compared with mild viremia ($P < 0.002$) and it was significantly higher in severe viremia if compared with moderate viremia ($P < 0.001$).

Importantly, a significant positive correlation was detected between HCV RNA and HCVcAg baseline values among all the studied cases ($P < 0.05$) with a correlation coefficient of 0.752, 0.976, and 1.00 respectively for mild, moderate, and severe viremia groups as shown in Table 3. The correlations of HCV RNA loads (IU/ml) with HCVcAg levels (Peiu/ml) including linear regression lines were illustrated in Fig. 3a–c.

For differentiation between mild and moderate viremia, HCVcAg proved sensitivity, specificity, PPV, NPV, and diagnostic accuracy of 87.5%, 85.7%, 77.8%, 92.3%, and 86.4% respectively when using a cutoff value

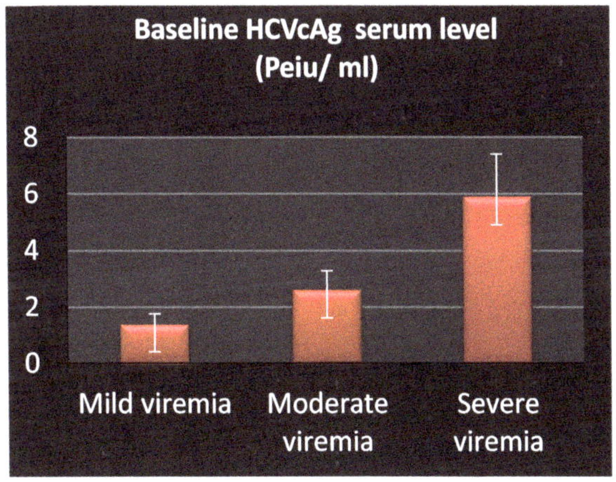

Fig. 2 Baseline HCVcAg levels (Peiu/mL)

Table 3 Correlation between baseline levels of HCVcAg (Peiu/ml) and HCV RNA (IU/ml) assays among the studied groups

Baseline HCV RNA (IU/ml)	Baseline HCVcAg (Peiu/ml)	
	r	*P* value
Group I: mild viremia group (No. = 140)	0.752	0.002*
Group II: moderate viremia group (No. = 80)	0.976	< 0.001**
Group III: severe viremia group (No. = 60)	1.00	< 0.001**

of 1.765 Peiu/ml. However, HCVcAg cutoff point of 3.42 Peiu/ml exhibited sensitivity, specificity, PPV, NPV, and diagnostic accuracy of 100%, 87.5%, 85.7%, 100%, and 92.9% respectively for differentiation between moderate and severe viremia (Table 4).

Regarding treatment response to the newly prescribed regimen of DAAs, 92.9% (260/280) of the studied cases achieved sustained virologic response (SVR-12), 3.6% (10/280) were non-responders with persistent viremia throughout the course of the study, and 3.6% (10/280) had recurrent viremia/relapse after treatment cessations as proved by RT-PCR results (Table 5).

Among patients who achieved SVR (260/280), HCVcAg was 100% (260/260) undetectable at both the 12th and 24th weeks. For the patients who proved non-response to anti-HCV treatment, HCVcAg was

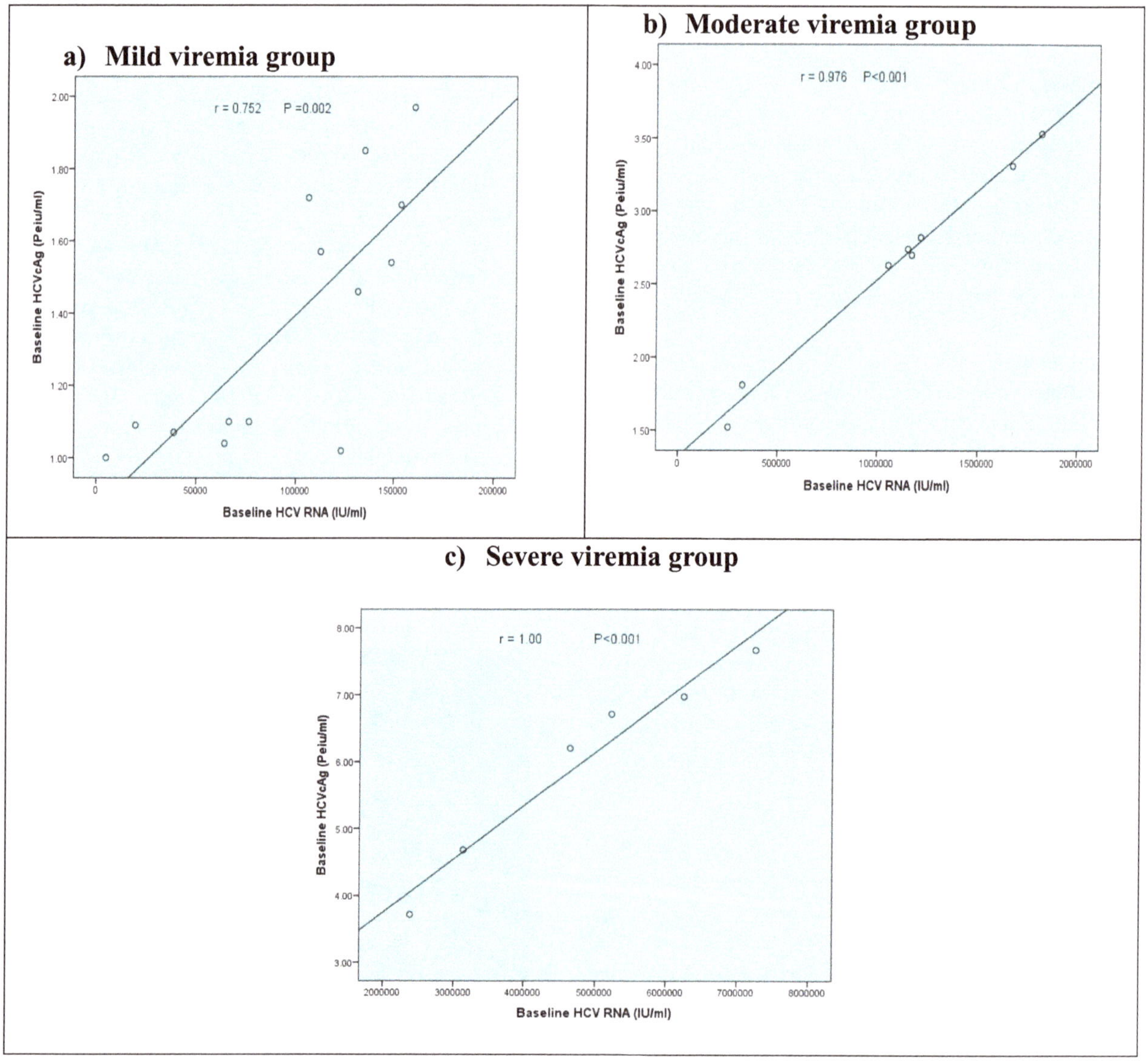

Fig. 3 a–c Correlation between baseline levels of HCVcAg (Peiu/ml) and HCV RNA (IU/ml) assays among the studied groups

Table 4 HCVcAg cutoff for differentiation between mild and moderate viremia

	AUC	Cutoff point	Sensitivity	Specificity	PPV	NPV	Accuracy
HCVcAg (Peiu/ml)	0.929	1.765	87.5%	85.7%	77.8%	92.3%	86.4%
HCVcAg cutoff for differentiation between moderate and severe viremia							
HCVcAg (Peiu/ml)	1.00	3.42	100%	87.5%	85.7%	100%	92.9%

continuously detectable at both the 12th and 24th weeks. However, for patients who developed recurrent viremia/ relapse, HCVcAg was undetectable at the 12th week and again became detectable at the 24th week post-treatment initiation (Table 6).

The degree of agreement between HCV RNA and HCVcAg results at the 12th and 24th weeks was 100% (Table 7). For evaluation of HCVcAg assay performance in prediction of treatment response at the 12th and 24th weeks, HCVcAg proved sensitivity, specificity, PPV, NPV, and accuracy of 100% (Table 8).

Discussion

HCV infection is a serious public health issue. Early detection and treatment are imperative to prevent its transmission. Limitations of anti-HCV and HCV RNA detection have restricted their applications in clinical practice [16].

HCVcAg has been proposed as an indirect marker of viral replication [16]. Recently, many assays have been developed for both qualitative and quantitative HCVcAg estimation, such as enzyme immunoassays (EIAs) or chemiluminescent immunoassays with an excellent correlation between HCVcAg concentrations and HCV RNA levels. These quantitative HCVcAg assays became promising alternatives to HCV nucleic acid-based techniques [17, 18].

In the current study, 280 patients with chronic HCV infection have been enrolled and arranged into mild, moderate, and severe viremia groups according to their HCV viral load. All studied individuals were prescribed the new regimen of anti-HCV treatment which included the new oral, interferon-free DAAs. The main targets were to correlate between baseline levels of both HCVcAg and HCV viremic load and to assess the utility of HCVcAg testing in the era of DAAs.

The recorded data denoted a highly significant statistical difference between the baseline values of both HCV RNA and HCVcAg among different viremia groups ($P < 0.001$). Furthermore, a significant positive correlation was detected between HCV RNA and HCVcAg baseline levels for all the studied cases ($P < 0.05$) (correlation coefficient; $r = 0.752$ for mild viremia, $r = 0.976$ for moderate viremia, and $r = 1.00$ for severe viremia). These finding agreed with previous reports by Soliman et al., Park et al., and Kim et al. [15, 19, 20] who confirmed excellent correlation to HCV RNA levels and that the kinetics of HCVcAg and viremia were almost similar. Thong et al. also postulated that in the overall cohort, HCVcAg levels significantly correlated with the corresponding HCV RNA levels ($r = 0.889$, $P < 0.001$). The authors recommended HCVcAg testing to be used as an alternative to HCV RNA assays in resource-limited settings [21].

Other previous studies involving other HCV genotypes demonstrated that detection of HCVcAg in serum or plasma is useful as an indirect marker of HCV replication due to the excellent correlation between HCVcAg and HCV RNA concentrations. In addition, HCVcAg assays, which are easier to perform than reverse transcription-PCR, also save time and are less expensive. HCVcAg is used currently to monitor patients undergoing antiviral therapy and to determine the clinical efficacy of such treatment [22–24].

Being closely related to HCV RNA as proved in current results, the present study involved analytical data that may support the use of HCVcAg as a prognostic marker for disease activity among HCV-infected patients and consequently to be implemented in clinical practice for the follow-up of treatment response. At a cutoff point of 1.765 Peiu/ml, HCVcAg was able to differentiate between mild and moderate viremia with sensitivity, specificity, PPV, NPV, and diagnostic accuracy of 87.5%, 85.7%, 77.8%, 92.3%, and 86.4%, respectively. However, HCVcAg cutoff point of 3.42 Peiu/ml exhibited sensitivity, specificity, PPV, NPV, and diagnostic accuracy of

Table 5 Treatment outcomes among the studied groups according to RT-PCR results

Treatment outcomes	Total cases (No. = 280)						Total (n = 280)		χ^2 test and P value
	Group I (n = 140),		Group II (n = 80)		Group III (n = 60),				
	No.	%	No.	%	No.	%	No.	%	
Responder/SVR (No. = 260)	130	92.9	70	87.5	60	100	260	92.9	Test = 3.56 $P = 0.47$
Non-responder (No. = 10)	10	7.1	0	0.0	0	0.0	10	3.6	
Relapse (No. = 10)	0	0.0	10	12.5	0	0.0	10	3.6	

Table 6 HCVcAg at baseline, the 12th week, and the 24th week regarding treatment response

Response of cases (No. = 280)	HCVcAg (Peiu/ml)				
	Baseline	At the 12th week		At the 24th week	
		Detectable	Undetectable	Detectable	Undetectable
Responder/SVR (No. = 260)	2.7 ± 2.1	0 0.0%	260 100%	0 0.0%	260 100%
Non-responder (No. = 10)	1.7	10 100%	0 0.0%	10 100%	0 0.0%
Relapse (No. = 10)	3.5	0 0.0%	10 100%	10 100%	0 0.0%

100%, 87.5%, 85.7%, 100%, and 92.9% respectively for differentiation between moderate and sever viremia. In another study by Sayed et al., the Roc curve showed that the best cutoff point between mild viremia patients and moderate viremia was found > 2.3 with a sensitivity of 81.25%, specificity of 100.0%, PPV of 100.0%, and NPV of 88.9%. While Roc curve for HCVcAg between moderate and severe viremia showed that the best cutoff point was > 4.2 with sensitivity of 87.5%, specificity of 93.75%, PPV of 87.5%, and NPV of 93.7% [25].

The introduction of DAAs therapies has revolutionized the treatment response of HCV. In this context, we explored the relevance of HCVcAg testing to evaluate the potential role in monitoring virologic response to the new regimen of protease inhibitor-based therapy. In the current work, 92.9% (260/280) of the studied cases achieved sustained virologic response, 3.6% (10/280) were non-responders with persistent viremia throughout the course of the study, and 3.6% (10/280) had recurrent viremia/relapse after completing treatment as proved by RT-PCR results. These results were almost comparable to the rates reported by Nouh et al. (95.8% of patients achieved SVR-12 and 4.2% were non-responders) [26]. Rockstroh et al. also postulated that advances in the treatment of HCV infection with DAAs have demonstrated over 90% cure rates, as defined by the SVR-12. With these therapies, high SVR rates can be obtained regardless of viral genotype, degree of liver fibrosis, or previous treatment history in the majority of patient groups [27].

Regarding relapse, in this study 3.6% of the enrolled patients had a relapse/recurrent viremia as proved by RT-PCR results after 3 months from completing treatment with the DAA combination therapy. Other studies conducted by Wang et al. and Rutter et al. revealed that about 13% of cases had relapse 3 months after completing treatment regimen with DAAs. They suggested that relapsed cases are probably attributed to emergence of treatment resistance-associated variants with reduced replication fitness compared with the wild type virus. If these resistance-associated variants cannot be eliminated by the required combination regimen, strains with reduced replication fitness may persist in low concentration and may account for late relapses [16, 28].

Interestingly, HCVcAg was able to detect 100% (260/260) of patients who achieved SVR-12, 100% (10/10) of those who were non-responders, and 100% (10/10) of patients who developed recurrent viremia/relapse during

Table 7 Degree of agreement between HCV RNA and HCVcAg results at the 12th and 24th week among the studied groups

HCV RNA at the 12th week					Total
			Positive	Negative	
HCVcAg at the 12th week	Positive	No.	10	0	10
		% (within HCV RNA at the 12th week)	100.0	.0	3.6
	Negative	No.	0	270	270
		% (within HCV RNA 12th week)	.0	100.0	96.4
Total		No.	10	270	280
		% (within HCV RNA 12th week)	100.0	100.0	100.0
HCV RNA at the 24th week					Total
			Positive	Negative	
HCVcAg at the 24th week	Positive	No.	20	0	20
		% (within HCV RNA at the 24th week)	100.0	.0	7.1
	Negative	No.	0	260	260
		% (within HCV RNA at the 24th week)	.0	100.0	92.9
Total		No.	20	260	280
		% (within HCV RNA at the 24th week)	100.0	100.0	100.0

Table 8 Evaluation of HCVcAg assay performance in prediction of treatment response at the 12th and 24th week among the studied groups

	Sensitivity	Specificity	PPV	NPV	Accuracy
HCVcAg at the 12th week (Peiu/ml)	100%	100%	100%	100%	100%
HCVcAg at the 24th week (Peiu/ml)	100%	100%	100%	100%	100%

post-treatment follow-up (sensitivity, specificity, PPV, NPV, and diagnostic accuracy of 100% in relation to PCR results). In the same field, Pischke et al. studied a group of patients who had received DAAs and concluded that early response to treatment could be assessed by the less-expensive HCVcAg assay with equal reliability as PCR testing; therefore, both assays allowed prediction of SVR-12 with the same accuracy [29]. Aghemo et al. also reported that concordance between the two tests in identifying patients who achieved SVR-12 was almost perfect where HCVcAg identified 97% of these patients [30]. In their study about the clinical utility of HCVcAg assay in the monitoring of DAAs for chronic hepatitis C, Lin et al. declared that the HCVcAg assay identified 99% of patients with SVR-12 and that both undetectability of serum HCVcAg and HCV RNA had a high positive predictive value at week 2 (98% vs. 100%) and at week 4 (97% vs. 99%) in predicting SVR-12 [8].

Regarding sensitivity and specificity of HCVcAg for assessment of post-treatment viremia, many studies were nearly parallel to our result; Arboledas et al. [31] reported that the sensitivity of HCVcAg test was 86.5% and Daniel et al. [32] showed 85.3% sensitivity. Meanwhile, Ergunay et al. [33] revealed 75.8% sensitivity. A group of studies recorded sensitivity of more than 90%, ranging from 93.26 to 96.3% as documented by Kotb et al. and Demircili et al. [34, 35]. Miedouge et al. reported that HCVcAg sensitivity was 100% [36].

In their studies, Kesli et al. and Demircili et al. [4, 35] showed results which were almost comparable to current results as regards specificity (100%). Ergunay et al. [33] revealed 95.1% specificity, while Miedouge et al. and Medici et al. respectively found 99.2% and 97.9% specificity for HCVcAg quantitative assays versus nucleic acid-based test [36, 37].

In the year 2018, the European Association for the Study of the Liver recommended that HCVcAg in serum or plasma is a marker of HCV replication that can be used instead of HCV RNA to diagnose acute or chronic HCV infection when HCV RNA assays are not available and/or not affordable. HCVcAg is an easy test with comparable sensitivity (> 90%) and satisfactory correlation with the HCV RNA. Quantification of HCVcAg is to be suggested as an attractive alternative to these expensive and demanding measurements [14].

Conclusions

HCVcAg displayed excellent sensitivity and specificity for detection of pre-treatment and post-treatment viremia in chronic HCV patients. HCVcAg successfully identified patients who achieved SVR from those with failed response and/or relapse after receiving the newly prescribed regimen of DAAs and should be considered for inclusion in routine laboratory testing. The technical feasibility of HCVcAg in diagnosis and treatment monitoring should improve access to care in areas where HCV RNA testing is not or hardly available. HCVcAg proved strong correlation with HCV RNA levels at mild, moderate, and sever viremia. We acknowledge that the results were analyzed with a relatively small cohort; therefore, to implement a practical policy in real-life settings, studies with larger cohorts are a must.

Abbreviations

HCV: Hepatitis C virus; HCVcAg: Hepatitis C virus core antigen; DAAs: Direct-acting antiviral drugs; SVR: Sustained virologic response; SOF: Sofosbuvir; DCV: Daclatasvir; RVN: Ribavirin

Acknowledgements

Not applicable.

Authors' contributions

AE contributed in the conception and design of the work and was the major contributor in writing, revision, and language polishing of the manuscript. GE contributed in performing the practical section of this work. ME, NE, and MZ contributed in the collection of samples and interpretation of the clinical and laboratory data. EE contributed in the revision of the work and corrected and edited the manuscript. All authors have read and approved the final manuscript.

Declarations

Ethics approval and consent to participate

Approval was obtained from the Ethics Committee of Faculty of Medicine, Menoufia University (No. 2311/14-8-2018). Informed written consent was obtained from each participant before enrollment in the study.

Competing interests

The authors declare no competing interests.

Author details

[1]Department of Medical Microbiology and Immunology, Faculty of Medicine, Menoufia University, Shibin El Kom, Egypt. [2]Department of Tropical Medicine, Faculty of Medicine, Menoufia University, Shibin El Kom, Egypt. [3]Department of Clinical Biochemistry and Molecular Diagnostics, National Liver Institute, Menoufia University, Shibin El Kom, Egypt. [4]Department of Hepatology and Gastroenterology, National Liver Institute, Menoufia University, Shibin El Kom, Egypt.

References

1. Zhijuan Fan MS, Junfeng Liu MS, Wang F, Jingmin Liu BS, Xian Ding BS, Liu S (2019) HCV core antigen is a useful predictor during pegylated-interferon/ribavirin therapy in patients with hepatitis C virus genotype 1b. Medicine 98:10(e14795)
2. El-Ghitany EM (2019) Hepatitis C virus infection in Egypt: current situation and future perspective. J High Institute Public Health 49(1):1–9. https://doi.org/10.21608/jhiph.2019.29460
3. National Institutes of Health (2002) NIH consensus statement on management of hepatitis C. NIH Consens State Sci Statements 19(3):1–46
4. Kesli R, Polat H, Terzi Y et al (2011) Comparison of a newly developed automated and quantitative hepatitis C virus (HCV) core antigen test with the HCV RNA assay for clinical usefulness in confirming anti-HCV results. J Clin Microbiol 49(12):4089–4093
5. Nguyen LT, Gray E, O'Leary A, Carr M, De Gascun CF (2016) The role of hepatitis C virus core antigen testing in the era of direct acting antiviral therapies: what we can learn from the protease inhibitors. PLoS One 11:e0163900
6. WHO Guidelines (2016) Guidelines for the screening care and treatment of persons with chronic hepatitis C infection: updated version. WHO Guidelines Approved by the Guidelines Review Committee, Geneva
7. Freiman M et al (2016) Hepatitis C core antigen testing for diagnosis of hepatitis C virus infection. A systematic review and meta-analysis. Ann. Intern. Med. 165(5):345–355. https://doi.org/10.7326/M16-0065
8. Lin SF, Tung SY, Wei KL, Chen CH, Hu TH, Shen CH, et al., (2020) Clinical utility of hepatitis C virus core antigen assay in the monitoring of direct-acting antivirals for chronic hepatitis C.PLOS ONE https://doi.org/https://doi.org/10.1371/journal.pone.0229994; Marsh 2020.
9. Hezode C, Fontaine H, Dorival C et al (2014) Effectiveness of telaprevir or boceprevir in treatment-experienced patients with HCV genotype 1 infection and cirrhosis. Gastroenterology 147(1):132–142. https://doi.org/10.1053/j.gastro.2014.03.051
10. Chronic hepatitis C virus infection: developing direct-acting antiviral drugs for treatment guidance for industry; U.S. Department of Health and Human Services Food and Drug Administration Center for Drug Evaluation and Research (CDER) November 2017; Clinical/Antimicrobial.
11. The American Association for the Study of Liver Diseases and the Infectious Diseases Society of America; AASLD & IDSA HCV (2018) Guidance Panel. Hepatitis C guidance 2018 update: AASLD-IDSA recommendations for testing, managing, and treating hepatitis C virus infection. Clin Infect Dis 67:1477–1492
12. HCV treatment protocol in Egypt (Supreme Council and National treatment programme of Hepatitis C updated Treatment Protocol December 2019; NCCVH).
13. Esmat G, Raziky ME, Nabeel MM, Maher R, Zakaria Z (2016) Seroprevalence of HCV among Cairo University students in Egypt. J Med Virol 88(8):1384–1387. https://doi.org/10.1002/jmv.24469
14. European Association for the Study of the Liver (EASL): Recommendations on the treatment of HCV hepatitis C: management of hepatitis C. J Hepatol, (2018); 69: 461–511. Pmid:2965033
15. Soliman HA, Hozayen WG, Mahmoud AM, Abo Seif MA, Fayed NA (2015) Significance of the hepatitis C virus core antigen testing as an alternative marker for hepatitis diagnosis in Egyptian patients. Eur Rev Med Pharmacol Sci 19(12):2240–2245
16. Wang L, Chen W, Xi W, Feng J, Dang P, Ma Y, Yu Y (2017) Utility of enzyme-linked immunosorbent assays to test core antigen in the diagnosis and antiviral therapy management of hepatitis C virus infections. J Med Virol. 89(7):1235–1240. https://doi.org/10.1002/jmv.24754
17. Kuo YH, Chang KC, Wang JH, Tsai PS, Hung SF, Hung CH, Chen CH, Lu SN (2012) Is hepatitis C virus core antigen an adequate marker for community screening? J Clin Microbiol 50:1989–1993
18. Alsiö A, Jannesson A, Langeland N, Pedersen C, Färkkilä M, Buhl MR, Mørch K, Westin J, Hellstrand K, Norkrans G et al (2012) Early quantification of HCV core antigen may help to determine the duration of therapy for chronic genotype 2 or 3 HCV infection. Eur J Clin Microbiol Infect Dis 31(7):1631–1635. https://doi.org/10.1007/s10096-011-1486-5
19. Park IY, Lee JH, Kim BS, Kim DY, Han KH, Kim HS (2010) New automated hepatitis C virus (HCV) core antigen assay as an alternative to real-time PCR for HCV RNA quantification. J Clin Microbiol 48:2253–2256
20. Kim MN, Kim HS, Kyung Kim JK, Kyung Kim B, Kim SU, Park JY, Kim DY, HoonAhn S, Han KH (2016) Clinical utility of a new automated hepatitis C virus core antigen assay for prediction of treatment response in patients with chronic hepatitis C. J Korean Med Sci 31(9):1431–1437. https://doi.org/10.3346/jkms.2016.31.9.1431
21. Thong VD, Akkarathamrongsin S, Avihingsanon A, Theamboonlers A, Poovorawan Y, Tangkijvanich P (2015) The correlation between hepatitis C core antigen and hepatitis C virus RNA levels with respect to human immunodeficiency virus status, hepatitis C virus genotype and interferon-lambda-4 polymorphism. Intervirology 58(2):73–79. https://doi.org/10.1159/000370070
22. Seme K, Poljak M, Babic DZ, Mocilnik T, Vince A (2005) The role of core antigen detection in management of hepatitis C: a critical review. J. Clin. Virol. 32(2):92–101. https://doi.org/10.1016/j.jcv.2004.10.005
23. Pérez-García A, Aguinaga A, Navascués A , Castilla J and Ezpeleta C (2019) Hepatitis C core antigen: diagnosis and monitoring of patients infected with hepatitis C virus. Int J Infect Dis: Volume 89, December Pages 131-136.
24. Lamoury FMJ , Soker A, Martinez D , Hajarizadeh B, Cunningham EB, Cunningham P et al., (2017) Hepatitis C virus core antigen: a simplified treatment monitoring tool, including for post-treatment relapse. J Clin Virol; Volume 92, July , Pages 32-38.
25. Sayed MM, El-Shafie AI, Hilal AF, Abdelsattar HA (2017) Can hepatitis C virus core antigen be used a reliable marker of viral load for hepatitis C virus infection in genotype 4? Egyptian liver journal.7 (1 and 2); 1-4.
26. Nouh MAE, Mohamed GE, Mohammed AMS, Ahmed REG (2020) Cost-effectiveness of HCV core antigen versus PCR for monitoring treatment response in DAAS-treated Egyptian patients. Afro-Egypt J Infect Endem Dis 10(2):174–182
27. Rockstroh JK, Jordan J, Feld J, Chevaliez S, Chengd K, Wedemeyere H, Sarrazin C, Maasoumy B, Hermand C, Hackett J, Daniel EC, Dawsond GJ, Clohertyd G, Pawlotsky JM (2017) HCV core antigen as an alternate test to HCV RNA for assessment of virologic responses to all-oral, interferon-free treatment in HCVgenotype 1 infected patients. J Virol Methods 245:14–18
28. Rutter K, Stättermayer AF, Ferenci P, Beinhardt S, Scherzer TM, Strassl R, Steindl-Munda P, Trauner M, Hofer H (2013) 896 Successful HCV eradication due to antiviral therapy is associated with improved long term outcome of patients with chronic hepatitis C. J Hepatol 1(58):S369
29. Pischke S, Polywka S, Proske VM, Lang M, Jordan S, Nashan B, Lohse AW, Sterneck M (2016) Course of hepatitis C virus (HCV) RNA and HCV core antigen testing are predictors for reaching sustained virologic response in liver transplant recipients undergoing sofosbuvir treatment in a real-life setting. Transplant Infect Dis 18(1):141–145. https://doi.org/10.1111/tid.12475
30. Aghemo A, Degasperi E, De Nicola S, Bono P, Orlandi A, D'Ambrosio R, Soffredini R, Perbellini R, Lunghi G, Colombo M (2016) Quantification of core antigen monitors efficacy of direct-acting antiviral agents in patients with chronic hepatitis C virus infection. Clin Gastroenterol Hepatol 14(9):1331–1336. https://doi.org/10.1016/j.cgh.2016.03.035
31. Arboledas JC, Guerrero IP, Rodríguez MJ, Martos ET, Pérez AB, León CC, Sánchez JF, Prieto MD, Porcuna NC, Mochón MD, Macías J (2017) Hepatitis C virus core antigen in the management of patients treated with new direct-acting antivirals. Diagnostic Microbiol Infect Dis 89(1):29–34. https://doi.org/10.1016/j.diagmicrobio.2017.06.006
32. Daniel HDJ, Vivekanandan P, Raghuraman S, Sridharan G, Chandy GM, Abraham P (2007) Significance of the hepatitis C virus (HCV) core antigen as an alternative plasma marker of active HCV infection. Indian J. Med. Microbiol. 25(1):37–42. https://doi.org/10.4103/0255-0857.31060
33. Ergünay K, Şener B, Alp A, Karakaya J, Hasçelik G (2011) Utility of a commercial quantitative hepatitis C virus core antigen assay in a diagnostic laboratory setting. Diagnostic Microbiol Infect Dis 70(4):486–491. https://doi.org/10.1016/j.diagmicrobio.2011.04.011
34. Kotb DN, Esmail MA, Abdelwahab SF, Abdel Hamid M (2017) Correlation between hepatitis C viral load and hepatitis C core antigenaemia among Egyptians. EMHJ 23(4):280–286. https://doi.org/10.26719/2017.23.4.280
35. Demircili ME, Ozdemir M, Feyzioglu B, Baysal B (2016) The efficiency of hepatitis C virus core antigen test in the diagnosis of hepatitis C infection. Viral Hepatitis J 22(1):18–22. https://doi.org/10.4274/vhd.78300
36. Miedouge M, Saune K, Kamar N, Rieu M, Rostaing L, Izopet J (2010) Analytical evaluation of HCV core antigen and interest for HCV screening in haemodialysis patients. J Clin Virol. 48:18–21
37. Medici MC, Furlini G, Rodella A, Fuertes A, Monachetti A, Calderaro A, Galli S, Terlenghi L, Olivares M, Bagnarelli P, Costantini A (2011) Hepatitis C virus core antigen: analytical performances, correlation with viremia and potential applications of a quantitative, automated immunoassay. J Clin Virol 51(4): 264–269. https://doi.org/10.1016/j.jcv.2011.05.003

8

IL-28B single nucleotide polymorphism as a predictor of hepatocellular carcinoma after treatment of chronic hepatitis C patients with direct acting antivirals

Nancy Abdel Fattah Ahmed[1*], Ahmed Shawky Hassan Ali[2], Rizk Ahmed El Baz[3] and Islam Abd El-Hamid El-Zayyadi[2]

Abstract

Background: Hepatitis C virus (HCV) infection is considered one of the main causes of chronic liver diseases. HCV is responsible for 25% of HCC cases worldwide. DAAs represent an important step for HCV eradication. The aim was to study the role of IL-28B single nucleotide polymorphism in the prediction of HCC in patients with HCV-related cirrhosis after DAAs.

Results: This study was done at Mansoura Specialized Hospital: 50 cases HCC after DAAs, 50 cases without HCC after DAAs, and 100 controls. SNPs of the IL-28B gene were genotyped. There was an insignificant difference between HCC patients and the cirrhotic group as regards genotypes (p value = 0.26) and alleles (p value = 0.77). A significant association in SNP of IL-28B between healthy individuals and the cirrhotic group was detected. C C genotype (28%) and C T (64%) genotype were more prevalent in the healthy group than in the cirrhotic group 20% and 52% respectively while T T genotype was more prevalent in cirrhotic patients (28%) than controls (8%). C allele was protective against cirrhosis with 60% distribution in healthy individuals and 46% in the cirrhotic group. T allele was more prevalent in cirrhotic (54%) than the normal group (40%)

Conclusion: Although IL-28B SNP had a role in HCV-related cirrhosis progression, it did not predict the probability for HCC development following DAAs.

Keywords: HCV, HCC, SNPs

Background

Hepatitis C virus (HCV) infection is considered one of the main causes of chronic liver diseases around the world. There are about 71 million chronically infected persons [1]. HCV is responsible for 27% of cases of cirrhosis and 25% of HCC cases worldwide [2]. Hepatocellular carcinoma (HCC) is the primary liver cancer derived from the hepatocytes [3]. DAAs represent uprising in HCV eradication [4]. The incidence of HCC is reduced in chronic hepatitis C genotype 4 patients with liver cirrhosis (F4) and advanced hepatic fibrosis (F3) who achieved SVR following DAAs treatment to 2.9% as compared with 5.3% in untreated patients [5]. Especially in absence of HCC risk factors, the recurrence incidence is decreased [6], also most recent articles found a reduced incidence, and the debate is near the end [7]. Unexpected high rate of HCC recurrence has been reported about 28.8% despite complete response to treatment [8]. IL-28B is a cytokine responsible for transcription of subsets of genes that play a crucial role in antiviral immune response [9]. Although the role of IL-

* Correspondence: ziad.emad90@yahoo.com
[1]Mansoura Specialized Medical Hospital, Internal Medicine Department Hepatology & Gastroenterology Unit, Faculty of Medicine, Mansoura University, Mansoura, Egypt
Full list of author information is available at the end of the article

28B SNP in HCC remains controversial, single nucleotide polymorphism of IL-28B can predict the response to DAAs with favorable and unfavorable genotypes [10].

Objectives

The objective is to study the role of IL-28B single nucleotide polymorphism in the prediction of HCC in patients with HCV-related cirrhosis after DAAs.

Methods

Study design

The present study was a cross-sectional study.

Settings

The study was conducted at Mansoura Specialized Medical Hospital.

Participants

This study included 50 cirrhotic patients due to HCV with a history of DAA therapy, 50 cirrhotic patients due to HCV with history of DAA therapy who developed HCC, 100 normal individuals neither infected by HCV nor had HCC as a control group, and all of them were from Mansoura Specialized Medical Hospital.

Variables

Inclusion criteria

Inclusion criteria include adult patients 18–65 years at Specialized Medical Hospital, Mansoura University inpatient and outpatient departments. They received DAAs therapy (sofosbuvir 400 mg once daily, daclatasvir 60 mg once daily, ribavirin 800–1200 mg) and SVR after 3 months of therapy or after 6 months of sofosbuvir and daclatasvir in patients who did not tolerate ribavirin.

Exclusion criteria

1. Co-infection with HBV or HIV.
2. Previous HCV treatment with interferon-based therapy.
3. Other etiologies of cirrhosis: autoimmune hepatitis, NASH, alcoholic, and other causes.
4. Known drug abuse.
5. Pregnant females.
6. Organ failure: heart failure, respiratory failure, renal failure.

Data sources/measurement

All selected patients were subjected to history taking and physical examination.

Laboratory and radiological investigations

These include complete blood count (CBC), serum albumin, total, direct bilirubin, INR, AST, ALT, creatinine, alpha fetoprotein, and IL28B gene polymorphism PCR.

Also, abdominal ultrasound, triphasic CT: HCC cases were diagnosed based on the arterial phase enhancement and washout during the portal venous phase. One case underwent liver biopsy after CT and MRI had been done without definite diagnosis of HCC and revealed undifferentiated carcinoma.

Bias

N/A

Study size

The study size is determined by the statistician.

Quantitative variables

N/A

Statistical methods

The collected data were coded and fed into the SPSS system (Statistical Package for Social Sciences) ver. 22

Results

Table 1 shows that groups are matched according to age and sex with male predominance in both cirrhotic and HCC(p value = 0.135, p value = 0.06), respectively

Table 2 shows significant increase in hepatic decompensation in the HCC group as regards encephalopathy, ascites, jaundice, and hematemesis (p value =0.008, p value =0.04, p value =0.001, and p value =0.023, respectively)

Table 3 shows significant lower serum albumin, Hgb, and platelets in HCC group with p value = 0.02, p value =0.03, and $p < 0.001$, respectively, and a significant higher AST, total, direct bilirubin, and INR in the HCC group with p value = 0.001,p= 0.005, p=0.02, and p= 0.009, respectively.

Table 4 shows a significant increase in Child B and C among the HCC group (p value < 0.001)

Table 5 shows the classification of HCC according to the number of lesions and BCLC, duration between end of treatment and HCC and associated PVT, and nodal and extrahepatic spread.

p1 difference between the control group and cirrhotic group, *p2* difference between the control group and HCC, *p3* difference between the cirrhotic and HCC cases

Table 6 shows an insignificant distribution in genotypes and alleles of IL-28B SNP between the HCC group and cirrhotic group and a significant distribution in genotypes and alleles between the control and cirrhotic groups.

Table 1 Demographic characteristics of the studied groups

	Control group *N*=100	Cirrhosis group *N*=50	HCC group *N*=50	Test of significance
Age/years				t=1.51
Mean±SD	57.92±7.40	55.24±5.42	57.08±6.74	p=0.135
Sex, *n* (%)				
Male	58 (58.0)	33 (66.0)	37 (74.0)	χ^2=5.70 p=0.06
Female	42 (42.0)	17 (34.0)	13 (26.0)	

*Statistically significant (if p< 0.05)

Table 7 shows that age and AFP are significant (p value = 0.002, p value = 0.009) respectively as predictors of HCC.

Table 8 shows a significant association between genotype and PVTT (P value = 0.02) and an insignificant association between genotype and other criteria of HCC cases

Participants

This study included 50 cirrhotic patients due to HCV with a history of DAA therapy, 50 cirrhotic patients due to HCV with a history of DAA therapy who developed HCC, and 100 normal individuals neither infected by HCV nor had HCC as a control group.

Descriptive data, outcome data, and main results

Descriptive data, outcome data, and main results are shown in Tables 1, 2, 3, 4, 5, 6, 7, and 8.

Other analyses

N/A

Key results

IL-28B SNP could not predict HCC development after DAAs.

IL-28 SNP had a significant role in the development of HCV-related cirrhosis.

AFP and age are strong predictors of HCC.

HCC leads to rapid deterioration of liver functions.

Close follow-up by US and AFP is recommended post DAAs specially in advanced fibrosis and cirrhosis.

Discussion

This work has great importance as prediction of post DAAS HCC is the headache association of such revolution in the treatment of HCV-related liver disease, reaffirming the role of IL-28B SNP in progression to and of cirrhosis is expected, and the results were surprising.

The present study includes 50 HCC patients post DAAs, 50 cirrhotic patients post DAAs without HCC, and 100 normal as a control.

In our study, the distribution of the polymorphisms between the HCC group and cirrhotic group was close in both, and no significant differences were found. In the HCC group, C C genotype, T T genotype, and C T genotype were 14%, 18%, and 68% while they represented 20%, 28%, and 52% respectively in cirrhotic group (p value =0.26). As regards alleles, there were no significant differences for C and T alleles between the HCC group (48%, 52%) and cirrhotic group (46%, 54%) (p value =0.77).

These results denote a lack of association between SNP of IL-28B and HCC post DAAs. Therefore, SNP of IL-28B cannot predict the emergence of HCC after DAAs.

Salum et al. [11] reported similar results of no significance was found in SNP of IL-28B in prediction of HCC post DAAs. They found C C, T T, and C T genotypes

Table 2 clinical presentation of the studied groups

	Cirrhosis group *N*=50(%)	HCC group *N*=50(%)	Test of significance
Hepatic encephalopathy	8 (16.0)	20 (40.0)	χ^2=7.14 p=0.008*
Ascites	17 (34.0)	27 (54.0)	χ^2=4.06 p=0.04*
Jaundice	11 (22.0)	26 (52.0)	χ^2=9.65 p=0.001*
Hematemesis	26 (52.0)	37 (74.0)	χ^2=5.19 p=0.023*
DM	20 (40.0)	18 (36.0)	χ^2=0.170 p=0.680

*Statistically significant (if p< 0.05)

Table 3 Laboratory results of the studied groups

	Cirrhosis group *N*=50	HCC group *N*=50	Test of significance
INR	1.49±0.37	1.29±0.34	*t*=2.68 *p*=0.009*
Albumin (g/dl)	3.12±0.49	2.83±0.77	*t*=2.29 *p*=0.024*
AST (IU/ml)	55.70±37.29	95.0±73.97	*z*=3.21 *p*=0.001*
ALT (IU/ml)	46.50±24.52	60.22±41.63	*z*=1.44 *p*=0.149
Platelet/cm (× 10^3)	106.22±42.06	88.02±39.54	*z*=2.23 *p*=0.001*
WBCs/cm	5.74±2.61	6.44±2.96	*z*=1.18 *p*=0.235
Hgb (g/dl)	9.11±0.97	9.71±1.73	*t*=2.12 *p*=0.036*
Creatinine (mg/dl)	1.11±0.37	1.18±0.49	*t*=0.851 *p*=0.397
Total bilirubin (mg/dl)	2.76±2.7	5.09±5.27	*z*=2.82 *p*=0.005*
Direct bilirubin (mg/dl)	1.67±2.06	3.15±3.6	*z*=2.19 *p*=0.028*

*Statistically significant (if $p < 0.05$)

were 31%, 6%, and 55% in HCC group while in cirrhotic group were 27%, 20%, and 26% (*p* value = 0.457). For alleles, they found in the HCC group C allele was 58% and T allele was 42%, while in the cirrhotic group, C allele was 53% and T alleles was 47% (*p* value = 0.31) which also refer to lack of significance between SNP of IL-28 and HCC post DAAs.

On the opposite side, Simili et al. [12] reported a significant association between SNP of IL-28 and HCC post DAAs. T T genotype was unfavorable and associated with a higher risk of HCC post DAAs (*p* value =0.024).

This conflict with the previous results is found as this study included a small number of HCC cases after DAAs of only 11 patients. Six of them had a history of HCC and were treated at least 6 months before DAAs, and 5 of them were without recurrence while a number of patients without recurrence in our study was 50 cases and in Salum et al. [11] was 65 patients.

Table 4 Child–Pugh score classification distribution among studied groups

	Cirrhosis group *N*=50 (%)	HCC group *N*=50 (%)	Test of significance
Child score			
A	34 (68.0)	6 (12.0)	χ^2=33.21 *P*< 0.001*
B	13 (26.0)	31 (62.0)	
C	3 (6.0)	13 (26.0)	

*Statistically significant (if $p < 0.05$)

HCV Genotype 4 is the most common genotype in Egypt while genotype 1a is the most common in Europe. Genotype distribution is important in predicting disease progression, response to therapy, progression of fibrosis, and a higher risk of HCC [13].

In our study, a significant association between SNP of IL-28B in healthy individuals and the cirrhotic group was detected (*p* value =0.004). A significant increase was observed in frequencies of IL-28B C C genotype in the healthy population (28%) than the cirrhotic group (20%) and in C T (64%) genotype in the healthy group than

Table 5 Characterization of HCC cases

Character	HCC group (*N*=50)
PVT	11 (22%)
Extrahepatic, LN spread	7 (14%)
Median period between EOT and HCC	18 m ± 6 m
Number of focal lesions	
Single	23 (46%)
2–3	12 (24%)
> 3	15 (30%)
BCLC	
Very early, early (0,A)	12 (24%)
Intermediate (B)	16 (32%)
Advanced (C)	4 (8%)
Terminal (D)	18 (36%)

Table 6 Genotypes and alleles distribution among studied groups

Polymorphism	Control group *N*=100 (%)	Cirrhosis group *N*=50 (%)	HCC group *N*=50 (%)	Test of significance	
TT	8 (8.0)	14 (28.0)	9 (18.0)	χ^2=13.12	p1=0.004*
CC	28 (28.0)	10 (20.0)	7 (14.0)	*p*=0.01*	p2=0.054
CT	64 (64.0)	26 (52.0)	34 (68.0)		p3=0.26
HWE	0.008*	0.741	0.126		
Allele	*n*=200	*N*=100	*N*=100		p1=0.02*
T	80 (40)	54 (54.0)	52 (52.0)	χ^2=6.87	p2=0.051
C	120 (60)	46 (46.0)	48 (48.0)	*p*=0.03*	p3=0.77

*Statistically significant (if $p < 0.05$)

the cirrhotic group (52%). On the other hand, T T genotype was more prevalent in cirrhotic patients (28%) than controls (8%).

As regards alleles, C allele appeared to be protective against cirrhosis with 60% distribution in healthy individuals and 46% in the cirrhotic group. T allele was more prevalent in cirrhotic (54%) than the normal group (40%) (*p* value =0.02)

A significant increase ($P < 0.0005$) was observed in frequencies of IL-28B C C genotypes in the healthy population than in the cirrhotic group (48%, 13%) respectively [14].

Attallah et al. [15] found that IL-28B T T genotype is more prevalent in patients with advanced fibrosis and cirrhosis among HCV genotype 4 Egyptian patients (*p* value ˂0.05).

Also, Fuente et al. [16] found TT genotype in IL28B polymorphism was highly prevalent in HCV cirrhotic patients but it did not directly influence hepatocarcinogenesis.

These similar results suggest the role of SNP IL-28 in HCV disease progression and liver cirrhosis.

Limitations

Transient elastography was not done as it is very expensive for our patients. Also, the relatively small number of patients was due to the difficulty in acceptance by patients to be included in a research study in addition to the high expense of the kits.

Table 7 Predictors of hepatocellular carcinoma among studied cases

	β	P value	AOR (95% CI)
Age/years	0.167	0.002	1.182 (1.06–1.32)
Albumin (g/dl)	− 0.542	0.363	0.582 (0.181–1.87)
AST (IU/ml)	0.006	0.370	1.006 (0.993–1.02)
AFP (ng/ml)	0.181	0.009	1.198 (1.05–1.37)
Hb (g/dl)	0.295	0.393	1.343 (0.683–2.64)
Total bilirubin (mg/dl)	− 1.093	0.314	0.335 (0.04–2.82)
Direct bilirubin (mg/dl)	1.337	0.349	3.809 (0.233–62.38)

*Statistically significant (if $p < 0.05$)

Interpretation

Our results should be interpreted with caution because of several limitations. We recruited 200 samples in this study; the sample size of each group was relatively small which may restrict its detailed subgroup analysis by the clinical index. All participants were all from Mansoura Specialized Medical Hospital which may not stand for all the Egyptian population.

Generalizability

The fundamental experiments should be further conducted to validate our results and explore the possible mechanism.

Table 8 Association between genotype and demographic and laboratory findings among studied HCC cases

	CC *N*=7	TT *N*=9	CT *N*=34	Test of significance
DM	3	6	9	*P*–0.245
Sex				
Male	5	10	22	*P*=0.73
Female	2	2	9	
AF				
> 400	4	2	14	*P*=0.356
≤400	3	7	20	
PVT	2	3	6	*P*=0.02*
Child				*P*=0.162
A	3	2	10	
B	2	2	17	
C	2	5	7	
Size				*P*=0.144
≤5	5	3	23	
> 5	2	6	11	
Number of lesions				
Single	4	2	10	*P*=0.468
≤3	2	3	15	
> 3	1	4	9	

Conclusion

Although IL-28B SNP had a role in HCV-related cirrhosis progression, it did not predict the probability for HCC development following DAAs. Further studies are recommended.

Abbreviations

HCV: Hepatitis C virus; HCC: Hepatocellular carcinoma; SNPs: Single nucleotide polymorphisms; AFP: Alpha fetoprotein; DAAs: Direct-acting antivirals; SVR: Sustained virologic response; HIV: Human immunodeficiency virus; HBV: Hepatitis B virus; PCR: Polymerase chain reaction; ALT: Alanine aminotransferase; AST: Aspartate transaminase; INR: International normalized ratio; CBC: Complete blood count; SPSS: Statistical Package for the Social Sciences; AUC: Area under the curve; CT: Computed tomography; AOR: Adjusted odds ratio; HWE: Hardy-Weinberg Equilibrium; JAK: Janus kinase; STAT: Signal transducer and activator of transcription proteins

Acknowledgements

Thanks to every person shared in this work and the National Committee for control of viral hepatitis for their great efforts.

Study design

The present study was cross-sectional in nature, and patients were selected from Mansoura Specialized Medical Hospital, Faculty of Medicine, Mansoura University.

Authors' contributions

The authors have read and approved the manuscript. NAFA (CA): idea of the study, design, and publishing. ASHA: literature search, clinical follow-up, and statistics. RAEB: laboratory studies. IAEE: manuscript review, editing, and data collection

Declarations

Ethics approval and consent to participate:

The study protocol was investigated and approved by the Medical Ethics Research Team, Faculty of Medicine, Mansoura University (code number MS. 18. 11.364). Every case, after guaranteeing privacy, has given informed written consent.

Competing interests

The authors declare that they have no competing interests.

Author details

[1]Mansoura Specialized Medical Hospital, Internal Medicine Department Hepatology & Gastroenterology Unit, Faculty of Medicine, Mansoura University, Mansoura, Egypt. [2]Specialized Medical Hospital,Internal Medicine Department, Faculty of Medicine, Mansoura University, Mansoura, Egypt. [3]Genetic Unit, Pediatric Hospital, Faculty of Medicine, Mansoura University, Mansoura, Egypt.

References

1. Ahmed NAF, Deiab AG, Hasan ASM, Abd Elbaky AMY (2020) Serum autotaxin levels in responders to HCV treatment by direct-acting antivirals. Egypt Liver J 10(1):1–4
2. Vescovo T, Refolo G, Vitagliano G, Fimia GM, Piacentini M (2016) Molecular mechanisms of hepatitis C virus–induced hepatocellular carcinoma. Clinical Microbiology and Infection 22(10):853–861. https://doi.org/10.1016/j.cmi.2016.07.019
3. Ozakyol A (2017) Global epidemiology of hepatocellular carcinoma (HCC epidemiology). Journal of gastrointestinal cancer 48(3):238–240. https://doi.org/10.1007/s12029-017-9959-0
4. Schinazi R, Halfon P, Marcellin P, Asselah T (2014) HCV direct-acting antiviral agents: the best interferon-free combinations. Liver International 34:69–78. https://doi.org/10.1111/liv.12423
5. Shiha, G., Mousa, N., Soliman, R., NNH Mikhail, N., Adel Elbasiony, M. and Khattab, M., 2020. Incidence of HCC in chronic hepatitis C patients with advanced hepatic fibrosis who achieved SVR following DAAs: a prospective study. J Viral Hepatitis, 27, 7, 671, 679, DOI: https://doi.org/10.1111/jvh.13276
6. Guarino M, Di Costanzo GG, Bruzzese D, Sessa A, etal (2020) Incidence of HCC recurrence after DAA treatment for HCV in a multicentre Italian cohort study. Liver Cancer Int 1(1):12–24. https://doi.org/10.1002/lci2.13
7. Muzica CM, Stanciu C, Huiban L, Singeap AM, Sfarti C, Zenovia S, Cojocariu C, Trifan A (2020) Hepatocellular carcinoma after direct-acting antiviral hepatitis C virus therapy: a debate near the end. World J Gastroenterol 26(43):6770
8. Conti F, Buonfiglioli F, Scuteri A, Crespi C, Bolondi L, Caraceni P, Foschi FG, Lenzi M, Mazzella G, Verucchi G, Andreone P (2016) Early occurrence and recurrence of hepatocellular carcinoma in HCV-related cirrhosis treated with direct-acting antivirals. J Hepatol 65(4):727–733. https://doi.org/10.1016/j.jhep.2016.06.015
9. Zhang Y, Zhu SL, Chen J, Li LQ (2016) Meta-analysis of associations of interleukin-28B polymorphisms rs8099917 and rs12979860 with development of hepatitis virus-related hepatocellular carcinoma. OncoTargets Ther 9:3249
10. Bazeed MMM, Elsheety AG, Bakeer MS, Saber MA, Mohammady EAN (2018) Comparison between clinical and biochemical versus interleukin 28B as a predictive factor of virological response to direct antiviral drugs without interferone in treatment of hepatitis C virus patients. Egypt J Hosp Med 73(10):7842–9.
11. Salum GM, Dawood RM, Abd el-Meguid, M., Ibrahim, N.E., Aziz, A.O.A. and El Awady, M.K. (2020) Correlation between IL28B/TLR4 genetic variants and HCC development with/without DAAs treatment in chronic HCV patients. Genes Dis 7(3):392–400. https://doi.org/10.1016/j.gendis.2019.05.004
12. Simili A, Mazzella G, Ravaioli F, Festi D, Bacchi-Reggiani ML, Porro A, Bazzoli F, Azzaroli F (2019) Interleukin 28 polymorphisms and hepatocellular carcinoma development after direct acting antiviral therapy for chronic hepatitis C. J Gastrointestinal Liver Dis 28(4):449–456. https://doi.org/10.15403/jgld-309
13. Goel A, Ahmed A, Waked I (2019) Clinical epidemiology of hepatitis C virus. In: Clinical Epidemiology of Chronic Liver Diseases. Springer, Cham, pp 149–170
14. El-Awady MK, Mostafa L, Tabll AA, Abdelhafez TH, El Din NGB, Zayed N, El Shenawy R, El Abd Y, Hasan RM, Zaghlol H, El Khayat H (2012) Association of IL28B SNP with progression of Egyptian HCV genotype 4 patients to end stage liver disease. Hepatitis Monthly 12(4):271
15. Attallah AM, Omran D, Marie MS, Abdelrazek M, Salama A, El Essawey R, Mobarak L, Maklad S, Omar A (2018) IL-28B rs12979860 polymorphism affect the course of chronic hepatitis and the development of HCC in Egyptian patients with hepatitis C type 4. British Journal of Biomedical Science 75(4): 157–162. https://doi.org/10.1080/09674845.2018.1489599
16. Fuente S, Citores MJ, Duca A, Cisneros E, Baños I, Vilches C, Cuervas-Mons V (2017) Interleukin-28B TT genotype is frequently found in patients with hepatitis C virus cirrhosis but does not influence hepatocarcinogenesis. Clin Exp Med 17(2):217–223. https://doi.org/10.1007/s10238-016-0418-1

9

The effect of hepatitis C virologic clearance on cardiovascular disease biomarker lipoprotein-associated phospholipase A2 and its relation to serum lipids

Amira Isaac[1], Basant Elmarashly[1*], Kadry El Saeed[1], Rasha Samir Mohamed[1], Shereen Abdelmonem Ibrahim[2] and Eslam Safwat[1]

Abstract

Background: Chronic hepatitis C virus (HCV) infection has been linked to cardiovascular disease (CVD). However, CVD risk prediction in chronic HCV-infected patients is problematic as the prevalence of different cardiac biomarkers in these patients is currently unknown. Serum lipids, which are routinely used in traditional CVD risk scores, may underestimate CVD risk in these patients, while non-hepatically produced biomarkers, including lipoprotein-associated phospholipase A2 (Lp-PLA2), may better reflect CVD risk. In this study, we aimed to evaluate the effect of sustained virologic response (SVR) on CVD risk, predicted by Lp-PLA2 mass in comparison with serum lipid levels.

Results: Ninety chronic HCV-infected patients were enrolled in this study. Serum Lp-PLA2 mass was measured before and after HCV treatment via direct-acting antivirals and compared with the changes in serum lipids and Framingham risk score (FRS). The Lp-PLA2 level was categorized into high (>235 ng/ml) or low predicted CVD risk (≤235 ng/ml). Mean Lp-PLA2 mass significantly decreased from 322.37 ± 79.15 ng/ml to 263.79 ± 51.804 ng/ml with SVR, and the number of high-risk patients significantly dropped from 82.22 to 60% after treatment. Total cholesterol, low-density lipoprotein, and high-density lipoprotein levels were low/optimal at baseline (170 ± 40.34 mg/dl, 71.98 ± 24.12 mg/dl, and 48.43 ± 6.79 mg/dl) and significantly increased with SVR (195.66 ± 55.68 mg/dl, 103.24 ± 46.57 mg/dl, and 53.91 ± 8.67 mg/dl). According to FRS, only 30% of patients were moderate/high risk at baseline and insignificantly declined to 28.89% post-treatment.

Conclusion: Lp-PLA2 may be a better predictor of CVD risk in chronic HCV-infected patients. Furthermore, SVR may reduce hepatic inflammation and consequently CVD risk.

Keywords: Hepatitis C, Cardiovascular disease, Lipoprotein-associated phospholipase A2, Serum lipids

Background

Hepatitis C virus (HCV) is one of the leading causes of liver cell failure and hepatocellular carcinoma (HCC). The pathological sequelae of HCV infection are not restricted to the liver but prevail in extra-hepatic tissues and organs, causing numerous HCV-associated co-morbidities that significantly increase morbidity and mortality, diminishing health-related quality of life [1]. HCV infection provokes fatty liver infiltration, insulin resistance (IR), type 2 diabetes mellitus (DM), and atherosclerosis [2], which are known complications of the metabolic syndrome, despite a paradoxically "protective" serum lipid profile characterized by optimal or low low-density lipoprotein (LDL) and total cholesterol levels [3]. The virus exerts these metabolic changes through its ability to affect hepatic lipid metabolism, interfere with

* Correspondence: b_elmarashly@med.asu.edu.eg
[1]Department of Internal Medicine, Gastroenterology and Hepatology Unit, Faculty of Medicine, Ain Shams University, Cairo 11566, Egypt
Full list of author information is available at the end of the article

insulin signaling, and directly infect the arterial wall causing chronic endothelial damage and systemic inflammation [2]. The development of DAAs has markedly improved treatment outcomes with SVR rates that could reach 90% or more [4]. HCV clearance has been shown to correct metabolic derangements such as IR and the consequences of direct infection of endothelial cells and monocytes [5]. However, an increase in serum cholesterol and LDL may be observed potentiating early atherosclerotic lesions and necessitating lipid-lowering therapy [6].

There are numerous biomarkers that enable risk stratification and consequently decision-making regarding the management of CVD. They can be grouped based on disease specificity, such as biomarkers of heart failure (brain natriuretic peptide and atrial natriuretic peptide) and of atherosclerotic coronary disease (troponin T or I, creatinine phosphokinase-MB), or they can be grouped according to the pathologic process they mediate, such as inflammation (high-sensitivity C-reactive protein [hsCRP], interleukin 6, fibrinogen, tumor necrosis factor-alpha), oxidative stress (isoprostanes), and metabolic biomarkers (lipoprotein (a), LDL, Lp-PLA2) [7].

Lp-PLA2, also known as platelet-activating factor acetylhydrolase, is mainly produced by macrophages and foam cells within atherosclerotic plaques, particularly in sites where leucocyte influx, cellular necrosis, and calcification are profound [8]. It promotes the pathogenesis of atherosclerosis through hydrolysis of oxidized phospholipids on modified LDL particles within the arterial intima [8]. Hence, the concentration of Lp-PLA2 and its by-product, lysophosphatidylcholine, in the coronary circulation reflects atheromatous plaque formation and a high risk of rupture [9]. Lp-PLA2 is characterized by its low biologic variability and high specificity for vascular inflammation, rather than systemic inflammation, and has a direct correlation with plaque inflammation making it a valuable biomarker reflecting CVD risk and a potential therapeutic target [10]. Based on several epidemiologic studies, an Lp-PLA2 level >235 ng/ml in healthy populations was found to signify a high risk for CVD [11]. Our aims were to measure serum lipid levels (hepatic CVD biomarkers) and Lp-PLA2 concentration (non-hepatic CVD biomarker) in chronic HCV-infected patients and explore the potential benefit of HCV treatment on cardiovascular outcomes, hypothesizing that SVR would be associated with a favorable reduction in the non-hepatic CVD biomarker and consequently CVD risk.

Methods

This study was conducted on 90 patients with chronic HCV infection who were eligible for antiviral treatment with DAAs, agreeable to regular follow-up. They were recruited from the National Committee for Control of Viral Hepatitis (NCCVH) regional center in Ain Shams University hospital during the period from May 2019 to April 2020, after approval of the Ain Shams University ethics committee was granted, and informed consents were taken from all patients.

All participants included in this study were 30 years or older, had no underlying CVD, had chronic HCV infection without concomitant hepatitis B virus (HBV) or human immunodeficiency virus (HIV) infection, had not previously undergone liver transplantation, had no history of HCC, had normal serum creatinine levels, were Child A or Child B7 according to Child-Pugh classification, were treatment-naïve, and were defined as "easy to treat" or "difficult to treat" (any of these criteria: total serum bilirubin ≥ 1.2 mg/dl, serum albumin ≤ 3.5 g/dl, INR ≥ 1.2, platelet count < 150,000/mm^3) as per the Egyptian NCCVH protocol, and accordingly administered an appropriate, personally tailored, DAA regimen for 3 months during the course of this study [12, 13]. All female patients were neither pregnant nor lactating throughout the course of this study.

For all patients, relevant history taking and clinical examination were conducted, and the following laboratory tests analyzed, using commercially available kits: alanine transaminase (ALT), aspartate transaminase (AST), serum albumin level, serum bilirubin level, international normalized ratio (INR), serum alpha-fetoprotein (AFP), complete blood count (CBC), quantitative HCV RNA assay, hepatitis B surface antigen (HBsAg) and HIV antibody, serum creatinine level and creatinine clearance, fasting blood glucose (FBG) and hemoglobin A1C (HbA1c), and lipid profile including LDL, HDL, and total cholesterol. Lp-PLA2 mass was measured using RayBio® Human Lp-PLA2 ELISA Kit. Twelve weeks after the end of treatment, HCV RNA was assessed to determine SVR, and Lp-PLA2 mass was measured and compared with serum lipids.

Furthermore, the Framingham CVD risk score (2008) was calculated for all patients before and after treatment and compared to the Lp-PLA2 level in terms of CVD risk predictability. Framingham risk score is an algorithm used to estimate the 10-year CVD risk of an individual, and it comprises six coronary risk factors, including sex, age, smoking history, systolic blood pressure, total cholesterol, and HDL levels. Individuals with low risk have 10% or less global CVD risk at 10 years, with intermediate risk 10–20%, and with high risk 20% or more [14].

Lastly, abdominal ultrasound and transient elastography were done for all patients before and after treatment to identify cirrhosis.

Lp-PLA2 mass assay was done by means of RayBio® Human Lp-PLA2 ELISA Kit, which is an in vitro enzyme-linked immunosorbent (ELISA) assay that employs an antibody specific for human Lp-PLA2 coated on a 96-well plate. Standards and samples were pipetted into the wells, and Lp-PLA2 present in a sample was bound to the wells by the immobilized antibody. The wells were washed, and biotinylated anti-human Lp-PLA2 antibody was added. After washing away the unbound biotinylated antibody, horseradish peroxidase (HRP)-conjugated streptavidin was pipetted to the wells. The wells were again washed, a tetramethylbenzidine (TMB) substrate solution was added, and color developed in proportion to the amount of Lp-PLA2 bound. The Stop Solution changed the color from blue to yellow, and the intensity of the color was measured at 450 nm. The mean absorbance for standards and samples was calculated, and the average zero standard optical density was subtracted. A standard curve was plotted on log-log graph paper, with standard concentration on the x-axis and absorbance on the y-axis. A best-fit straight line through the standard points was drawn. The minimum detectable dose of human Lp-PLA2 (the analyte concentration resulting in an absorbance that is 2 SD higher than that of the blank) was determined to be 8.1 ng/ml.

Statistical analysis

The collected data were coded, tabulated, and statistically analyzed using IBM SPSS statistics (Statistical Package for Social Sciences) software version 20. Quantitative data were expressed as mean ± SD (standard deviation) for normally distributed data. Qualitative data were presented as numbers and percentages.

In quantitative data, Student's t-test was used to compare two independent groups with normally distributed data and paired t-test in cases of two dependent groups with normally distributed data. Analysis of variance (ANOVA) (F) test was used to compare between more than two independent groups with normally distributed data, followed by post hoc analysis to compare between every two groups. In qualitative data, inferential analyses for independent variables were done using the chi-square (X^2) test for differences between proportions. Correlations were done using the Pearson correlation coefficient test (r). The receiver operating characteristic (ROC) curve was constructed to obtain the most sensitive and specific cut-off values for different parameters to discriminate patients with high CVD risk from those with low CVD risk. The level of significance was determined by the p-value where $p < 0.05$ is significant, <0.01 is highly significant, and otherwise is insignificant.

Results

Total studied patients comprised 55 males (61.11%) and 35 females (38.89%), with ages ranging from 30 to 68 years old (mean 46.88 ± 10.61 years). Per abdominal ultrasound and transient elastography, 22 patients were found to have liver cirrhosis. Amongst cirrhotic patients, 9/22 (40.91%) were Child A5, 12/22 (54.55%) were Child A6, and 1/22 (4.55%) was Child B7, as per the Child-Pugh score. "Easy to treat" patients (50%), as per NCCV H guidelines, were given sofosbuvir (SOF) and daclatasvir (DCV) while "difficult to treat" patients (50%) were administered SOF, DCV, and ribavirin (RBV). Twelve weeks after the end of treatment, SVR was observed in 86/90 patients (96.6%). Four of 90 patients (4.4%) had not achieved SVR, with no statistical significance between their pre-treatment and post-treatment HCV RNA levels ($p = 0.068$).

Baseline characteristics of the study cohort regarding demographic data, the prevalence of different CVD risk factors, Child score, and fibrosis stage are summarized in Table 1.

A comparison between cirrhotic and non-cirrhotic patients regarding baseline biochemical parameters and FRS is highlighted in Table 2 and demonstrates that most of the studied parameters were statistically significant between both groups, except AST, hemoglobin level, Lp-PLA2 mass, and Framingham risk score ($p > 0.05$). Notably, total cholesterol level, LDL, and HDL levels were significantly lower in cirrhotic patients as compared to non-cirrhotic patients ($p < 0.001$). There was no statistically significant difference in abdominal ultrasound findings ($p = 0.84$), liver stiffness score ($p = 0.596$), and Child-Pugh score of cirrhotic patients ($p = 0.181$) after treatment as compared to baseline.

A statistically significant increase in serum total cholesterol, LDL, and HDL was observed in patients who achieved SVR ($p < 0.001$) 12 weeks after the end of treatment, while no or insignificant change was observed in non-SVR patients ($p = 0.391$, $p = 0.115$, $p = 0.444$) (Tables 3 and 4).

Furthermore, our study demonstrated a significant decrease in Lp-PLA2 concentration after DAA therapy, in patients who experienced SVR (263.79 ± 51.804 ng/ml vs. 322.37 ± 79.15 ng/ml) ($p < 0.001$). On the contrary, patients who did not achieve SVR experienced a non-significant rise in post-treatment Lp-PLA2 concentration (392.25 ± 88.733 ng/ml vs. 370 ± 98.668 ng/ml) ($p = 0.198$) (Tables 3 and 4).

The Lp-PLA2 level was analyzed as a continuous variable and categorized into high (>235 ng/ml) or low predicted CVD risk (≤235 ng/ml). There is a significant decline in the number of patients classified as high risk, after treatment with DAAs, from 74/90 (82.22%) to 54/90 (60%), with a consequent rise in the number of low-risk patients from 16/90 (17.78%) to 36/90 (40%) post-treatment ($p = 0.002$). Notably, no statistically significant difference in baseline Lp-PLA2 concentration has been shown between cirrhotic and non-cirrhotic patients ($p = 0.463$) (Table 2).

Framingham risk score, designed to predict 10-year CVD risk, was calculated for all patients before and after

Table 1 Baseline characteristics of all studied patients

Descriptive data		
Age (years), mean ± SD (range)		46.878 ± 10.605 (30–68)
BMI (kg/m^2), mean ± SD (range)		26.232 ± 2.140 (21–31)
Gender, n (%)	Male	55 (61.11%)
	Female	35 (38.89%)
Smoking, n (%)	Smoker	18 (20%)
	Non-smoker	72 (80%)
Hypertension, n (%)	Hypertensive	15 (16.67%)
	Normotensive	75 (83.33%)
Diabetes mellitus, n (%)	Diabetic	7 (7.78%)
	Pre-diabetic	13 (14.44%)
	Non-diabetic	70 (77.78%)
FBG (mg/dl), mean ± SD (range)		89.989 ± 15.786 (66–135)
HbA1c (%), mean ± SD (range)		5.420 ± 0.609 (4.1–7)
Child score, n (%)	A5	9 (40.91%) 9 (45%)
	A6	12 (54.55%) 10 (50%)
	B7	1 (4.55%) 1 (5%)
Fibrosis stage, n (%)	F0	16 (17.78%)
	F1	39 (43.33%)
	F2	10 (11.11%)
	F3	3 (3.33%)
	F4	22 (24.44%)
DAA regimen, n (%)	SOF/DCV	45 (50%)
	SOF/DCV/RBV	45 (50%)
HCV RNA (IU/ml), median (IQR)		2,253,000 (573,662.25–4,000, 000)

Abbreviations: *SD*, standard deviation; *n*, number; *BMI*, body mass index; *DAA*, direct-acting antiviral; *SOF*, sofosbuvir; *DCV*, daclatasvir; *RBV*, ribavirin; *FBG*, fasting blood glucose; *HCV*, hepatitis C virus; *RNA*, ribonucleic acid; *IQR*, interquartile range

HCV treatment, and patients were accordingly stratified into low-, moderate-, and high-risk groups. At baseline, 14/90 (15.56%) were classified as high risk, 13/90 (14.44%) as moderate risk, and 63/90 (70%) as low risk. There was no significant difference in calculated risk scores and risk stratification into each group after treatment as compared to baseline (p = 0.976).

Regarding different CVD risk factors, gender had a statistically significant impact on Lp-PLA2 level where men had significantly higher levels than women ($p < 0.001$). Also, significantly higher levels were noted amongst hypertensive patients, diabetic patients, and smokers (p < 0.001, 0.008, <0.001, respectively). Using post hoc analysis, a significant difference in Lp-PLA2 levels between diabetic and non-diabetic patients (p = 0.015) was noted. In addition, "difficult to treat" patients administered SOF/DCV/RBV were found to have significantly higher levels of Lp-PLA2 as opposed to "easy to treat patients" given SOF/DCV (p = 0.006) (Table 5).

Pre-treatment Lp-PLA2 concentration showed a statistically significant positive correlation with age, BMI, FBG, HbA1c, and Framingham score and a statistically significant negative correlation with serum albumin and platelet count. In addition, post-treatment Lp-PLA2 level shows a significant positive correlation with age, BMI, FBG, HbA1c, AST, and both liver stiffness score and Framingham risk score. On the other hand, there is a significant negative correlation with HDL, serum albumin, and platelet count (Table 6).

Finally, our study demonstrated the diagnostic performance of the best cut-off values of baseline AST, ALT, serum albumin, platelet count, and liver stiffness score in differentiating between high and low CVD risk, as defined by an Lp-PLA2 cut-off value of >235 ng/ml. At a cut-off value of >29 IU/l for AST, the sensitivity was 78.38% and specificity 43.75% with an accuracy of 57.5%, and at a cut-off value of >28 IU/l for ALT, the sensitivity was slightly higher (82.43%), yet the specificity was much lower (31.25%) with slightly less accuracy of 52%. A liver stiffness score of >6.3 kPa provides a relatively better specificity of 75% and accuracy of 62.2%. At a cut-off value of ≤261,000/μl for platelet count, the sensitivity was 79.73% and specificity 56.25% with an accuracy of 71.8%. Last but not least, at a cut-off value of ≤3.7 g/dl for serum albumin, the sensitivity in discriminating high from low CVD risk was the lowest (37.84%) amongst the five parameters analyzed, yet specificity was the highest (93.75%) with an accuracy of 63.7% (Fig. 1).

Discussion

HCV infection increases CVD risk through several mechanisms, including insulin resistance, hepatic steatosis, and increased chronic inflammation and immune activation [15].

There are countless risk score calculators and charts that aim to predict 10-year CVD risk in the general population. However, serum lipids, which are incorporated in most CVD risk scores, including the Framingham risk score, are reduced in the setting of chronic liver disease and may therefore underestimate CVD risk in infected persons [16]. This highlights the need for alternative means to estimate CVD risk in chronic HCV-infected patients and the validation of non-hepatically produced CVD biomarkers for this purpose.

Lipoprotein-associated phospholipase A2 (Lp-PLA2) is a novel inflammatory marker that has been found to be a CVD risk marker independent of traditional risk factors, including LDL and hsCRP [17]. It is characterized by high vascular endothelial specificity and low biovariability [18].

Regarding changes in serum lipids, this study illustrates low or optimal levels of baseline total cholesterol, LDL, and HDL with a statistically significant increase after SVR

Table 2 Comparison between cirrhotic and non-cirrhotic patients regarding baseline patients' age, biochemical parameters, and Framingham risk score

Baseline parameter	Cirrhotic patients (n = 22)	Non-cirrhotic patients (n = 68)	Student's t-test	
			t	p
Age (years)	51.045 ± 10.781	45.529 ± 10.267	2.164	0.033
AST (IU/l)	55.955 ± 35.77	45.971 ± 24.985	1.457	0.149
ALT (IU/l)	70.909 ± 50.675	48.824 ± 33.663	2.344	0.021
Albumin (g/dl)	3.653 ± 0.487	4.05 ± 0.393	−3.881	<0.001
Total bilirubin (mg/dl)	0.94 ± 0.524	0.698 ± 0.308	2.663	0.009
Direct bilirubin (mg/dl)	0.464 ± 0.233	0.349 ± 0.234	2.012	0.047
INR	1.165 ± 0.156	1.087 ± 0.114	2.546	0.013
Hemoglobin (g/dl)	13.136 ± 1.593	13.557 ± 1.548	−1.101	0.274
Total leucocyte count (10^3/μl)	5.695 ± 1.861	7.150 ± 2.487	−2.520	0.014
Platelet count (10^3/μl)	159.727 ± 71.748	219.044 ± 80.611	−3.077	0.003
LDL (mg/dl)	39.001 ± 7.528	80.397 ± 19.489	−9.701	<0.001
Total cholesterol (mg/dl)	122.409 ± 29.156	182.103 ± 33.774	−7.436	<0.001
HDL (mg/dl)	40.136 ± 5.375	50.544 ± 5.462	−7.798	<0.001
Lp-PLA2 (ng/ml)	335.455 ± 74.345	320.941 ± 82.023	0.737	0.463
Framingham risk score	10.323 ± 9.921	8.175 ± 8.205	1.013	0.314

Abbreviations: *n*, number; *AST*, aspartate transaminase; *ALT*, alanine transaminase; *INR*, international normalized ratio; *LDL*, low-density lipoprotein; *HDL*, high-density lipoprotein; *Lp-PLA2*, lipoprotein-associated phospholipase A2

achievement ($p < 0.001$), regardless of fibrosis, compared to non-SVR patients, who experienced an insignificant change in their lipid profile parameters 12 weeks after the end of treatment. It is apparent that successful eradication of HCV promotes normalization of the cellular function of hepatocytes improving hepatic lipid production. This highlights the strong association between HCV and lipid levels. A limitation associated with this finding is that the present study did not assess the diet, physical activity level, waist circumference, and family history of patients, which are crucial factors that influence lipid metabolism.

Notably, lipid profile components were found to be significantly lower in cirrhotic patients, a finding which is in accordance with several other studies that demonstrated similar results [19–22]. It is apparent that successful eradication of HCV promotes normalization of the cellular function of hepatocytes improving hepatic lipid production, reflecting the strong association and interaction between HCV and lipid levels. A limitation associated with this finding is that the present study did not assess the dietary habits, physical activity, waist circumference, and family history of patients, which are crucial factors that influence lipid metabolism.

On the other hand, the current study demonstrated a significant decrease in Lp-PLA2 concentration after DAA therapy in patients who experienced SVR, while patients who did not achieve SVR experienced a rise in Lp-PLA2, yet this increase was of no statistical significance. This finding is in accordance with a study conducted by Chew et al. [23]. It is a distinct finding that might be explained by the ongoing HCV viremia, which in turn augments hepatic inflammation, and promotes further systemic immune activation and inflammation.

As per the Framingham risk score, 70% of patients were defined as low risk, with only 30% classified as moderate/high risk at baseline. Furthermore, there was no significant difference in calculated risk scores and risk stratification into each group after treatment as compared to baseline, indicating a lack of any correlation between HCV clearance and this score.

Table 3 Comparison between pre-treatment and post-treatment lipid profile and Lp-PLA2 in patients who achieved SVR (n = 86)

Lipid parameter	Time		Paired t-test	
	Pre-treatment	12 weeks post-treatment	t	p
LDL (mg/dl)	71.977 ± 24.126 (26–130)	103.244 ± 46.570 (44–203)	−9.395	<0.001
Total cholesterol (mg/dl)	170 ± 40.344 (80–278)	195.663 ± 55.678 (92–311)	−8.764	<0.001
HDL (mg/dl)	48.43 ± 6.785 (31–60)	53.907 ± 8.674 (37–71)	−10.1	<0.001
Lp-PLA2 (ng/ml)	322.372 ± 79.146 (189–498)	263.791 ± 51.804 (166–412)	13.829	<0.001

Abbreviations: *n*, number; *LDL*, low-density lipoprotein; *HDL*, high-density lipoprotein; *Lp-PLA2*, lipoprotein-associated phospholipase A2

Table 4 Comparison between pre-treatment and post-treatment lipid profile and Lp-PLA2 in patients who failed to achieve SVR (n = 4)

Lipid parameter	Time		Paired t-test	
	Pre-treatment	12 weeks post-treatment	t	p
LDL (mg/dl)	33.75 ± 4.573 (27–37)	36.5 ± 4.655 (30–41)	−2.200	0.115
Total cholesterol (mg/dl)	114 ± 32.527 (87–158)	117.5 ± 28.361 (88–153)	−1.000	0.391
HDL (mg/dl)	38.75 ± 6.702 (32–48)	37.25 ± 5.123 (30–42)	0.878	0.444
Lp-PLA2 (ng/ml)	370 ± 98.668 (260–474)	392.25 ± 88.733 (319–500)	−1.648	0.198

Abbreviations: *n*, number; *LDL*, low-density lipoprotein; *HDL*, high-density lipoprotein; *Lp-PLA2*, lipoprotein-associated phospholipase A2

On the contrary, using a cut-off value of >235 ng/ml for Lp-PLA2 mass, 17.78% of patients were found to be low risk, with 82.2% of patients identified as high risk at baseline. A significant decline in the number of patients classified as high risk was observed after treatment with DAAs, from 82.2 to 60%, with a consequent rise in the number of low-risk patients to 40% post-treatment (p = 0.002). Comparable results were demonstrated by Chew et al., who conducted a study comprising 54 HCV/HIV co-infected patients administered peginterferon (PEG)/ ribavirin (RBV) for 72 weeks. At baseline, there was no difference in CVD risk class by Lp-PLA2 level, whereas, after treatment, Lp-PLA2 levels decreased, although not statistically significantly, amongst SVRs (median change = −17.5 ng/ml [IQR, −67.0 to 47.0]) but not non-SVRs (median change = 9.50 ng/ml [IQR, −49.0 to 67.0]). There was a statistically significant difference in CVD risk class distribution by Lp-PLA2 level at 24 weeks after the end of treatment, with 25 of 27 (93%) of the non-SVR group in the high-risk category compared with 17 of 27 (63%) of the SVR group (p = 0.021) [23]. Another study conducted by Chew et al. aimed to predict CVD risk in HCV-infected and HCV non-infected patients using the Framingham risk score. In unadjusted analyses, the Framingham risk score was similar between both groups (p = 0.192), while adjusting for CVD risk factors overlooked by the Framingham risk score (age, race, BMI, chronic kidney disease, drug and alcohol use, and HIV status), HCV infection was associated with minimally lower risk score (p < 0.001) [24]. This suggests that the Framingham risk score may underestimate CVD risk in these patients, which is in accordance with our study.

A lack of association of Lp-PLA2 with the degree of liver disease was evident in the present study as the difference in Lp-PLA2 concentration between cirrhotic and non-cirrhotic patients was statistically insignificant (S = 0.463), suggesting that it may be less confounded by hepatic dysfunction as opposed to hepatically produced CVD biomarkers.

Lp-PLA2 concentration was found to show a significant positive correlation with age, smoking, BMI, hypertension, diabetes, FBG, and HbA1c level. Gender differences in Lp-PLA2 levels were also found; men had significantly higher levels than women (358.018 ± 77.133 vs. 271.8 ± 51.467 ng/ml; p < 0.001). Lower Lp-PLA2 levels in women could be explained by the fact that estrogen hormone causes down-regulation of Lp-PLA2 expression due to lower concentrations of LDL cholesterol in women or estrogen-related decrease in platelet-activating factor acetylhydrolase activity [25]. Of note,

Table 5 Relationship between baseline Lp-PLA2 and gender, smoking, hypertension, diabetes, and ease of treatment

Parameter		Lp-PLA2 (ng/ml)	t-test or ANOVA			
			t or F	p		
Gender	**Male** (n = 55)	358.018 ± 77.133	5.832	<0.001		
	Female (n = 35)	271.8 ± 51.467				
Smoking	**Smoker** (n = 18)	444.833 ± 26.425	10.83	<0.001		
	Non-smoker (n = 72)	294.403 ± 57.237				
Hypertension	**Hypertensive** (n = 15)	396.8 ± 69.548	4.17	<0.001		
	Normotensive (n = 75)	310.027 ± 74.298				
Diabetes	**Diabetic** (n = 7)	398 ± 51.095	5.171	0.008†	**D&P**	0.440‡
	Pre-diabetic (n = 13)	353.923 ± 86.238			**D&N**	0.015‡
	Non-diabetic (n = 70)	311.671 ± 76.597			**P&N**	0.167‡
Ease of treatment	**Easy to treat** (n = 45)	301.444 ± 78.506	−2.837	0.006		
	Difficult to treat (n = 45)	347.533 ± 75.582				

†ANOVA (F) test, ‡post hoc test

Abbreviations: *n*, number; *Lp-PLA2*, lipoprotein-associated phospholipase A2; *D*, diabetic; *P*, pre-diabetic; *N*, non-diabetic

Table 6 Correlation between Lp-PLA2 level and socio-clinical parameters, Framingham risk score (2008), and liver stiffness score at baseline and at 12 weeks post-treatment

Studied parameter	Lp-PLA2 (ng/ml)			
	Pre-treatment correlations		Post-treatment correlations	
	r	p	R	p
Age	0.350	0.001	0.409	<0.001
BMI (kg/m^2)	0.331	0.001	0.258	0.014
FBG (mg/dl)	0.353	0.001	0.412	<0.001
HbA1c	0.332	0.001	0.403	<0.001
Platelets (10^3/ l)	−0.225	0.033	−0.229	0.03
AST (IU/l)	0.188	0.076	0.296	0.005
ALT (IU/l)	0.099	0.355	0.033	0.76
Albumin (g/dl)	−0.336	0.001	−0.31	0.003
LDL (mg/dl)	0.142	0.182	0.197	0.062
Total cholesterol (mg/dl)	0.077	0.468	0.043	0.689
HDL (mg/dl)	−0.096	0.366	−0.284	0.007
Framingham score	0.669	<0.001	0.677	<0.001
Liver stiffness score (kPa)	0.157	0.139	0.276	0.008

Abbreviations: *Lp-PLA2*, lipoprotein-associated phospholipase A2; *BMI*, body mass index; *FBG*, fasting blood glucose; *HbA1c*, hemoglobin A1c; *AST*, aspartate transaminase; *ALT*, alanine transaminase; *LDL*, low-density lipoprotein; *HDL*, high-density lipoprotein

estrogen replacement therapy could significantly reduce Lp-PLA2 activity in healthy post-menopausal women [26], while administration of steroids with progesterone-like activity increases Lp-PLA2 activity [27]. Additionally, smoking may increase the carrier (LDL) and the substrate (oxidized LDL) for Lp-PLA2 [28].

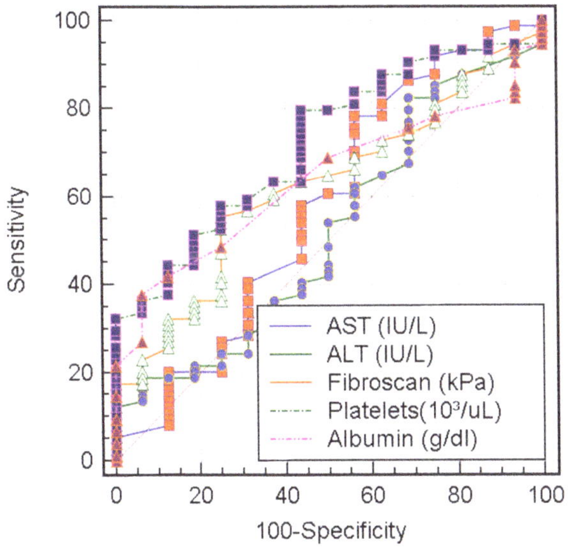

Fig. 1 ROC curve of the best cut-off value of baseline AST, ALT, liver stiffness score, platelet count, and serum albumin in discriminating high CVD risk (Lp-PLA2 > 235 ng/ml) from low CVD risk (Lp-PLA2 ≤ 235 ng/ml). Abbreviations: AST, aspartate transaminase; ALT, alanine transaminase; ROC, receiver operating characteristic; CVD, cardiovascular disease; Lp-PLA2, lipoprotein-associated phospholipase A2

Finally, our study demonstrates the diagnostic performance of the best cut-off values of baseline AST, ALT, serum albumin, platelet count, and liver stiffness score in the prediction of cardiovascular disease risk in chronic HCV-infected patients. A cut-off value of >28 IU/l for ALT yielded the highest sensitivity (82.43%) in predicting CVD risk, while an albumin level ≤3.7 g/dl was most specific (93.75%) with the highest positive predictive value (96.6%).

We have to declare that the interpretation of the favorable changes in Lp-PLA2 mass was hindered by the lack of validation of the biomarker for CVD risk prediction in the context of HCV infection and the inability to correlate biomarker levels with hard outcomes such as CVD events or valid alternative means. Despite these limitations, our data remain informative, and further investigation that aims to test the predictive utility of both non-hepatic and hepatic CVD biomarkers and quantifying the potential benefit of HCV treatment on CVD is warranted.

Conclusion

Traditional risk score calculators incorporating hepatically produced biomarkers, such as Framingham risk score, may underestimate CVD risk in HCV-infected patients, while Lp-PLA2 may provide a better estimate of CVD risk as it is a non-hepatically produced biomarker with no relation to liver disease severity. Furthermore, HCV clearance may reduce CVD risk as perpetuated by the significant reduction in Lp-PLA2 levels after DAA therapy and SVR.

Abbreviations
AFP: Alpha-fetoprotein; ALT: Alanine transaminase; ANOVA: Analysis of variance; AST: Aspartate transaminase; CBC: Complete blood count; CVD: Cardiovascular disease; DCV: Daclatasvir; DM: Diabetes mellitus; ELISA: Enzyme-linked immunosorbent assay; FBG: Fasting blood glucose; HbA1c: Hemoglobin A1c; HBsAg: Hepatitis B surface antigen; HBV: Hepatitis B virus; HCC: Hepatocellular carcinoma; HCV: Hepatitis C virus; HIV: Human immunodeficiency virus; HRP: Horseradish peroxidase; hsCRP: High-sensitivity C-reactive protein; INR: International normalized ratio; IQR: Interquartile range; IR: Insulin resistance; LDL: Low-density lipoprotein; Lp-PLA2: Lipoprotein-associated phospholipase A2; NCCVH: National Committee for Control of Viral Hepatitis; PEG: Peginterferon; RBV: Ribavirin; RNA: Ribonucleic acid; ROC: Receiver operator characteristic; SD: Standard deviation; SOF: Sofosbuvir; SVR: Sustained virologic response; TMB: Tetramethylbenzidine

Acknowledgements
The authors express their gratitude to the staff members of the Clinical Pathology and Internal Medicine (gastroenterology and hepatology unit) departments at Ain Shams University Hospital, Cairo, Egypt.

Authors' contributions
AI proposed the research subject, conducted a final revision of the gathered data, and shared in writing the manuscript. BE shared in the data acquisition and revision and drafting of the manuscript, besides being the corresponding author. KE made a substantial contribution in writing the manuscript and revising it critically for important intellectual content. RSM contributed to the study by revising and drafting the work and participated in writing the manuscript. SAI revised the laboratory analysis, tabulated the data, and helped in the statistical analysisS of the collected data. ES shared in the data collection, revision, and interpretation of the statistical analysis of all data and in writing the manuscript. All authors have read and approved the submitted version of the manuscript. Each author agreed to be personally accountable for their own contributions and ensured that questions related to the accuracy or integrity of any part of the work are appropriately investigated and resolved.

Declarations

Ethics approval and consent to participate
The study was performed according to the ethical standards for human experimentation and in accordance with the ethical principles of the 1975 Declaration of Helsinki. Patients included in the study signed an informed written consent to participate. All procedures performed in this study were in accordance with the standards of the Research Ethics Committee (REC) of the Faculty of Medicine, Ain Shams University (FWA 000017585).

Competing interests
The authors declare that they have no competing interests.

Author details
[1]Department of Internal Medicine, Gastroenterology and Hepatology Unit, Faculty of Medicine, Ain Shams University, Cairo 11566, Egypt. [2]Department of Clinical Pathology, Faculty of Medicine, Ain Shams University, Cairo 11566, Egypt.

References
1. Negro F (2014) Facts and fictions of HCV and comorbidities: steatosis, diabetes mellitus, and cardiovascular diseases. J Hepatol. 61(1):S69–S78. https://doi.org/10.1016/j.jhep.2014.08.003
2. Kralj D, Virović Jukić L, Stojsavljević S, Duvnjak M, Smolić M, Čurčić IB (2016) Hepatitis C virus, insulin resistance, and steatosis. J Clin Transl Hepatol 4(1): 66–75. https://doi.org/10.14218/JCTH.2015.00051
3. El Sagheer G, Soliman E, Ahmad A, Hamdy L (2018) Study of changes in lipid profile and insulin resistance in Egyptian patients with chronic hepatitis C genotype 4 in the era of DAAs. Libyan J Med. 13(1):1435124. https://doi.org/10.1080/19932820.2018.1435124
4. Kohli A, Shaffer A, Sherman A, Kottilil S (2014) Treatment of hepatitis C: a systematic review. JAMA. 312(6):631–640. https://doi.org/10.1001/jama.2014.7085
5. Meissner EG, Lee YJ, Osinusi A, Sims Z, Qin J, Sturdevant D, McHutchison J, Subramanian M, Sampson M, Naggie S, Patel K, Remaley AT, Masur H, Kottilil S (2015) Effect of sofosbuvir and ribavirin treatment on peripheral and hepatic lipid metabolism in chronic hepatitis C virus, genotype 1-infected patients. Hepatology. 61(3):790–801. https://doi.org/10.1002/hep.27424
6. Corey KE, Kane E, Munroe C, Barlow LL, Zheng H, Chung RT (2009) Hepatitis C virus infection and its clearance alter circulating lipids: implications for long-term follow-up. Hepatology. 50(4):1030–1037. https://doi.org/10.1002/hep.23219
7. Dhingra R, Vasan RS (2017) Biomarkers in cardiovascular disease: statistical assessment and section on key novel heart failure biomarkers. Trends Cardiovasc Med. 27(2):123–133. https://doi.org/10.1016/j.tcm.2016.07.005
8. Bhatti S, Hakeem A, Cilingiroglu M (2010) Lp-PLA(2) as a marker of cardiovascular diseases. Curr Atheroscler Rep. 12(2):140–144. https://doi.org/10.1007/s11883-010-0095-6
9. Lavi S, McConnell JP, Rihal CS et al (2007) Local production of lipoprotein-associated phospholipase A2 and lysophosphatidylcholine in the coronary circulation: association with early coronary atherosclerosis and endothelial dysfunction in humans. Circulation. 115(21):2715–2721. https://doi.org/10.1161/CIRCULATIONAHA.106.671420
10. Cojocaru M, Cojocaru IM, Silosi I (2010) Lipoprotein-associated phospholipase A2 as a predictive biomarker of sub-clinical inflammation in cardiovascular diseases. Maedica (Bucur). 5(1):51–55
11. Lanman RB, Wolfert RL, Fleming JK, Jaffe AS, Roberts WL, Warnick GR, McConnell JP (2006) Lipoprotein-associated phospholipase A2: review and recommendation of a clinical cut point for adults. Prev Cardiol. 9(3):138–143. https://doi.org/10.1111/j.1520-037x.2006.05547.x
12. Elsharkawy A, Fouad R, El Akel W et al (2017) Sofosbuvir-based treatment regimens: real life results of 14 409 chronic HCV genotype 4 patients in Egypt. Aliment Pharmacol Ther. 45(5):681–687. https://doi.org/10.1111/apt.13923
13. El-Akel W, El-Sayed MH, El Kassas M et al (2017) National treatment programme of hepatitis C in Egypt: hepatitis C virus model of care. S. 24(4): 262–267. https://doi.org/10.1111/jvh.12668
14. D'Agostino RB Sr, Vasan RS, Pencina MJ, Wolf PA, Cobain M, Massaro JM, Kannel WB (2008) General cardiovascular risk profile for use in primary care: the Framingham Heart Study. Circulation. 117(6):743–753. https://doi.org/10.1161/CIRCULATIONAHA.107.699579
15. Babiker A, Jeudy J, Kligerman S, Khambaty M, Shah A, Bagchi S (2017) Risk of cardiovascular disease due to chronic hepatitis C infection: a review. J Clin Transl Hepatol. 5(4):343–362. https://doi.org/10.14218/JCTH.2017.00021
16. Butt AA, Yan P, Simon TG, Chung RT, Abou-Samra AB, ERCHIVES study team (2015) Changes in circulating lipids level over time after acquiring HCV infection: results from ERCHIVES. BMC Infect Dis 15(1):510. https://doi.org/10.1186/s12879-015-1268-2
17. Ali M, Madjid M (2009) Lipoprotein-associated phospholipase A2: a cardiovascular risk predictor and a potential therapeutic target. Future Cardiol. 5(2):159–173. https://doi.org/10.2217/14796678.5.2.159
18. Zalewski A, Macphee C (2005) Role of lipoprotein-associated phospholipase A2 in atherosclerosis: biology, epidemiology, and possible therapeutic target. Arterioscler Thromb Vasc Biol. 25(5):923–931. https://doi.org/10.1161/01.ATV.0000160551.21962.a7
19. Kuo YH, Chuang TW, Hung CH, Chen CH, Wang JH, Hu TH, Lu SN, Lee CM (2011) Reversal of hypolipidemia in chronic hepatitis C patients after

successful antiviral therapy. J Formos Med Assoc. 110(6):363–371. https://doi.org/10.1016/S0929-6646(11)60054-5

20. Nagano T, Seki N, Tomita Y, Sugita T, Aida Y, Itagaki M, Sutoh S, Abe H, Tsubota A, Aizawa Y (2015) Impact of chronic hepatitis C virus genotype 1b infection on triglyceride concentration in serum lipoprotein fractions. Int J Mol Sci 16(9):20576–20594. https://doi.org/10.3390/ijms160920576
21. Dai CY, Chuang WL, Ho CK, Hsieh MY, Huang JF, Lee LP, Hou NJ, Lin ZY, Chen SC, Hsieh MY, Wang LY, Tsai JF, Chang WY, Yu ML (2008) Associations between hepatitis C viremia and low serum triglyceride and cholesterol levels: a community-based study. J Hepatol. 49(1):9–16. https://doi.org/10.1016/j.jhep.2008.03.016
22. Jang ES, Won JE, Jung JI, Lee SH, Kim JW, Jeong SH (2011) The effect of antiviral therapy on serum cholesterol levels in chronic hepatitis C. Gut Liver. 5(3):356–362. https://doi.org/10.5009/gnl.2011.5.3.356
23. Chew KW, Hua L, Bhattacharya D et al (2014) The effect of hepatitis C virologic clearance on cardiovascular disease biomarkers in human immunodeficiency virus/hepatitis C virus coinfection. Open Forum Infect Dis 1(3):ofu104. https://doi.org/10.1093/ofid/ofu104
24. Chew KW, Bhattacharya D, McGinnis KA et al (2015) Short communication: Coronary heart disease risk by Framingham Risk Score in hepatitis C and HIV/hepatitis C-coinfected persons. AIDS Res Hum Retroviruses. 31(7):718–722. https://doi.org/10.1089/AID.2014.0284
25. Miyaura S, Maki N, Byrd W, Johnston JM (1991) The hormonal regulation of platelet-activating factor acetylhydrolase activity in plasma. Lipids. 26(12):1015–1020. https://doi.org/10.1007/BF02536494
26. Yoshimura T, Ohshige A, Maeda T, Ito M, Okamura H (1999) Estrogen replacement therapy decreases platelet-activating factor-acetylhydrolase activity in post-menopausal women. Maturitas. 31(3):249–253. https://doi.org/10.1016/s0378-5122(99)00004-3
27. Ohshige A, Ito M, Koyama H, Maeda T, Yoshimura T, Okamura H (1994) Effects of estrogen and progesterone on platelet-activating factor acetylhydrolase activity in ovariectomised rats. Artery. 21(4):234–242
28. Yanbaeva DG, Dentener MA, Creutzberg EC, Wesseling G, Wouters EF (2007) Systemic effects of smoking. *Chest*. 131(5):1557–1566. https://doi.org/10.1378/chest.06-2179

10

The expression of microRNA-331-3p and microRNA-23b3 in Egyptian patients with early-stage hepatocellular carcinoma in hepatitis C-related liver cirrhosis

Reham A. Aboelwafa[1], Walid Ismail Ellakany[2], Marwa A. Gamaleldin[1] and Marwa A. Saad[3*]

Abstract

Background: Hepatocellular carcinoma and hepatitis C are strongly associated. The current work aimed to study the expression levels of microRNA-331-3p and microRNA-23b-3p as propable biomarkers for detecting liver cancer (HCC) at its early stages in patients with HCV-related liver cirrhosis. The current prospective study included two hundred participants, divided into three groups: group I, 100 patients with HCV-related liver cirrhosis; group II, 50 HCC patients at early stages; and group III, 50 apparentlyhealthy controls. All patients had routine laboratory workup and ultrasound hepatic assessment. Values of microRNA-331-3p and microRNA-23b-3p were measured by real-time quantitative PCR.

Results: Levels of miR-331-3p were significantly higher in HCC patients than in cirrhotic patients and controls ($p < 0.001$), while levels of miR-23b-3p were significantly lower in HCC patients compared to cirrhotics and controls ($p < 0.001$). ROC curve revealed that miR-23b-3p had 80% sensitivity and 74% specificity, miR-331-3p had 66% sensitivity and 61% specificity, and AFP had 64% sensitivity and 61% specificity of 61% in discrimination between HCC patients from controls.

Conclusion: Serum miR-23b-3p is a more effective predictor than miR-331-3p and AFP for the development of hepatocellular carcinoma in hepatitis C (HCV)-related cirrhotic patients.

Keywords: miR-331-3p, miR-23b-3p, HCV, HCC, Egyptian, Liver cirrhosis

Background

Hepatocellular carcinoma (HCC) is a universal health problem. HCC represents the sixth most common cancer worldwide [1], and the fourth common cancer in Egypt [2]. HCV promotes cirrhosis, which is found in 80–90% of patients with HCC [3]. Prospective studies have shown a significant increase in the incidence of HCC among HCV-infected cohorts, compared to HCV-negative cohorts. HCV-induced HCC development is a multi-step process that may progress over 20–40 years [4]. HCV is an RNA virus with limited integration of its genetic material into the host's genome. Therefore, the carcinogenic potential of HCV is generally assumed to be linked to the indirect mechanisms [5].

MicroRNAs (miRNAs) are a class of small 18-23-nucleotides that have a role in different biological functions including proliferation, differentiation, and apoptosis [6]. Abnormal miRNA expression has been implicated in the pathogenesis of various cancers [7]. Discovery that microRNAs are detected in patients' sera raised the assumption that these serum biomarkers can be used as a less invasive screening or diagnostic tools [8]. miR-331-3p is one of the most upregulated miRNAs that promote proliferation, migration, and invasion of

* Correspondence: marwa.saad@alexmed.edu.eg
[3]Internal medicine department, Faculty of Medicine, Alexandria University, Alexandria, Egypt
Full list of author information is available at the end of the article

the tumor cells, including HCC [9]. miR-23b-3p was identified as a tumor suppressor that downregulated in different classes of human malignant tumors [10].

microRNA-331-3p and microRNA-23b-3p expression in hepatic carcinoma was examined in some studies [11, 12].

The current work aimed to determine the potentiality of serum miR-331-3p and miR-23b-3p as screening biomarkers for early stages of liver cancer in patients with HCV-related hepatic cirrhosis.

Methods

The current prospective study involved 150 patients out of 2140 patients who attended the tropical medicine, hepatology, oncology, and general medicine outpatient clinics in the Alexandria University Hospital (Alexandria, Egypt) in the period from December 2017 till January 2020. The control group involved 50 apparently healthy volunteers.

The proposal was explained to all participants, and they signed a written consent. The proposal was accepted by the committee of ethics (Faculty of medicine, University of Alexandria).

Exclusion criteria included patients with coinfections with hepatitis B virus (HBV) or HIV, organ transplantation, autoimmune disease or use of immunosuppressant or antiviral drugs, diabetes mellitus, Schistosoma, and other malignant comorbidities.

All participants were subjected to full history taking, thorough clinical examination, laboratory investigations including complete blood picture, liver transaminases (alanine aminotransferase (ALT), and aspartate aminotransferase (AST)), serum albumin, total bilirubin, and alpha-fetoprotein, and abdominal ultrasonography.

Two hundred participants were divided into three groups: group I, 100 patients with HCV-related liver cirrhosis; group II, 50 patients with early-stage hepatocellular carcinoma (HCC); and group III, 50 healthy controls.

Ultrasound examinations were performed by experienced ultra-sonographers in the Radiology Department of the main Alexandria University Hospital. Items to be observed in ultrasound examination were determination of the liver size, nodularity of the liver surface, the coarseness of the parenchyma, size of lymph nodes around the hepatic artery, patency and flow of veins and arteries, and probable hepatocellular carcinoma.

HCV antibody testing was done by using a commercial recombinant immunoblot assay and confirmed by real-time quantitative HCV RNA PCR (more than 15 IU/ml).

All the HCC patients were diagnosed by abdominal ultrasound and alpha-fetoprotein [13]. Triphasic CT scan examination and Barcelona clinic liver cancers (BCLC) [25] staging was done for the selection of group II patients. Based on BCLC; patients at a very early stage (stage 0) and early stage (stage A) were selected as candidates for study with single tumors less than 2 cm or multinodular tumor less than 3 cm in size, with the absence of clinically relevant portal hypertension.

Real-time quantitative PCR for miR-331-3p and miR-23b expression levels

Total RNA including microRNA was immediately isolated from plasma samples using miRNeasy Mini Kit (Qiagen, Maryland, USA) according to manufacturers' instructions. The concentration and purity of the extracted total RNA were assisted using NanoDrop2000 Spectrophotometer (Thermo Scientific, USA). Single-stranded cDNA was synthesized from purified RNA samples using the Taqman miRNA reverse transcription Kit (Applied Biosystems, USA) for RNA reverse transcription according to the manufacturer's protocol. The real-time amplification was performed using TaqMan MicroRNA assays for miR-331-3p, miR-23-3p, and TaqMan Fast Advanced Mater Mix (Applied Biosystems, USA) on the RotorGene Q Real-Time PCR System (Qiagen, Germany). RNU6 was used as endogenous references; its expression was stable in all the samples and independent of the analyzed variables. The relative expression levels were determined using the $2^{-\Delta\Delta CT}$ method.

Statistical analysis

Data were fed to the computer and analyzed using IBM SPSS software package version 20.0. (Armonk, NY: IBM Corp). The Kolmogorov- Smirnov was used to verify the normality of distribution of variables. Comparisons between groups for categorical variables were assessed using the Chi-square test. ANOVA was used for comparing the four studied groups and followed by post hoc test (Tukey) for pairwise comparison. While Kruskal-Wallis test was used to compare different groups for abnormally distributed quantitative variables and followed by post hoc test (Dunn's for multiple comparisons test) for pairwise comparison. The significance of the obtained results was judged at the 5% level.

Results

The current study involved 200 participants divided into the following groups: group I, 100 patients with HCV-related liver cirrhosis; group II, 50 HCC patients at an early stage (16 patients (32%) were BCLC stage 0 and 34 patients (68%) were BCLC stage A); and group III, 50 apparently healthy controls.

The mean age of group I was 47.4 ± 9.7years, group II was 50.6 ± 5.2years, and of group III was 47.5 ± 9.3years with no significant difference between the three groups (p = 0.086) (Table 1).

Table 1 Comparison between the three studied groups according to the demographic data, laboratory investigations, and serum concentrations of miR-331-3p and miR-23b-3p

	Group I (HCV-related liver cirrhosis) (n = 100)	Group II (HCC group) (n = 50) (16 stage 0 BCLC, 34 stage A BCLC)	Group III (healthy controls) (n = 50)	Test of Sig.	p
Age (years)					
Mean ± SD	47.4 ± 9.7	50.6 ± 5.2	47.5 ± 9.3	F = 2.489	0.086
Median (min.–max.)	49(25–61)	51(41–59)	48(32–63)		
Gender					
Male	79 (79%)	40 (80%)	35 (70%)	χ^2 = 1.863	0.394
Female	21 (21%)	10 (20%)	15 (30%)		
ALT (IU/L)					
Mean ± SD	59.7 ± 35.1	60.4 ± 26.3	19.0 ± 7.7	H = 72.496*	< 0.001*
Median (min.–max.)	56.5[a] (8.4–165)	48[a] (33–127)	18.4[b] (5.8–38.1)		
AST (IU/L)					
Mean ± SD	53.2 ± 30.1	55.3 ± 24.8	18.7 ± 6.3	H = 84.833*	< 0.001*
Median (min.–max.)	45.5[a] (6.9–155)	44.5[a] (30–119)	17.6[b] (6.4–30.2)		
Total bilirubin (mg/dl)					
Mean ± SD	1.2 ± 0.6	1.1 ± 0.4	0.7 ± 0.3	H = 25.660*	< 0.001*
Median (min.–max.)	1.1[a] (0.2–2.8)	1[a] (0.4–2)	0.8[b] (0.1–1.2)		
Albumin (g/dl)					
Mean ± SD	3.9[b] ± 3.1	3.6[c] ± 2.6	4.3[a] ± 4.8	F = 46.804*	< 0.001*
Median (min.–max.)	4.0 (3.3–4.5)	3.6 (3.2–4.0)	4.2 (3.4–5.2)		
Hemoglobin (g/dl)					
Mean ± SD	13.6[a] ± 1.8	12.2[b] ± 1.3	14.1[a] ± 1.1	F = 22.005*	< 0.001*
Median (min.–max.)	13.9 (8.5–16.4)	12.0 (10.0–15.0)	14.4 (12.1–15.9)		
Total leukocytic count (× 10^9)					
Mean ± SD	5.2[b] ± 1	4.2[c] ± 1.1	6.7[a] ± 1.8	F = 51.129*	< 0.001*
Median (min.–max.)	5.1 (3.5–7.1)	4 (2.4–6.3)	6.5 (4.3–10.2)		
Platelet count (× 10^9)					
Mean ± SD	160.9[a] ± 46.8	130.2[c] ± 21.5	223.1[b] ± 44.1	F = 67.135*	< 0.001*
Median (min.–max.)	158 (63–254)	134.5 (91–162)	238.5 (126–358)		
AFP (ng/ml)					
Mean ± SD	140.3 ± 45.2	183.1 ± 77	1.0 ± 0.4	H = 117.964*	< 0.001*
Median (min.–max.)	138[b] (1.8–240)	196[a] (58–287)	1[c] (0.2–1.9)		
miR-331-3p ($2^{-\Delta CT}$)					
Mean ± SD	2.2 ± 1.3	7.6 ± 10	1.1 ± 0.5	H = 69.738*	< 0.001*
Median (min.–max.)	1.98[b] (0.1–7.8)	3.8[a] (0.1–41)	1[c] (0.1–3.2)		
miR-23b-3p ($2^{-\Delta CT}$)					
Mean ± SD	0.9 ± 0.8	0.3 ± 0.3	1.5 ± 1.1	H = 54.230*	< 0.001*
Median (min.–max.)	0.8[b] (− 0.98 to 3.2)	0.2[c] (0–1.7)	1.3[a] (− 1 to 3.8)		

χ^2 chi-square test, *F* F for ANOVA test, *H* H for Kruskal-Wallis test, *p* p-value for comparing between the studied groups
Means/median with common letters are not significant (i.e., means with different letters are significant)
*Statistically significant at p ≤ 0.05

Group I comprised of 79 males (79%) and 21 females (21%), group II comprised of 40 males (80%) and 10 females (20%), and group III comprised of 35 males (70%) and 15 females (30%), with no statistically significant difference between the three studied groups ($p = 0.394$) (Table 1).

As regards results of peripheral blood picture, levels of serum transaminases, total bilirubin levels, and serum albumin levels, all were summarized in Table 1.

The mean of AFP was significantly higher in group II than in groups I and III. Furthermore, it was significantly higher in group II than group III ($P < 0.001$ and $P < 0.001$, respectively) (Table 1).

Regarding miR-331-3p expression, plasma levels were significantly higher in group II compared to group I and III ($p < 0.001$ and $P < 0.001$, respectively). Also, a high statistically significant difference was observed between groups (II and III, $p < 0.001$) (Table 1).

On the contrary, miR-23b-3p expression levels were significantly lower in group II compared to group I, and both were significantly lower than the controls ($p < 0.001$) (Table 1).

Further analysis of plasma levels of miRNAs in group II revealed that the mean of miR-331-3p in stage 0 HCC was 8.1 ± 10.3, while it was 7.3 ± 10.1 in patients with stage A, with no statistical difference could be detected between both groups ($p = 0.967$). Regarding miR-23b-3p, its mean in patients with stage 0 HCC was 0.21 ± 0.22, while it was 0.31 ± 0.37, with no statistical difference between both groups ($p = 0.371$) (Table 2).

Using ROC curves to determine the diagnostic accuracy of AFP, miR-331-3p, and miR-23-3p in differentiating patients with early stages of hepatic cancer from patients with HCV-related liver cirrhosis revealed that values of AFP more than 148 ng/ml had a 64% sensitivity and 61% specificity to differentiate early carcinoma patients from cirrhotic ones (Fig. 1). Values of miR-331-3p more than 2.18 had a 66% sensitivity and 61% specificity to differentiate patients with early stages of HCC (Fig. 2). Regarding miR-23b-3p, values less than or equal to 0.36 had an 80% sensitivity and 74% specificity to diagnose HCC at its early stages (Fig. 3). Combining AFP (ng/ml) and miR-331-3p (Fig. 4) gave sensitivity of 76% and specificity of 65%. Combining AFP (ng/ml) & miR-23b-3p (Fig. 5) gave sensitivity of 82% and specificity of 69%. While the sensitivity and specificity of combining the three parameters (Fig. 6) were 86% and 64%, respectively (Table 3).

Discussion

Hepatitis C virus (HCV) is one of the main carcinogens for hepatocellular carcinoma (HCC) [14]. It infects around 71 million people around the world [15]. The HCV infects the liver leading to HCC [16]. And while around 399,000 patients died from HCV in 2016, only around 19% knew about their infection status [16]. And although AFP has been always used to diagnose HCC, it is neither specific nor sensitive [12]. Therefore, it is crucial to look for new predictive markers of HCC as early as possible to improve the patients' prognosis.

miRNAs are small non-coding RNA molecules that are composed of 21–23 nucleotides that affect target gene expression by negatively controlling post-transcriptional gene expression [16, 17]. They are highly tissue-specific and can withstand severe conditions like extreme temperature and low pH, making them highly stable in the serum or plasma samples and, therefore, qualifying them as perfect noninvasive markers for early HCC diagnosis [12].

Several studies identified a microRNA panel to distinguish HCV-related HCC from liver cirrhosis [18–20]. In a recent study, it was discovered that there are four miRNAs, including MiR-331-3p that significantly increased in HCC and two miRNAs including miR-23b-3p that significantly decreased in HCC patients compared to liver cirrhosis. Those six miRNAs have been found in the studies to effectively discriminate the HCC from liver cirrhosis and healthy controls [21].

In our study, miR-331-3p was shown to significantly increase in patients with early stages HCC compared to cirrhotic patients. Similar results were also reported by a previous study on HCC tissues that detected overexpression of miR-331-3p in the HCC cells and proved that it helped proliferation and spread of HCC via suppressing

Table 2 Plasma concentrations of miR-331-3p and miR-23b-3p in group II (n = 50)

	BCLC stage		U	p
	Stage 0 (n = 16)	Stage A (n = 34)		
miR-331-3p ($2^{-\Delta CT}$)				
Mean ± SD	8.1 ± 10.3	7.3 ± 10.1	270.0	0.967
Median (min.–max.)	3.8 (1.3–36.2)	3.7 (0.1–41)		
miR-23b-3p ($2^{-\Delta CT}$)				
Mean ± SD	0.21 ± 0.22	0.31 ± 0.37	229.0	0.371
Median (min.–max.)	0.14 (0.01–0.8)	0.18 (0.02–1.7)		

U Mann-Whitney test, *p* p value for comparing between BCLC stage and serum concentrations of miR-331-3p and miR-23b-3p

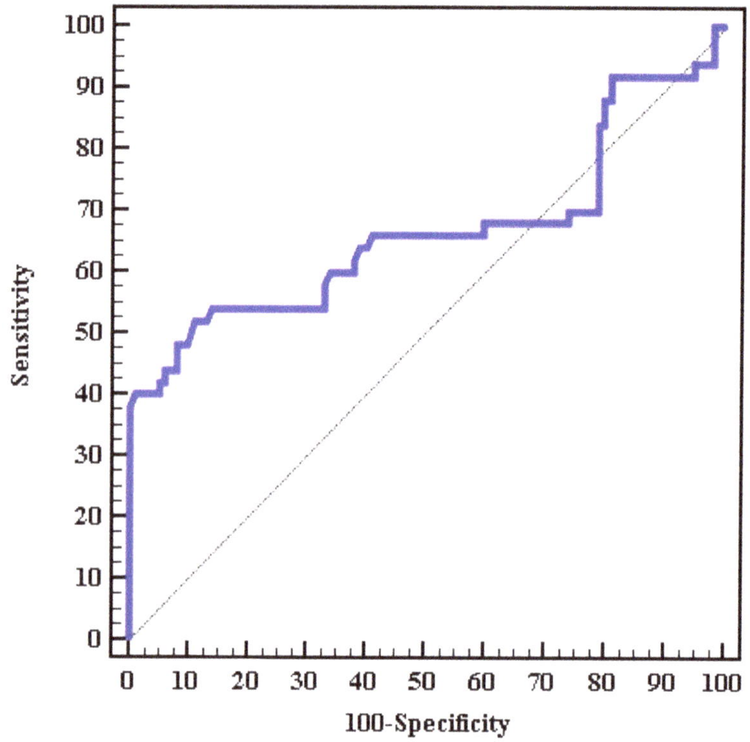

Fig. 1 ROC curve for AFP (ng/ml) to predict early-stage HCC patients (group II) from HCV-related cirrhosis (group I)

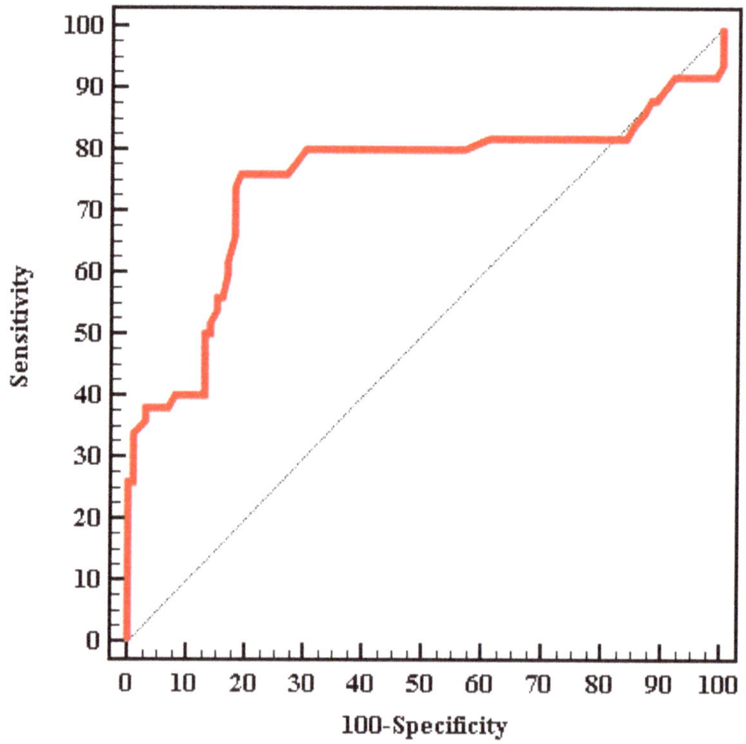

Fig. 2 ROC curve for miR-331-3p to predict Early-stage HCC patients (group II) from HCV-related cirrhosis (group I)

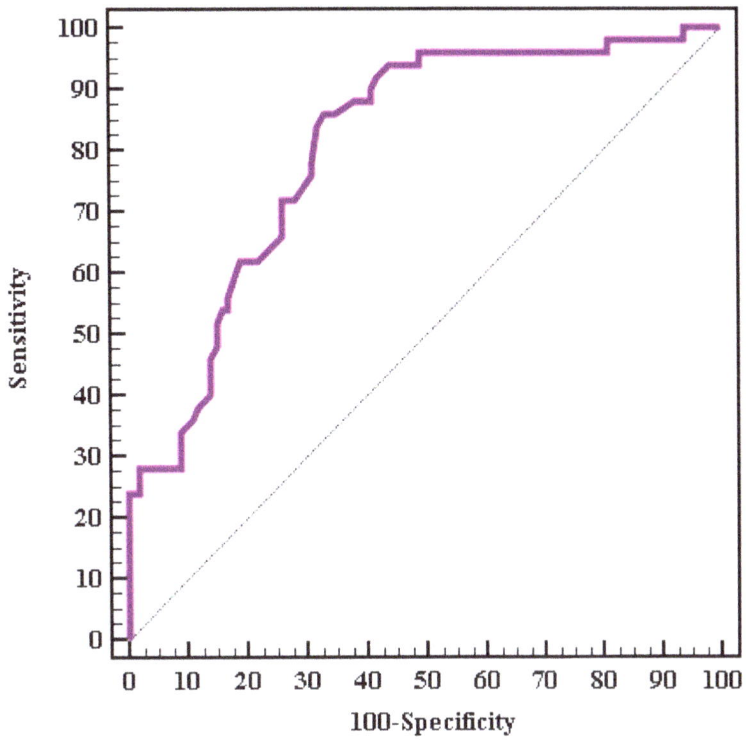

Fig. 3 ROC curve for miR-23b-3p to predict early-stage HCC patients (group II) from HCV-related cirrhosis (group I)

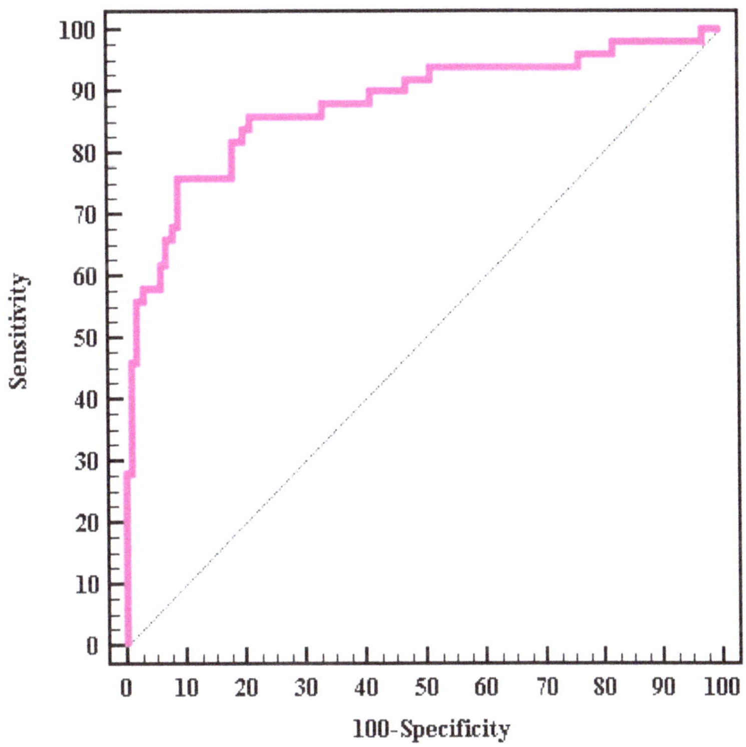

Fig. 4 ROC curve for the combination of AFP and miR-331-3p to predict early-stage HCC patients (group II) from HCV-related cirrhosis (group I)

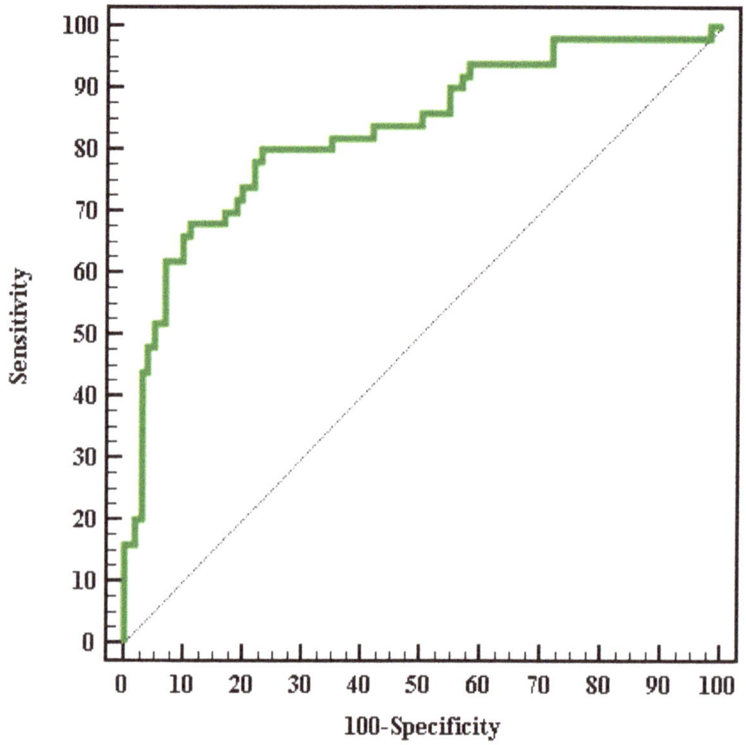

Fig. 5 ROC curve for the combination of AFP and miR-23b-3p to predict early-stage HCC patients (group II) from HCV-related cirrhosis (group I)

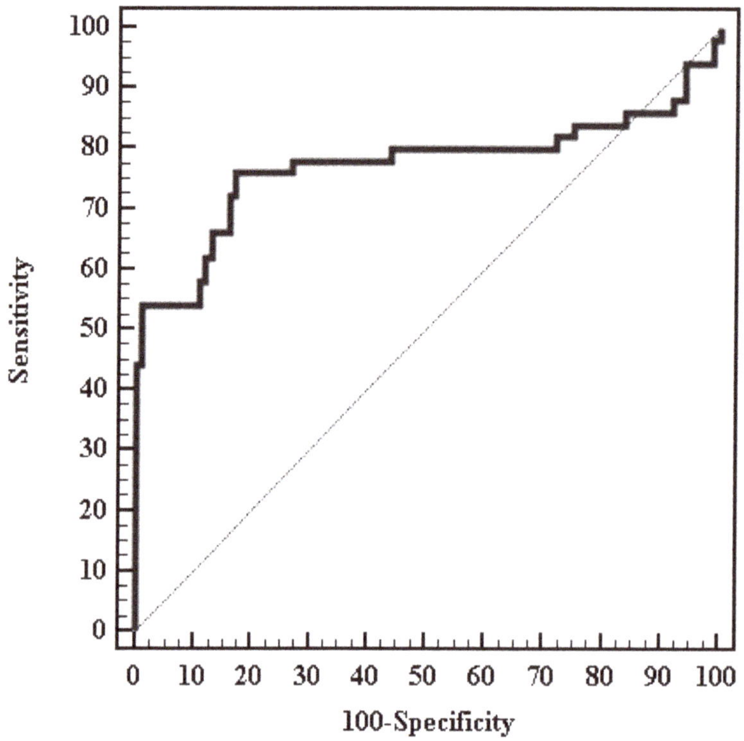

Fig. 6 ROC curve for the combination of AFP, miR-331-3p, and miR-23b-3p to predict early-stage HCC patients (group II) from HCV-related cirrhosis (group I)

Table 3 Agreement (sensitivity, specificity) for AFP, miR-331-3p, and miR-23b-3p for diagnosing early-stage HCC patients

	AUC	p	95% CI	Cut-off	Sensitivity	Specificity	PPV	NPV
AFP (ng/ml)	0.665	0.001*	0.557–0.772	> 148	64.0	61.0	45.1	77.2
miR-331-3p	0.703	< 0.001*	0.602–0.803	> 2.18	66.0	61.0	45.8	78.2
miR-23b-3p	0.781	< 0.001*	0.706–0.856	≤ 0.36	80.0	74.0	60.6	88.1
AFP (ng/ml) and miR-331-3p	0.773	< 0.001*	0.678–0.868		76.0	65.0	52.1	84.4
AFP (ng/ml) and miR-23b-3p	0.814	< 0.001*	0.746–0.883		82.0	69.0	56.9	88.5
AFP (ng/ml) and miR-331-3p and miR-23b-3p	0.854	< 0.001*	0.791–0.916		86.0	64.0	54.4	90.1

AUS area under a curve, *NPV* negative predictive value, *p value* probability value, *PPV* positive predictive value, *CI* confidence intervals
*Statistically significant at $p \leq 0.05$

leucine-rich repeat protein phosphatase mediated dephosphorylation of protein kinase B [22]. These results were consistent with Chen et al. [23] results who found that serum miR-331-3p significantly increased in HCC compared to patients with benign hepatic tumors and was associated with poor HCC prognosis. In the current study, comparison between patients with stage 0 HCC and stage A regarding levels of miR331-3p did not show significant difference.

miR-23b-3p showed a significant decrease in the plasma of patients with early HCC compared to cirrhotic patients. These results are consistent with those results reported previously by Cao et al. who stated that miR-23b-3p was downregulated in HCC tissue cells [24]. Despite the miR-23b-3p in tissues has been identified as a diagnostic molecular marker and a possible therapeutic target for patients with HCC [13], its serum concentrations have not been thoroughly researched in many studies before.

On further analysis, the diagnostic sensitivities and specificities of both miR 331 3p and mi-23b-3p had been calculated using the ROC curves. According to the ROC curves data, it was shown that mi-23b-3p had the best sensitivity (80%) and specificity (74%). In a study by Sun et al., miR-23b-3p had better sensitivity compared to miR-331-3p, but contrary to our results miR-331-3p showed the highest specificity [12].

Conclusion

Serum miR-23b-3p is a more effective predictor than miR-331-3p and AFP for the development of hepatocellular carcinoma in cirrhotic HCV patients. The usual marker used in the clinical practice to predict HCC is AFP, but our results revealed that miR-23b-3p has a greater sensitivity and specificity than AFP. The cost-effectiveness as well as the benefits depends on the price of the kit and the number of the samples to be done.

Limitation of the study

Small sample size and future studies should be done in large number of patients to verify our results.

Abbreviation

AFP: Alpha-fetoprotein; ALT: Alanine aminotransferase; AST: Aspartate aminotransferase; EMT: Epithelial-mesenchymal transformation; HBV: Hepatitis B virus; HCC: Hepatocellular carcinoma; HCV: Hepatitis C virus; HIV: Human immunodeficiency virus; miRNAs: Microribonucleic acid; Pyk2: Proline-rich tyrosine kinase 2

Acknowledgements

We sincerely thank all patients and healthy volunteers for their participation in the current study. We also thank Mr. Amgad Hamza for revising the statistical analysis of the results.

Authors' contributions

All authors have contributed to the current work. R.A. and M.G. had performed laboratory investigations of the participants, analysis, and interpretation of the data. W.E. contributed substantially to the conception and design of the study, acquisition of data, and analyzed and interpreted the data. M.S. contributed to the acquisition of data, drafted the manuscript, and critical revision of the manuscript. All the authors approved the final version submitted for publication and take responsibility for the statements made in the published article.

Declarations

Ethics approval and consent to participate

The proposal of the current study was approved by the ethical committee of the Faculty of Medicine—Alexandria University (the approval number is not available). Informed written consent was signed by all participants or their caregivers before the study. The committee's reference number is not available. The current study is original and has not been published elsewhere in any form or language (partially or in full). Results of the current study were presented, honestly, and without fabrication, falsification, or inappropriate data manipulation. No data, text, or theories by others are presented as if they were the author's own ("plagiarism").

Competing interests

The authors declare that they have no competing interests.

Author details

[1]Clinical Pathology Department, Faculty of Medicine, Alexandria University, Alexandria, Egypt. [2]Tropical medicine Department, Faculty of Medicine, Alexandria University, Alexandria, Egypt. [3]Internal medicine department, Faculty of Medicine, Alexandria University, Alexandria, Egypt.

References

1. Forner A, Reig M, Bruix J (2018) Hepatocellular carcinoma. Lancet. 391(10127):1301–1314. https://doi.org/10.1016/S0140-6736(18)30010-2
2. Rashed WM, Kandeil MAM, Mahmoud MO, Ezzat S (2020) Hepatocellular carcinoma (HCC) in Egypt: a comprehensive overview. J Egypt Natl Canc Inst. 32(1):5. https://doi.org/10.1186/s43046-020-0016-x
3. El-Serag HB (2012) Epidemiology of viral hepatitis and hepatocellular carcinoma. Gastroenterology 142((6)):1264–73. e1
4. Goossens N, Hoshida Y (2015) Hepatitis C virus-induced hepatocellular carcinoma. Clin Mol Hepatol. 21(2):105–114. https://doi.org/10.3350/cmh.2015.21.2.105
5. Billerbeck E, de Jong Y, Dorner M, de la Fuente C, Ploss A (2013) Animal models for hepatitis C. Curr Top Microbiol Immunol. 369:49–86. https://doi.org/10.1007/978-3-642-27340-7_3
6. Gao B, Ning S, Li J, Liu H, Wei W, Wu F et al (2015) Integrated analysis of differentially expressed mRNAs and miRNAs between hepatocellular carcinoma and their matched adjacent normal liver tissues. Oncol Rep. 34(1):325–333. https://doi.org/10.3892/or.2015.3968
7. Hironaka-Mitsuhashi A, Matsuzaki J, Takahashi RU, Yoshida M, Nezu Y, Yamamoto Y et al (2017) A tissue microRNA signature that predicts the prognosis of breast cancer in young women. PLoS One. 12(11):e0187638. https://doi.org/10.1371/journal.pone.0187638
8. Yokoi A, Yoshioka Y, Hirakawa A, Yamamoto Y, Ishikawa M, Ikeda SI,2017 Kato T, Niimi K, Kajiyama H, Kikkawa F, Ochiya T A combination of circulating miRNAs for the early detection of ovarian cancer. Oncotarget. ;8(52):89811-89823, doi: https://doi.org/10.18632/oncotarget.20688.
9. Papadopoulos EI, Papachristopoulou G, Ardavanis A, Scorilas A (2018) A comprehensive clinicopathological evaluation of the differential expression of microRNA-331 in breast tumors and its diagnostic significance. Clin Biochem. 60:24–32. https://doi.org/10.1016/j.clinbiochem.2018.07.008
10. Jiang W, Min J, Sui X, Qian Y, Liu Y, Liu Z, Zhou H, Li X, Gong Y (2015) MicroRNA-26a-5p and microRNA-23b-3p up-regulate peroxiredoxin III in acute myeloid leukemia. Leuk Lymphoma. 56(2):460–471. https://doi.org/10.3109/10428194.2014.924115
11. He RQ, Wu PR, Xiang XL, Yang X, Liang HW, Qiu XH, Yang LH, Peng ZG, Chen G (2018) Downregulated miR-23b-3p expression acts as a predictor of hepatocellular carcinoma progression: a study based on public data and RT-qPCR verification. Int J Mol Med. 41(5):2813–2831. https://doi.org/10.3892/ijmm.2018.3513
12. Sun Q, Li J, Jin B, Wang T, Gu J (2020) Evaluation of miR-331-3p and miR-23b-3p as serum biomarkers for hepatitis c virus-related hepatocellular carcinoma at early stage. Clin Res Hepatol Gastroenterol. 44(1):21–28. https://doi.org/10.1016/j.clinre.2019.03.011
13. He RQ, Wu PR, Xiang XL, Yang X, Liang HW, Qiu XH, Yang LH, Peng ZG, Chen G (2018) Downregulated miR-23b-3p expression acts as a predictor of hepatocellular carcinoma progression: a study based on public data and RT-qPCR verification. Int J Mol Med. 41(5):2813–2831. https://doi.org/10.3892/ijmm.2018.3513
14. Axley P, Ahmed Z, Ravi S, Singal AK (2018) Hepatitis C virus and hepatocellular carcinoma: a narrative review. J Clin Transl Hepatol. 6(1):79–84. https://doi.org/10.14218/JCTH.2017.00067
15. Mason LM, Duffell E, Veldhuijzen IK, Petriti U, Bunge EM, Tavoschi L (2019) Hepatitis B and C prevalence and incidence in key population groups with multiple risk factors in the EU/EEA: a systematic review, Euro Surveill. 24((30))
16. Lorini S, Gragnani L, Zignego AL (2020) The relevance of MicroRNAs in the pathogenesis and prognosis of HCV-disease: the emergent role of miR-17-92 in cryoglobulinemic vasculitis. Viruses 12((12))
17. Inui M, Martello G, Piccolo S (2010) MicroRNA control of signal transduction. Nat Rev Mol Cell Biol. 11(4):252–263. https://doi.org/10.1038/nrm2868
18. Elemeery MN, Badr AN, Mohamed MA, Ghareeb DA (2017) Validation of a serum microRNA panel as biomarkers for early diagnosis of hepatocellular carcinoma post-hepatitis C infection in Egyptian patients. World J Gastroenterol. 23(21):3864–3875. https://doi.org/10.3748/wjg.v23.i21.3864
19. Zekri AN, Youssef AS, El-Desouky ED, Ahmed OS, Lotfy MM, Nassar AA et al (2016) Serum microRNA panels as potential biomarkers for early detection of hepatocellular carcinoma on top of HCV infection. Tumour Biol. 37(9): 12273–12286. https://doi.org/10.1007/s13277-016-5097-8
20. El-Abd NE, Fawzy NA, El-Sheikh SM, Soliman ME (2015) Circulating miRNA-122, miRNA-199a, and miRNA-16 as biomarkers for early detection of hepatocellular carcinoma in Egyptian patients with chronic hepatitis C virus infection. Mol Diagn Ther. 19(4):213–220. https://doi.org/10.1007/s40291-015-0148-1
21. Li J, Jin B, Wang T, Li W, Wang Z, Zhang H, Song Y, Li N (2019) Serum microRNA expression profiling identifies serum biomarkers for HCV-related hepatocellular carcinoma. Cancer Biomark. 26(4):501–512. https://doi.org/10.3233/CBM-181970
22. Chang RM, Yang H, Fang F, Xu JF, Yang LY (2014) MicroRNA-331-3p promotes proliferation and metastasis of hepatocellular carcinoma by targeting PH domain and leucine-rich repeat protein phosphatase. Hepatology. 60(4):1251–1263. https://doi.org/10.1002/hep.27221
23. Chen L, Chu F, Cao Y, Shao J, Wang F (2015) Serum miR-182 and miR-331-3p as diagnostic and prognostic markers in patients with hepatocellular carcinoma. Tumour Biol. 36(10):7439–7447. https://doi.org/10.1007/s13277-015-3430-2
24. Cao J, Liu J, Long J, Fu J, Huang L, Li J et al (2017) microRNA-23b suppresses epithelial-mesenchymal transition (EMT) and metastasis in hepatocellular carcinoma via targeting Pyk2. Biomed Pharmacother 89:642–650

11

Evaluation of HCV-related liver fibrosis post-successful DAA therapy

Nermine Ehsan[1], Dina Sweed[1*] and Maha Elsabaawy[2]

Abstract

Background: The rapidly developing era of direct-acting antiviral regimens (DAAs) for more than one hepatitis C virus (HCV) genotype had certainly alleviated HCV burden all over the world. Liver fibrosis is the major dramatic complication of HCV infection, and its progression leads to cirrhosis, liver failure, and hepatocellular carcinoma. The impact of DAAs on liver fibrosis had been debatably evaluated with undetermined resolution.

Main body: The aim of this review is to accurately revise the effects of DAA regimens on liver fibrosis which can either be regression, progression, or non-significant association. Liver fibrosis regression is a genuine fact assured by many retrospective and prospective clinical studies. Evaluation could be concluded early post-therapy reflecting the dynamic nature of the process.

Conclusions: The ideal application of DAA regimens in treating HCV has to be accomplished with efficient non-invasive markers in differentiating proper fibrosis evaluation from necroinflammation consequences. Liver biopsy is the gold standard that visualizes the dynamic of fibrosis regression.

Keywords: Direct-acting antivirals, Hepatitis C virus, Liver fibrosis, Sustained viral response

Background

The advent of DAA therapies against HCV infection is considered by many as the most momentous scientific event taking place in the last few years [1]. Before the developing era of DAAs, HCV infection represented more than 70% of chronic liver disease morbidity and mortality especially in countries with high HCV burden [2]. Nowadays, the outstanding results of DAA therapies had tardily listed HCV in newly reported etiologies of liver diseases [1]. However, the encumbrance of HCV-related liver fibrosis progressing to cirrhosis, hepatocellular carcinoma, and decompensated liver disease is still ensuing [3]. The foreseeable end of these HCV-related disorders is linked to the death of the last untreatable case, which is expected to be by 2030 [2]. Nevertheless, the most important question is: are these therapies capable of regressing fibrosis or even stopping the progression of this definite dynamic process?

* Correspondence: dr.dinasweed@yahoo.com
[1]Pathology Department, National Liver Institute, Menofia University, Shibin El-Kom 32511, Egypt
Full list of author information is available at the end of the article

Main text

Does fibrosis really regress?

Remodeling of liver vascular and regaining the normal lobular architecture upon removal of the incriminating factor is the ultimate hope of liver researchers. As a rule, removing the offender is the most accurate way of reaching a resolution [4]. Accordingly, liver fibrosis—at a certain point—is capable of regression by directly eliminating the cause. Reportedly, on well-targeted early treated autoimmune hepatitis, or hepatitis B virus (HBV) infection, regression of fibrosis was a possible prospective [4].

Liver fibrosis is crucially linked to the evolution of certain inflammatory cascades, activated cells, and fibrogenic cytokines [5]. Likewise, in fibrosis regression, the convoluted process of fibrosis regression is reported to be simultaneous with deactivated myofibroblasts, mounting of collagenases enzymes, fibrillar cellular matrix degradation, ending with cell death (senescence and apoptosis of activated stellate cells), and resorption of fibrous septa [6]. Concerning cirrhosis, a more complex end-stage fibrosis, it comprises angiogenesis, necroinflammation, innate immunity, oxidative stress, tissue hypoxia, and bacterial translocation [7]. Accordingly, regression of fibrosis rather than cirrhosis is considered as a likely prospective. Nevertheless, liver fibrosis regression is not guaranteed to take place on treating the offending agent. Many factors had been demarcated to be of influence on the occurrence of fibrosis regression process: individual's age, genetic and epigenetic factors, and rate of fibrosis progression (slow or rapid fibrosis), or disease-related factors like etiology and staging of chronic liver disease [8–12].

For liver fibrosis to be evitable, interference should be at a certain time; otherwise, no regression is predictable. The point of no return is that at which liver fibrosis progression is inevitable [13]. The cause might be structural extensive crosslinks developed in collagen, the fibrotic bands consisting mainly of fibrillar collagen, as the collagen bands mature. Some of these crosslinks are irreversible and cannot be degraded by the normal collagenases representing a point of unavoidable fibrosis progression [13].

Evaluation of fibrosis

In the era of interferon (IFN), liver biopsy was the most accountable determinant of treatment decision as a precise measure of liver fibrosis [14].

The contemporary protocols of DAA HCV therapies had adopted reliance on non-invasiveness [15, 16]. The currently handled non-invasive hybrid clinical and laboratory scores of liver fibrosis had performed poorly inaccurate, with failure to distinguish the stages of the dynamic evolutions of liver fibrosis. Moreover, the performance of the more advanced imaging measures that assess liver stiffness (LS) with a fibroscan device like transient elastography (TE), shear wave (SW), acoustic radiation force impulse elastography (ARFI), and magnetic resonance elastography (MRE) [15, 16]. Eventually, there is no perfect one test solution, as serum markers are good at the ends but too soft in the middle. It was found that to be more effective, several tests have to be used together, such as 2 biomarker tests or one biomarker and an elastography test [17].. Despite the high costs, tuning to MRI elastography is said to be promising [18].

The substantial necessity of a widely available accurate, reproductive, and dynamic measure of liver fibrosis progression, and likewise regression, is still representing an unmet need in hepatology research.

It is noteworthy to mention that the difference between liver fibrosis stages is a qualitative rather than a quantitative linear measure, as the amounts of deposited collagens in each stage are not the multiple of the previous stage [19]. Accordingly, more collagenases are needed in late fibrosis stages than earlier ones [9]. Similarly, the non-linearity of collagen deposition in relation to the time interval is evidently clear. Notably, the changes in LS measurement in advanced stages might be within the same stage of fibrosis for the wide included range of numbers [20].

Histopathological features of fibrosis regression

There was no consensus for the proposed histological scoring system for chronic viral hepatitis post-treatment. Histological evaluations are better performed on paired liver biopsies: one obtained before initiation of the therapy and the other at least 6 months after the end of treatment (EOT). In the previous studies, regression was defined as a decrease of at least one point in either METAVIR or histology activity index (HAI) score from baseline to post-treatment evaluation [21, 22].

Fibrosis stage was assessed using the four stages METAVIR fibrosis scoring system [23]. Subsequently, stage 4 cirrhosis was further subdivided into three subgroups based on the thickness of fibrous septa and the size of the nodules that properly correlated with the clinical stage as well as the risk of hepatocellular carcinoma recurrence after curative resection. Stage 4A is characterized by mild cirrhosis with thin septa (definite or probable), stage 4B is moderate cirrhosis showing at occasional broad fibrous septa, and stage 4C refers to severe cirrhosis in which at least one very broad septum or many micronodules are present [24, 25]. The grade of necro-inflammatory activity was assessed using the HAI criteria with a maximum score of HAI is 18 [26].

Hepatic repair complex is another scoring system that depends on the presence of relevant histological findings that implies a regression of cirrhosis. This system relied on the histological findings of perforated delicate septa, isolated thick collagen fibers, thin periportal fibrous spikes, hepatic vein remnants with prolapsed hepatocytes, split septa interrupted by clusters or cords of hepatocytes, and aberrant parenchymal veins [27].

The Beijing classification, P-I-R Score (predominantly regressive, indeterminate, and predominantly progressive), is a unique method that provides a dynamic evaluation of the fibrosis course progression versus regression. This system was proposed by Sun et al., in the evaluation of chronic HBV pre- and post-therapy [28]. Fibrosis was assessed using routine hematoxylin and eosin, reticulin, and trichrome stains. The cases were sub-classified into predominantly progressive fibrosis in which most fibrous septa were broad, with loosely aggregated pale stained collagen infiltrated by inflammatory cells and ductular reactions; indeterminate fibrosis midway between progressive and regressive fibrosis; and predominantly regressive in which most fibrous septa showed thin, dense, and acellular stroma lack capillary vascular proliferation and staining deeply on trichrome stain.

Since liver cirrhosis is a heterogeneous process, future efforts are recommended to incorporate features of regression and validate a staging system for better assessment of fibrosis and necro-inflammation regression in chronic liver diseases [29].

Advancement of the digital pathology and the application of morphometry in the assessment of collagen proportionate area (CPA) was impressive in the detection of fibrosis regression post-HCV treatment [30]. In addition, second harmonic generation/two-photon excitation fluorescence (SHG/TPEF), a quantitative assessment of liver fibrosis width, assumed to be the most predictive feature indicative of fibrosis regression [31, 32].

Fibrosis regression in recovered HCV patients

Fibrosis regression evaluation post-treating HCV should be done only after at least 1 year of achieving sustained virological response (SVR). Earlier performed studies should not be significantly considered for their inaccurate conclusions.

In the IFN era

Liver biopsy was the gold standard relied on for proper pretreatment staging of liver fibrosis and treatment decisions. Most studies performed for post-treatment evaluation of fibrosis were dependent on paired liver biopsies [14].

The remarkable, pooled study of Poynard et al. tested the effect of different types of IFN containing regimens on liver fibrosis and even cirrhosis. The study enrolled 4493 patients from four randomized trials of pegylated (PEG) IFN alfa-2b (IFN α2b) alone, in combination with ribavirin (RBV), or of combined IFN α2b and (RBV) [33–36]. At the initial biopsy, 75% had no significant fibrosis while 25% had significant fibrosis with the mean METAVIR fibrosis stage ranging from 1.3 to 1.5. The SVR rate varied significantly from 5 to 63% according to the regimen. In patients with SVR, there was less fibrosis progression (7% versus 17% and 21% in relapsers and non-responders, respectively). However, independent of achieving an SVR, young patients (< 40 years old) with low body mass index (less than 27) and who had a low fibrosis stage at baseline are at low risk of fibrosis progression. A paired biopsy was available from 3010 patients with a 20-month mean duration between the biopsies. The histological response showed improvement in the fibrosis stage in 55% of patients, no change in 31%, and an upstage in 14% of the cases. In addition, fibrosis progression was the worst in patients treated with IFN for 24 weeks. The second biopsy stated that cirrhosis was observed in 6% versus 10% of patients treated with reinforced regimens compared to non-treated patients. Even more, nearly half of the treated patients showed a reversal of cirrhosis; however, the difference was a one-stage change [37]. Another study enrolled 150 patients who achieved SVR after a combinational treatment therapy of IFN α2b and RBV. Pre-treatment liver biopsies highlighted the stage of fibrosis to be stage 2 and 6 in 77% and 11%, respectively. A 5-year follow-up documented a noteworthy fibrosis regression in about 81.5%. Of the 12 patients with advanced fibrosis/cirrhosis, ten had decreased fibrosis scores in a range of two points or greater [38]. However, a large long-term (10 years) observational study assessing the regression of fibrosis on IFN-treated HCV patients relying on non-invasive liver fibrosis parameters (APRI score and FIB4 formula) had also addressed remarkable regression proven in those with SVR achievement [39].

In DAA era

The advent of DAA therapies was associated with the prevalence of the non-invasive measures of liver fibrosis staging and had eliminated the role of liver biopsy [40]. Accordingly, most studies searching for fibrosis regression are currently dependable on paired or bi-paired non-invasive measures [15–19]. In a study carried by Knop et al. on 54 cirrhotic patients revealed a reduction of LS in 88% and 57% of DAA-treated patients after 6 months of achieving SVR using TE and AFRI techniques, respectively [41]. Based on the non-invasive scores, liver transplant recipients were also evaluated for fibrosis reversal on a 3-month interval of DAA therapy of HCV [42]. Martini et al. monitored 125 post-transplanted patients treated with DAAs using TE and found a stepwise decline of LS from 20.4 to 17.5 to 14.0 kPa at 6 and 12 months, respectively [43]. Another study on 112 patients received IFN/DAAs post-transplantation and followed up for 1 year demonstrated that a nearly 43.2% and 72–85% of cirrhotic and remaining stages patients showed histological evidence of fibrosis regression at least 1-metavir stage, respectively [44]. A 6-month interval study performed on 51 post-transplant patients followed up for 1 year after achieving SVR using SW, TE, and ARFI showed at least a 20% decrease in LS compared with baseline [45]. Despite the short-term follow-up, Elraziky et al. in their study which was dependent on TE, PRI, and FIB 4 in the assessment of fibrosis revealed fibrosis regression in 27.5% of patients 3 months after SVR. Treated cirrhotic patients experienced fibrosis regression irrespective of their therapy regimens, whereas fibrosis regression was dependent on achieving SVR in cirrhotic patients [46]. A similar prospective study adopting SW was performed serially for 6 months post-treatment pledging the assumption of early regression post-DAA therapies [47]. An 18-month study had evaluated the changes in LS through TE, APRI, and FIB4 scores following DAA therapies, revealing a significant alleviation of liver stiffness among SVR achievers [48]. ARFI was the nominated measure of LS in the study of Chen et al., who reported a significant decrease in fibrosis measures on 24 weeks post-treatment follow-up [49]. Nearly 25.5% of cirrhotic patients followed up for 1 year declined to 18.1% on TE [50]. Prakash et al. demonstrated that 39% of cirrhotic patients declined to < 2.67 on FIB 4 monitoring technique [51]. The most promising MRE had been adopted for a short-term study of assessing fibrosis regression coinciding with SVR detecting. Surprisingly, a significant reduction in the fibrosis burden was evidenced by an acute lessening in liver T1, T2, and T2* and a liver perfusion upsurge [18].

Soliman et al. had assessed the degree of fibrosis regression through TE, in a 1-year interval, and had substantially confined the role of DAAs in regression of fibrosis either with or without IFNs [12]. Another 1-year comparative retrospective Egyptian study had delineated a higher rate of regression of fibrosis in DAAs successfully treated cases (52.5%) than those who were responsive to IFN treatment (23.3%). In this study, reliance was based on TE for the DAA-treated group versus liver biopsy in the IFN group [52].

However, all these studies have raised a significant concern about the credibility of all used parameters in genuine assessment of fibrosis regression, or these are the penalties of alleviated necroinflammation following the direct viral effects of these drugs. So, despite the marvelous achievement of the therapeutic goal of DAAs, more meticulous judging measures are still needed for better appraisal of the proposed residual liver disease burden following the end of therapy. Assumptions had to be delineated for planning better strategies directed to HCV-related liver disease burden complete elimination.

Hepatocellular carcinoma (HCC) post-DAA versus IFN regimens

A meta-analysis of twelve studies showed a reduction in HCC risk of 76% in patients achieving SVR following IFN therapy [53]. On the other hand, conflicting data appeared regarding the risk of HCC occurrence and recurrence post-DAAs treatment. Three studies reported that DAA-induced SVR did not reduce the occurrence and recurrence of HCC; however, these studies were small-size, single-centered of short-term follow-up cohorts [54–56]. The possible explanation is that a rapid HCV suppression mediated immunological changes and induced a more aggressive HCC. Furthermore, HBV reactivation in the setting of DAA use has been reported which may co-operate in HCC development [57]. The follow-up of 344 cirrhotic patients without HCC treated with DAAs for 6 months revealed the occurrence of HCC in 9/285 patients (3.2%) and recurrence in 17/59 patients (28.8%). Conti et al. assumed the high HCC risk was related to the Child-Pugh class and prior HCC history rather than HCV genotype or DAA regimen [55]. Other reports suggested the risk of HCC was 9% within 6 months and 7.4% within 12 months follow-up [54, 56]. In contrast, large cohort studies have demonstrated a reduced risk of HCC in patients achieving SVR post-DAA regimen [58–60]. The risk of HCC was 1.2% among 22, 500 patients treated with DAAs of which 0.8% had achieved SVR. The main co-factors for the development of HCC in that study were liver cirrhosis and failure of achieving SVR [58]. In a retrospective study including more than 60,000 HCV patients treated with antiviral therapy either DAAs, IFN-based regimens, or combined regimens, achievement of SVR was the main factor associated with low HCC risk regardless of the antiviral regimen [60]. A systematic meta-analysis of 26 observational studies on HCC occurrence following different anti-viral therapies (IFN = 17, DAAs = 9 studies) reported higher HCC risk in DAA-treated patients compared to IFN. However, the higher risk was alleviated after adjustment for study follow-up and age. DAA-treated patients were older and had a short follow-up duration [61]. Additionally, in a large cohort of 17,836 HCV-infected either treated with IFN or DAAs revealed a significantly higher HCC incidence rate than IFN treated patients. DAA-treated patients were of older age with elevated serum AFP and had liver cirrhosis, the main risk factors for HCC occurrence. A sub-analysis in cirrhotic patients showed a high risk of HCC in untreated patients with an equal risk in both treated patients [59]. Mariño et al. reported a 3.73% risk of developing HCC in 1123 cirrhotic patients treated with DAAs; the risk was higher in patients without SVR, who had more severe diseases (Child B or C, decompensation or high liver stiffness) and atypical nodules [62].

The risk of HCC recurrence occurred at a similar rate in patients treated with DAA or IFN regimens after adjustment of the cofactors [61, 63, 64]. The cumulative incidence of HCC recurrence was dependent on the achievement of SVR in both arms of treatment [63]. Moreover, in a study including 149 liver-transplanted candidates who underwent initial complete response to loco-regional therapies for HCV-related HCC, DAA therapy was associated with reduced risk of waitlist dropout due to tumor progression or death [65]. However, in a prospective cohort that included 333 successfully treated HCC patients, divided into 60 patients who received DAAs and 273 patients who were DAA-untreated after HCC ablation, a higher risk of HCC recurrence appeared in post-DAA-treated patients versus untreated patients. In addition, the risk was higher in patients treated with transarterial chemoembolization rather than curative measures. The main cofounders affecting HCC recurrence were age, male gender, mean tumor size, and the time interval between complete HCC ablation and occurrence of HCC recurrence [66].

Fibrosis regression and the risk of HCC

In a study by Crissien et al. five patients developed HCC after SVR over the emerging 5 years; two of them experienced fibrosis regression by TE [67]. In addition, Chekuri et al. suggested that fibrosis regression reached its plateau about 1 year after SVR [68]. Moreover, the fibrosis regression does not exclude the development of HCC years after treatment [67, 68]. Therefore, due to the lack of sufficient information about the possible risk of HCC reduction after SVR with the DAAs, patients, particularly with advanced fibrosis namely F3/F4, should undergo a regular screening of HCC [69].

Conclusions

DAA regimens represent a breakthrough of this century. DAAs have demonstrated genuine significant impacts on all HCV-related health hazards, initially sourced from liver fibrosis regression which is considered the milestone of chronic liver disease with its complications. It was assumed that the more time passed, the more significant reported changes on fibrosis appeared. However, DAAs have proved high accuracy in the early distinguishing of dynamic fibrosis regression changes. However, proper judging on the effect of DAA therapies of HCV on liver disease burden should be more furtherly evaluated on large-scale cohorts, along with longer durations. The unmet need of a single reproductive test equating the accuracy of liver biopsy for evaluating fibrosis rather than necroinflammation should be the urge of upcoming research.

Abbreviations

ARFI: Acoustic radiation force impulse elastography; CPA: Collagen proportionate area; DAAs: Direct-acting antiviral regimens; EOT: End of treatment; HAI: Histology activity index; HCV: Hepatitis C virus; LS: Liver stiffness; MRE: Magnetic resonance elastography; P-I-R Score: Progressive, indeterminate, and regressive score; SHG/TPEF: Second harmonic generation/two-photon excitation fluorescence; SVR: Sustained virological response; SW: Shear wave; TE: Transient elastography; HCC: Hepatocellular carcinoma

Acknowledgements

Not applicable.

Authors' contributions

All authors of this paper have participated in its drafting and approved the final version submitted. NE and DS wrote the pathological part. MS wrote the hepatology part. All authors acquired and interpreted the collected data. NE and MS revised and edited the final version.

Declarations

Ethics approval and consent to participate

Not applicable.

Competing interests

The authors declare that they have no competing interests.

Author details

Pathology Department, National Liver Institute, Menofia University, Shibin El-Kom 32511, Egypt. [2]Hepatology and Gastroenterology Department, National Liver Institute, Menofia University, Shibin El-Kom, Egypt.

References

1. Musa NI, Mohamed IE, Abohalima AS (2020) Impact of treating chronic hepatitis C infection with direct-acting antivirals on the risk of hepatocellular carcinoma recurrence. Egyptian Liver J 10(1):26. https://doi.org/10.1186/s43066-020-00035-x
2. Gomaa A, Allam N, Elsharkawy A, El Kassas M, Waked I (2017) Hepatitis C infection in Egypt: prevalence, impact and management strategies. Hepat Med 9:17–25. https://doi.org/10.2147/HMER.S113681
3. Meringer H, Shibolet O, Deutsch L (2019) Hepatocellular carcinoma in the post-hepatitis C virus era: should we change the paradigm? World J Gastroenterol 25(29):3929–3940. https://doi.org/10.3748/wjg.v25.i29.3929
4. Zoubek ME, Trautwein C, Strnad P (2017) Reversal of liver fibrosis: from fiction to reality. Best Pract Res Clin Gastroenterol 31(2):129–141. https://doi.org/https://doi.org/10.1016/j.bpg.2017.04.005
5. Pinzani M (2015) Pathophysiology of liver fibrosis. Dig Dis 33(4):492–497. https://doi.org/10.1159/000374096
6. Povero D, Busletta C, Novo E, di Bonzo LV, Cannito S, Paternostro C, Parola M (2010) Liver fibrosis: a dynamic and potentially reversible process. Histol Histopathol 25(8):1075–1091. https://doi.org/10.14670/hh-25.1075
7. Saffioti F, Pinzani M (2016) Development and regression of cirrhosis. Dig Dis 34(4):374–381. https://doi.org/10.1159/000444550
8. Freeman AJ, Dore GJ, Law MG, Thorpe M, Von Overbeck J, Lloyd AR, Marinos G, Kaldor JM (2001) Estimating progression to cirrhosis in chronic hepatitis C virus infection. Hepatology 34(4):809–816. https://doi.org/10.1053/jhep.2001.27831
9. Arthur MJP (2002) Reversibility of liver fibrosis and cirrhosis following treatment for hepatitis C. Gastroenterology 122(5):1525–1528. https://doi.org/10.1053/gast.2002.33367
10. Thein H-H, Yi Q, Dore GJ, Krahn MD (2008) Estimation of stage-specific fibrosis progression rates in chronic hepatitis C virus infection: a meta-analysis and meta-regression. Hepatology 48(2):418–431. https://doi.org/10.1002/hep.22375
11. Tachi Y, Hirai T, Ishizu Y, Honda T, Kuzuya T, Hayashi K, Ishigami M, Goto H (2016) α-Fetoprotein levels after interferon therapy predict regression of liver fibrosis in patients with sustained virological response. J Gastroenterol Hepatol 31(5):1001–1008. https://doi.org/10.1111/jgh.13245
12. Hanan S, Dina Z, Marwa S, Manal H, Rehab B, Nehad H, Amal S, Sherief A-E (2020) Predictors for fibrosis regression in chronic HCV patients after the treatment with DAAS: results of a real-world cohort study. Endocr Metab Immune Disord Drug Targets 20(1):104–111. https://doi.org/10.2174/1871530319666190826150344
13. Sun M, Kisseleva T (2015) Reversibility of liver fibrosis. Clin Res Hepatol Gastroenterol 39(Suppl 1 (0 1)):S60–S63. https://doi.org/10.1016/j.clinre.2015.06.015
14. Ellis EL, Mann DA (2012) Clinical evidence for the regression of liver fibrosis. J Hepatol 56(5):1171–1180. https://doi.org/10.1016/j.jhep.2011.09.024
15. Abdelsameea E, Alsebaey A, Abdel-Razek W, Ehsan N, Morad W, Salama M, Waked I (2020) Elastography and serum markers of fibrosis versus liver

biopsy in 1270 Egyptian patients with hepatitis C. Eur J Gastroenterol Hepatol 32(12):1553–1558. https://doi.org/10.1097/MEG.0000000000001672
16. Sigrist RMS, Liau J, Kaffas AE, Chammas MC, Willmann JK (2017) Ultrasound elastography: review of techniques and clinical applications. Theranostics 7(5):1303–1329. https://doi.org/10.7150/thno.18650
17. Nallagangula KS, Nagaraj SK, Venkataswamy L, Chandrappa M (2017) Liver fibrosis: a compilation on the biomarkers status and their significance during disease progression. Future Sci OA 4(1):FSO250. https://doi.org/10.4155/fsoa-2017-0083
18. Bradley C, Scott RA, Cox E, Palaniyappan N, Thomson BJ, Ryder SD, Irving WL, Aithal GP, Guha IN, Francis S (2019) Short-term changes observed in multiparametric liver MRI following therapy with direct-acting antivirals in chronic hepatitis C virus patients. Eur Radiol 29(6):3100–3107. https://doi.org/10.1007/s00330-018-5788-1
19. Masugi Y, Abe T, Tsujikawa H, Effendi K, Hashiguchi A, Abe M, Imai Y, Hino K, Hige S, Kawanaka M, Yamada G, Kage M, Korenaga M, Hiasa Y, Mizokami M, Sakamoto M (2017) Quantitative assessment of liver fibrosis reveals a nonlinear association with fibrosis stage in nonalcoholic fatty liver disease. Hepatol Commun 2(1):58–68. https://doi.org/10.1002/hep4.1121
20. Castéra L, Vergniol J, Foucher J, Le Bail B, Chanteloup E, Haaser M, Darriet M, Couzigou P, de Lédinghen V (2005) Prospective comparison of transient elastography, Fibrotest, APRI, and liver biopsy for the assessment of fibrosis in chronic hepatitis C. Gastroenterology 128(2):343–350. https://doi.org/10.1053/j.gastro.2004.11.018
21. Cheng C-H, Chu C-Y, Chen H-L, Lin IT, Wu C-H, Lee Y-K, Hu P-J, Bair M-J (2020) Direct-acting antiviral therapy of chronic hepatitis C improves liver fibrosis, assessed by histological examination and laboratory markers. J Formos Med Assoc doi:https://doi.org/https://doi.org/10.1016/j.jfma.2020.11.018, 120, 5, 1259, 1268
22. Sun Y-M, Chen S-Y, You H (2020) Regression of liver fibrosis: evidence and challenges. Chin Med J 133(14):1696–1702. https://doi.org/10.1097/CM9.0000000000000835
23. Bedossa P, Poynard T (1996) An algorithm for the grading of activity in chronic hepatitis C. Hepatology 24 (2):289-293. https://doi.org/10.1002/hep.510240201
24. Kim MY, Cho MY, Baik SK, Park HJ, Jeon HK, Im CK, Won CS, Kim JW, Kim HS, Kwon SO, Eom MS, Cha SH, Kim YJ, Chang SJ, Lee SS (2011) Histological subclassification of cirrhosis using the Laennec fibrosis scoring system correlates with clinical stage and grade of portal hypertension. J Hepatol 55(5):1004–1009. https://doi.org/10.1016/j.jhep.2011.02.012
25. Kim SU, Oh HJ, Wanless IR, Lee S, Han K-H, Park YN (2012) The Laennec staging system for histological sub-classification of cirrhosis is useful for stratification of prognosis in patients with liver cirrhosis. J Hepatol 57(3):556–563. https://doi.org/10.1016/j.jhep.2012.04.029
26. Ishak K, Baptista A, Bianchi L, Callea F, De Groote J, Gudat F, Denk H, Desmet V, Korb G, MacSween RNM, Phillips MJ, Portmann BG, Poulsen H, Scheuer PJ, Schmid M, Thaler H (1995) Histological grading and staging of chronic hepatitis. J Hepatol 22(6):696–699. https://doi.org/10.1016/0168-8278(95)80226-6
27. Wanless IR, Nakashima E, Sherman M (2000) Regression of human cirrhosis. Morphologic features and the genesis of incomplete septal cirrhosis. Archiv Pathol Lab Medicine 124(11):1599–1607. https://doi.org/10.1043/0003-9985(2000)124<1599:rohc>2.0.co;2
28. Sun Y, Zhou J, Wang L, Wu X, Chen Y, Piao H, Lu L, Jiang W, Xu Y, Feng B, Nan Y, Xie W, Chen G, Zheng H, Li H, Ding H, Liu H, Lv F, Shao C, Wang T, Ou X, Wang B, Chen S, Wee A, Theise ND, You H, Jia J (2017) New classification of liver biopsy assessment for fibrosis in chronic hepatitis B patients before and after treatment. Hepatology 65 (5):1438-1450. https://doi.org/10.1002/hep.29009
29. Lo RC, Kim H (2017) Histopathological evaluation of liver fibrosis and cirrhosis regression. Clin Mol Hepatol 23(4):302–307. https://doi.org/10.3350/cmh.2017.0078
30. D'Ambrosio R, Aghemo A, Rumi MG, Ronchi G, Donato MF, Paradis V, Colombo M, Bedossa P (2012) A morphometric and immunohistochemical study to assess the benefit of a sustained virological response in hepatitis C virus patients with cirrhosis. Hepatology 56 (2):532-543. https://doi.org/10.1002/hep.25606
31. Wang B, Sun Y, Zhou J, Wu X, Chen S, Wu S, Liu H, Wang T, Ou X, Jia J, You H (2018) Advanced septa size quantitation determines the evaluation of histological fibrosis outcome in chronic hepatitis B patients. Mod Pathol 31(10):1567–1577. https://doi.org/10.1038/s41379-018-0059-x
32. Sun Y, Zhou J, Wu X, Chen Y, Piao H, Lu L, Ding H, Nan Y, Jiang W, Wang T, Liu H, Ou X, Wee A, Theise ND, Jia J, You H (2018) Quantitative assessment of liver fibrosis (qFibrosis) reveals precise outcomes in Ishak "stable" patients on anti-HBV therapy. Sci Rep 8(1):2989–2989. https://doi.org/10.1038/s41598-018-21179-2
33. McHutchison JG, Gordon SC, Schiff ER, Shiffman ML, Lee WM, Rustgi VK, Goodman ZD, Ling M-H, Cort S, Albrecht JK (1998) Interferon alfa-2b alone or in combination with ribavirin as initial treatment for chronic hepatitis C. N Engl J Med 339(21):1485–1492. https://doi.org/10.1056/NEJM199811193392101
34. Poynard T, Marcellin P, Lee SS, Niederau C, Minuk GS, Ideo G, Bain V, Heathcote J, Zeuzem S, Trepo C, Albrecht J (1998) Randomised trial of interferon α2b plus ribavirin for 48 weeks or for 24 weeks versus interferon α2b plus placebo for 48 weeks for treatment of chronic infection with hepatitis C virus. Lancet 352(9138):1426–1432. https://doi.org/10.1016/S0140-6736(98)07124-4
35. Lindsay KL, Trepo C, Heintges T, Shiffman ML, Gordon SC, Hoefs JC, Schiff ER, Goodman ZD, Laughlin M, Yao R, Albrecht JK (2001) A randomized, double-blind trial comparing pegylated interferon alfa-2b to interferon alfa-2b as initial treatment for chronic hepatitis C. Hepatology 34(2):395–403. https://doi.org/10.1053/jhep.2001.26371
36. Manns MP, McHutchison JG, Gordon SC, Rustgi VK, Shiffman M, Reindollar R, Goodman ZD, Koury K, Ling M-H, Albrecht JK (2001) Peginterferon alfa-2b plus ribavirin compared with interferon alfa-2b plus ribavirin for initial treatment of chronic hepatitis C: a randomised trial. Lancet 358(9286):958–965. https://doi.org/10.1016/S0140-6736(01)06102-5
37. Poynard T, McHutchison J, Manns M, Trepo C, Lindsay K, Goodman Z, Ling MH, Albrecht J (2002) Impact of pegylated interferon alfa-2b and ribavirin on liver fibrosis in patients with chronic hepatitis C. Gastroenterology 122(5):1303–1313. https://doi.org/10.1053/gast.2002.33023
38. George SL, Bacon BR, Brunt EM, Mihindukulasuriya KL, Hoffmann J, Di Bisceglie AM (2009) Clinical, virologic, histologic, and biochemical outcomes after successful HCV therapy: a 5-year follow-up of 150 patients. Hepatology (Baltimore, Md) 49(3):729–738. https://doi.org/10.1002/hep.22694
39. Lu M, Li J, Zhang T, Rupp LB, Trudeau S, Holmberg SD, Moorman AC, Spradling PR, Teshale EH, Xu F, Boscarino JA, Schmidt MA, Vijayadeva V, Gordon SC, Chronic Hepatitis Cohort Study I (2016) Serum biomarkers indicate long-term reduction in liver fibrosis in patients with sustained virological response to treatment for HCV infection. Clin Gastroenterol Hepatol 14(7):1044–1055.e1043. https://doi.org/10.1016/j.cgh.2016.01.009
40. Lucero C, Brown RS Jr (2016) Noninvasive measures of liver fibrosis and severity of liver disease. Gastroenterol Hepatol (N Y) 12(1):33–40
41. Knop V, Hoppe D, Welzel T, Vermehren J, Herrmann E, Vermehren A, Friedrich-Rust M, Sarrazin C, Zeuzem S, Welker MW (2016) Regression of fibrosis and portal hypertension in HCV-associated cirrhosis and sustained virologic response after interferon-free antiviral therapy. J Viral Hepat 23(12):994–1002. https://doi.org/10.1111/jvh.12578
42. Iacob S, Cerban R, Pietrareanu C, Ester C, Iacob R, Gheorghe C, Popescu I, Gheorghe L (2018) 100% sustained virological response and fibrosis improvement in real-life use of direct acting antivirals in genotype-1b recurrent hepatitis C following liver transplantation. J Gastrointestinal Liver Dis: JGLD 27(2):139–144. https://doi.org/10.15403/jgld.2014.1121.272.100
43. Martini S, Sacco M, Strona S, Arese D, Tandoi F, Dell Olio D, Stradella D, Cocchis D, Mirabella S, Rizza G, Magistroni P, Moschini P, Ottobrelli A, Amoroso A, Rizzetto M, Salizzoni M, Saracco GM, Romagnoli R (2017) Impact of viral eradication with sofosbuvir-based therapy on the outcome of post-transplant hepatitis C with severe fibrosis. Liver Int 37 (1):62-70. https://doi.org/10.1111/liv.13193
44. Mauro E, Crespo G, Montironi C, Londoño M-C, Hernández-Gea V, Ruiz P, Sastre L, Lombardo J, Mariño Z, Díaz A, Colmenero J, Rimola A, Garcia-Pagán JC, Brunet M, Forns X, Navasa M (2018) Portal pressure and liver stiffness measurements in the prediction of fibrosis regression after sustained virological response in recurrent hepatitis C. Hepatology 67 (5):1683-1694. https://doi.org/10.1002/hep.29557
45. Alem SA, Said M, Anwar I, Abdellatif Z, Elbaz T, Eletreby R, AbouElKhair M, El-Serafy M, Mogawer S, El-Amir M, El-Shazly M, Hosny A, Yosry A (2018) Improvement of liver stiffness measurement, acoustic radiation force impulse measurements, and noninvasive fibrosis markers after direct-acting antivirals for hepatitis C virus G4 recurrence post living donor liver transplantation: Egyptian cohort. J Med Virol 90(9):1508–1515. https://doi.org/10.1002/jmv.25210

46. El-Raziky M, Khairy M, Fouad A, Salama A, Elsharkawy A, Tantawy O (2018) Effect of direct-acting agents on fibrosis regression in chronic hepatitis C virus patients' treatment compared with interferon-containing regimens. J Interf Cytokine Res 38(3):129–136. https://doi.org/10.1089/jir.2017.0137
47. Kohla MAS, Fayoumi AE, Akl M, Abdelkareem M, Elsakhawy M, Waheed S, Abozeid M (2020) Early fibrosis regression by shear wave elastography after successful direct-acting anti-HCV therapy. Clin Exp Med 20(1):143–148. https://doi.org/10.1007/s10238-019-00597-0
48. Omar H, Said M, Eletreby R, Mehrez M, Bassam M, Abdellatif Z, Hosny A, Megawer S, El Amir M, Yosry A (2018) Longitudinal assessment of hepatic fibrosis in responders to direct-acting antivirals for recurrent hepatitis C after liver transplantation using noninvasive methods. Clin Transpl 32(8):e13334. https://doi.org/https://doi.org/10.1111/ctr.13334
49. Chen S-H, Lai H-C, Chiang IP, Su W-P, Lin C-H, Kao J-T, Chuang P-H, Hsu W-F, Wang H-W, Chen H-Y, Huang G-T, Peng C-Y (2018) Changes in liver stiffness measurement using acoustic radiation force impulse elastography after antiviral therapy in patients with chronic hepatitis C. PLoS One 13(1): e0190455–e0190455. https://doi.org/10.1371/journal.pone.0190455
50. Rout G, Nayak B, Patel AH, Gunjan D, Singh V, Kedia S, Shalimar (2019) Therapy with oral directly acting agents in hepatitis C infection is associated with reduction in fibrosis and increase in hepatic steatosis on transient elastography. J Clin Exp Hepatol 9(2):207–214. https://doi.org/10.1016/j.jceh.2018.06.009
51. Prakash S, Rockey DC (2020) 1006 predictors of poor fibrosis regression after direct acting antiviral therapy in patients with chronic hepatitis C and cirrhosis. Gastroenterology 158(6):S-1302–S-1303. https://doi.org/10.1016/S0016-5085(20)33918-4
52. Abdelsameea E, Alsebaey A, Abdel-Samiee M, Abdel-Razek W, Salama M, Waked I (2020) Direct acting antivirals are associated with more liver stiffness regression than pegylated interferon therapy in chronic hepatitis C patients. Expert Review of Anti-infective Therapy:1-7. doi:https://doi.org/10.1080/14787210.2021.1864326
53. Morgan RL, Baack B, Smith BD, Yartel A, Pitasi M, Falck-Ytter Y (2013) Eradication of hepatitis C virus infection and the development of hepatocellular carcinoma. Ann Intern Med 158(5_Part_1):329–337. https://doi.org/10.7326/0003-4819-158-5-201303050-00005
54. Reig M, Mariño Z, Perelló C, Iñarrairaegui M, Ribeiro A, Lens S, Díaz A, Vilana R, Darnell A, Varela M, Sangro B, Calleja JL, Forns X, Bruix J (2016) Unexpected high rate of early tumor recurrence in patients with HCV-related HCC undergoing interferon-free therapy. J Hepatol 65(4):719–726. https://doi.org/10.1016/j.jhep.2016.04.008
55. Conti F, Buonfiglioli F, Scuteri A, Crespi C, Bolondi L, Caraceni P, Foschi FG, Lenzi M, Mazzella G, Verucchi G, Andreone P, Brillanti S (2016) Early occurrence and recurrence of hepatocellular carcinoma in HCV-related cirrhosis treated with direct-acting antivirals. J Hepatol 65(4):727–733. https://doi.org/10.1016/j.jhep.2016.06.015
56. Cardoso H, Vale AM, Rodrigues S, Gonçalves R, Albuquerque A, Pereira P, Lopes S, Silva M, Andrade P, Morais R, Coelho R, Macedo G (2016) High incidence of hepatocellular carcinoma following successful interferon-free antiviral therapy for hepatitis C associated cirrhosis. J Hepatol 65(5):1070–1071. https://doi.org/10.1016/j.jhep.2016.07.027
57. Bersoff-Matcha SJ, Cao K, Jason M, Ajao A, Jones SC, Meyer T, Brinker A (2017) Hepatitis B virus reactivation associated with direct-acting antiviral therapy for chronic hepatitis C virus: a review of cases reported to the U.S. Food and Drug Administration adverse event reporting system. Ann Intern Med 166(11):792–798. https://doi.org/10.7326/M17-0377
58. Kanwal F, Kramer J, Asch SM, Chayanupatkul M, Cao Y, El-Serag HB (2017) Risk of hepatocellular cancer in HCV patients treated with direct-acting antiviral agents. Gastroenterology 153(4):996–1005.e1001. https://doi.org/10.1053/j.gastro.2017.06.012
59. Li DK, Ren Y, Fierer DS, Rutledge S, Shaikh OS, Lo Re Iii V, Simon T, Abou-Samra A-B, Chung RT, Butt AA (2018) The short-term incidence of hepatocellular carcinoma is not increased after hepatitis C treatment with direct-acting antivirals: an ERCHIVES study. Hepatology 67 (6):2244-2253. doi: https://doi.org/https://doi.org/10.1002/hep.29707
60. Ioannou GN, Green PK, Berry K (2017) HCV eradication induced by direct-acting antiviral agents reduces the risk of hepatocellular carcinoma. Journal of Hepatology:S0168-8278(0117)32273-32270. doi:https://doi.org/10.1016/j.jhep.2017.08.030
61. Waziry R, Hajarizadeh B, Grebely J, Amin J, Law M, Danta M, George J, Dore GJ (2017) Hepatocellular carcinoma risk following direct-acting antiviral HCV therapy: a systematic review, meta-analyses, and meta-regression. J Hepatol 67(6):1204–1212. https://doi.org/10.1016/j.jhep.2017.07.025
62. Mariño Z, Darnell A, Lens S, Sapena V, Díaz A, Belmonte E, Perelló C, Calleja JL, Varela M, Rodriguez M, Rodriguez de Lope C, Llerena S, Torras X, Gallego A, Sala M, Morillas RM, Minguez B, Llaneras J, Coll S, Carrion JA, Iñarrairaegui M, Sangro B, Vilana R, Sole M, Ayuso C, Ríos J, Forns X, Bruix J, Reig M (2019) Time association between hepatitis C therapy and hepatocellular carcinoma emergence in cirrhosis: relevance of non-characterized nodules. J Hepatol 70(5):874–884. https://doi.org/10.1016/j.jhep.2019.01.005
63. Nagata H, Nakagawa M, Asahina Y, Sato A, Asano Y, Tsunoda T, Miyoshi M, Kaneko S, Otani S, Kawai-Kitahata F, Murakawa M, Nitta S, Itsui Y, Azuma S, Kakinuma S, Nouchi T, Sakai H, Tomita M, Watanabe M (2017) Effect of interferon-based and -free therapy on early occurrence and recurrence of hepatocellular carcinoma in chronic hepatitis C. J Hepatol 67(5):933–939. https://doi.org/10.1016/j.jhep.2017.05.028
64. Nishibatake Kinoshita M, Minami T, Tateishi R, Wake T, Nakagomi R, Fujiwara N, Sato M, Uchino K, Enooku K, Nakagawa H, Asaoka Y, Shiina S, Koike K (2019) Impact of direct-acting antivirals on early recurrence of HCV-related HCC: comparison with interferon-based therapy. J Hepatol 70(1):78–86. https://doi.org/10.1016/j.jhep.2018.09.029
65. Huang AC, Mehta N, Dodge JL, Yao FY, Terrault NA (2018) Direct-acting antivirals do not increase the risk of hepatocellular carcinoma recurrence after local-regional therapy or liver transplant waitlist dropout. Hepatology (Baltimore, Md) 68(2):449–461. https://doi.org/10.1002/hep.29855
66. Lithy RM, Elbaz T, H. Abdelmaksoud A, M. Nabil M, Rashed N, Omran D, Kaseb AO, O. Abdelaziz A, I. Shousha H (2020) Survival and recurrence rates of hepatocellular carcinoma after treatment of chronic hepatitis C using direct acting antivirals. Eur J Gastroenterol Hepatol. https://doi.org/10.1097/MEG.0000000000001972. Online ahead of print
67. Crissien A, Minteer W, Pan J, Frenette C, Pockros P (2015) Regression of advanced fibrosis or cirrhosis measured by elastography in patients with chronic hepatitis C who achieved sustained virologic response after treatment for HCV (Abstract 108). Presented at the 66th Annual Meeting of the American Association for the Study of Liver Diseases Boston, MA
68. Chekuri S, Nickerson J, Bichoupan K, Sefcik R, Doobay K, Chang S, DelBello D, Harty A, Dieterich DT, Perumalswami PV, Branch AD (2016) Liver stiffness decreases rapidly in response to successful hepatitis C treatment and then plateaus. PLoS One 11(7):e0159413–e0159413. https://doi.org/10.1371/journal.pone.0159413
69. Khan R, Velpari S, Koppe S (2018) All patients with advanced fibrosis should continue to be screened for hepatocellular carcinoma after sustained virological response of hepatitis C virus. Clin Liver Dis (Hoboken) 12(5):137–139. https://doi.org/10.1002/cld.707

12

Survival benefits of adding simvastatin to standard therapy for secondary prevention of bleeding esophageal varices in patients with hepatitis C-related liver cirrhosis

Helmy Elshazly[1], Hasan Zaghlah[1], El-Sayed Tharwa[1], Ahmed Abuamer[1], Dina Nor-Eldin[2], Reem El Sheemy[3] and Mohamed El Kassas[4*]

Abstract

Background: The combination of endoscopic band ligation and beta-blockers is the standard of care treatment for secondary prevention of variceal bleeding; however, rebleeding still occurs with associated high mortality. Simvastatin (a lipid-lowering agent) was found to reduce portal hypertension and decrease hepatic fibrosis. This study aimed to assess the effect of adding simvastatin to the standard therapy to prevent variceal rebleeding and its impact on survival in patients with liver cirrhosis.

Results: This single-center randomized controlled clinical trial included 80 patients with cirrhosis receiving the standard secondary prophylaxis for variceal bleeding composed of endoscopic variceal ligation and non-selective β-blockers (either propranolol or carvedilol). Two weeks after the first attack of hematemesis, patients were randomized into two groups: group I who received the standard therapy (40 patients) and group II who administered simvastatin (20 mg daily for 2 weeks and 40 mg daily after that). Patients were followed up for 1 year. The primary endpoints were rebleeding and overall survival. Thirty patients of group I completed the study while ten patients died during the follow-up period. The simvastatin group showed a significantly better overall 1-year survival (3 deaths during follow-up) compared to the control group (37/40, 92.5% vs. 30/40; 75%) (*p*-value 0.034); however, this was lacking in Child C patients. No similar difference was present in rebleeding rates between the two groups (5/40, 12.5% vs. 3/40, 7.5%) (*p*-value 0.456) in groups I and II, respectively.

Conclusions: Adding simvastatin to the standard therapy in secondary prevention of variceal bleeding could be associated with survival benefits in patients with Child A and B cirrhosis, while was incapable of reducing rebleeding.

Keywords: Bleeding varices, Beta-blockers, Egypt, Hematemesis, Cirrhosis, Secondary prevention, Simvastatin, Statins, Portal hypertension, Prophylaxis

* Correspondence: m_elkassas@yahoo.com
[4]Endemic Medicine Department, Faculty of Medicine, Helwan University, Ain Helwan, Cairo 11795, Egypt
Full list of author information is available at the end of the article

Background

Liver cirrhosis is considered the most common cause of portal hypertension (PHT) [1]. Increased portal inflow and increased outflow resistance are associated with the development of PHT [2]. Liver transplantation is indicated in patients with advanced cirrhosis complicated by PHT; furthermore, morbidity and mortality are augmented in these patients [3, 4]. PHT management's ideal drug should decrease portal pressure by lowering intrahepatic vascular resistance while maintaining or increasing hepatic blood flow [3]. Moreover, it should improve liver function through its antifibrotic effects, and it should be able to increase nitric oxide bioavailability in the liver to help fulfill many of these requirements [3, 5–8]. Currently, the available therapies for PHT are based on the use of β-adrenergic blockers, with or without organic nitrates, and allow achievement of the target hemodynamic response in less than half of patients.

Moreover, about 30% of patients may have contraindications or may not tolerate β-blockers [9]. Statins such as simvastatin are used mainly for cardiovascular diseases and metabolic syndrome. They exert multiple pleiotropic effects and can be used safely in patients with chronic liver diseases [10]. Statins can have anti-inflammatory and antifibrotic effects in patients with liver cirrhosis through many proposed mechanisms [11–14]. Some reports showed survival benefits and improvement in liver profile with simvastatin use [14, 15]. Moreover, an improvement in PHT, reduction in hepatocellular carcinoma (HCC) incidence, and delays in hepatic decompensation have been associated with the use of statins in patients with liver cirrhosis [15, 16].

We aimed to assess the effect of adding simvastatin to the standard therapy used to prevent variceal rebleeding and to evaluate its impact on survival in patients with HCV-related liver cirrhosis. Statins have a long history of being safe and tolerable medications. Because this family of drugs is generic and inexpensive, there will be few barriers to general acceptance of statins' role in preventing bleeding in patients with esophageal varices if the theory is validated.

Methods

This prospective single-center randomized control study was conducted in the National Liver Institute Hospital, Menoufia, Egypt, between June 2017 and January 2019. The target population of this study was patients with cirrhosis as diagnosed by abdominal ultrasonography and furtherly confirmed and stratified by the Child-Turcotte-Pugh score (CTP score), who recovered from the first attack of variceal bleeding. The sample size and power analysis were calculated using the Epi-Info software statistical package created by the World Health Organization and Center for Disease Control and Prevention, Atlanta, GA, USA, version 2002. The criteria used for sample size calculations were 95% confidence limit and 80% power of the study. The sample size was estimated as 40 subjects in each study group, with a total sample size of 80 participants.

Within 2 weeks of the index hematemesis episode, patients were randomized into two groups (by using closed envelops) that was previously generated with a specialized software:

Group 1 (control group) included 40 patients who received the standard secondary prophylaxis of variceal bleeding composed of endoscopic variceal band ligation and non-selective β-blockers (NSBB): either propranolol or carvedilol.

Group 2 included 40 patients who received simvastatin in addition to the previous standard secondary prophylaxis of variceal bleeding. Simvastatin was given in a dose of 20 mg daily for 2 weeks and 40 mg daily after that.

The inclusion criteria were age between 18 and 80 years, evidence of liver cirrhosis, and first attack of variceal bleeding within the previous 2 weeks. The exclusion criteria included pregnancy or lactation, hepatocellular

Table 1 Baseline characteristics in both groups

			Range	Mean ± S.D	*t* test	*p*-value
Age		Group I	33–63	47.48 ± 7.36	0.030	0.863
		Group II	33–65	47.75 ± 6.82		
Sex			Group I	Group II	Total	
Male		*N*	22	30	52	
		%	55.0%	75.0%	65.0%	
Female		*N*	18	10	28	
		%	45.0%	25.0%	35.0%	
Total		*N*	40	40	80	
		%	100.0%	100.0%	100.0%	
Chi-square	X^2	3.516				
	p-value	0.0610.061				

carcinoma, creatinine above 2 mg/dL, CTP score > 13, contraindication for statins, previous portosystemic shunt, bleeding gastric varices, thrombosed portal vein or portal vein malformations, previous treatment with the standard of care prophylaxis (before the index episode), and previous exposure to statins within 1 month of randomization.

All recruited patients received the standard secondary prophylaxis of variceal bleeding (endoscopic variceal band ligation and NSBB). Medical prophylaxis (NSBB) started after a week of the index hematemesis episode, with either propranolol or carvedilol. Doses of NSBB were increased gradually to the maximum tolerated dose. After having the initial endoscopic band ligation session, scheduled endoscopic follow-up was arranged 2 to 4 weeks after and repeated until reporting variceal eradication. Patients were followed up regularly after 2 weeks of randomization; at months 3, 6, and 9; and at the end of the follow-up year. Other concomitant medications of the study patients were maintained during the follow-up period. Upper GI endoscopy was the standard gold method used in diagnosing and staging gastroesophageal varices (GOVs) (small varices < 5 mm and large varices > 5 mm).

Results

The current study included 80 patients with cirrhosis and PHT (40 in each group). Regarding the cause of cirrhosis, 77 patients were hepatitis C virus (HCV)-positive, two were hepatitis B virus (HBV)-positive, and one had combined HCV and HBV infections. There was no statistically significant difference between the two groups regarding age, sex, clinical features, and medical history (hypertension, diabetes mellitus, and diuretics therapy history). Baseline characteristics in both groups are detailed in Table 1.

Also, no significant difference was encountered in the CTP score between the two studied groups (Table 2).

Table 2 Comparison of the Child-Pugh score classification of the studied groups

Child score			Group I	Group II	Total
A		*N*	8	9	17
		%	20.0%	22.5%	21.3%
B		*N*	21	19	40
		%	52.5%	47.5%	50.0%
C		*N*	11	12	23
		%	27.5%	30.0%	28.8%
Total		*N*	40	40	80
		%	100.0%	100.0%	100.0%
Chi-square	X^2	0.202			
	p-value	0.904			

Table 3 Endoscopic finding of the two studied groups

Endoscope			Group I	Group II	X^2	*p*-value
15 days	Grade 2	*N*	21	24	2.237	0.327
		%	52.5%	60.0%		
	Grade 3	*N*	13	14		
		%	32.5%	35.0%		
	Grade 4	*N*	6	2		
		%	15.0%	5.0%		
3 months	Grade 2	*N*	22	31	5.901	0.052
		%	55.0%	77.5%		
	Grade 3	*N*	12	8		
		%	30.0%	20.0%		
	Grade 4	*N*	6	1		
		%	15.0%	2.5%		
6 months	Grade 2	*N*	27	33	5.667	0.059
		%	67.5%	82.5%		
	Grade 3	*N*	8	7		
		%	20.0%	17.5%		
	Grade 4	*N*	5	0		
		%	12.5%	.0%		
9 months	Grade 2	*N*	32	35	3.134	0.209
		%	80.0%	87.5%		
	Grade 3	*N*	5	5		
		%	12.5%	12.5%		
	Grade 4	*N*	3	0		
		%	7.5%	.0%		
12 months	Grade 2	*N*	32	35	3.134	0.209
		%	80.0%	87.5%		
	Grade 3	*N*	5	5		
		%	12.5%	12.5%		
	Grade 4	*N*	3	0		
		%	7.5%	0%		

Also, no statistically significant difference between the two groups was present in baseline laboratory analysis (blood picture indices, liver and kidney function tests, INR). After having the initial endoscopic band ligation session, scheduled endoscopic follow-up was performed at 2–4 weeks after; at months 3, 6, and 9; and at the end of the follow-up year. Detailed follow-up results of the performed endoscopies are reported in Table 3.

Statistically significant survival benefits were observed in the simvastatin group (37/40; 92.5%) as compared to the control group (30/40; 75.0%) (*p*-value = 0.034). Upon stratifying the patients according to CTP score, there was a significant difference in survival in patients with CTP A & B classes ($p < 0.05$), while no survival benefits were found in CTP class C patients, as shown in Fig. 1. All reported deaths in both groups were linked to events

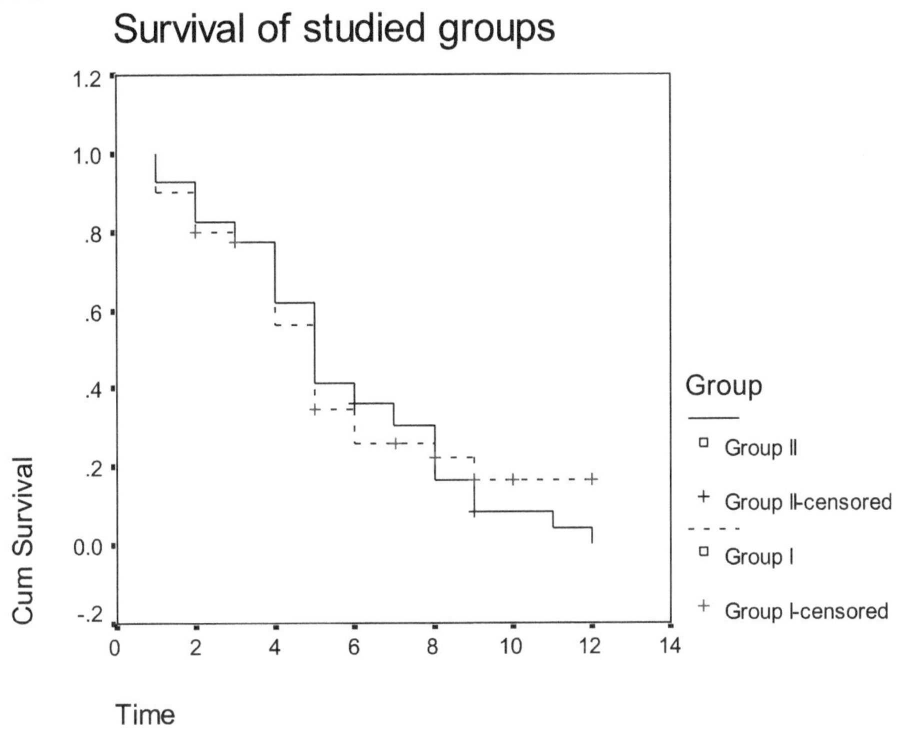

Fig. 1 Survival of the studied groups

related to the existing liver disease including encephalopathy and bleeding episodes. Meanwhile, no significant difference was present in rebleeding rates between the two groups, as 5 cases in group 1 experienced bleeding attacks (12.5%), compared to 3 cases in group II (7.5%) (p-value 0.456). A highly significant difference was noted in the incidence of hepatic encephalopathy (HE) between group I (15/40) and group II (0/40) ($p < 0.05$); however, this effect was not present in multivariate analysis (Table 4). No significant difference was observed in the occurrence of adverse events during the study between the two groups as regards diarrhea (5% and 10%) and worsening of ascites (17.5% and 22.5%) in groups I and II, respectively; however, myalgia was more frequent in the simvastatin group (5% in group I and 20% in group II, p-value 0.043). Multivariate analysis was performed to test simvastatin's effect and confirmed that only survival was affected and no statistical differences between the 2 groups in other factors like the presence of encephalopathy, myalgia, and Child score of the studied patients (Table 4).

Table 4 Multivariate analysis of the effect of simvastatin in improving the survival

	Multivariate	
	OR (95% CI)	p-value
Encephalopathy	0.725 (0.352–1.652)	0.998
Survival	0.136 (0.020–0.916)	0.040*
Myalgia	5.812 (0.658–51.361)	0.113
Child score	4.419 (0.874–22.341)	0.072

Discussion

In the current study, there was a significant reduction in the incidence of HE episodes in the simvastatin group (0/40), compared to the control group (15/40), and this is in accordance with the finding of studies which showed survival benefits and improvement in liver functions with simvastatin [14, 15]. Improvement in PHT, reduction in the incidence of HCC, and delays in hepatic decompensation have been associated with statin therapy among patients with cirrhosis [15, 16]. In our study, there was no significant difference between the two groups concerning INR, albumin level, total bilirubin, AST, and ALT, and this comes with an agreement with the findings in most of the studies discussing the impact of statins on the liver biochemical profile [17–19]. Statins are known to decrease Rho-kinase activity in activated hepatic stellate cells [11]. Besides, statins have anti-inflammatory, immunomodulatory, and antioxidant properties [12]. Simvastatin is also known to induce Krüppel-like factor 2, which improves liver fibrosis and PHT by increasing nitric oxide bioavailability [13, 14]. Generally, conflicting reports are available in the literature regarding liver function changes with statin use, with an insignificant risk of elevated transaminases [20, 21]. No significant difference was observed in the adverse effects noted during the study between the two groups in terms of diarrhea or worsening of ascites; however, there was a significant difference between the two study groups in myalgia, while other studies found no significant difference in adverse effect in the term of diarrhea, ascites, and myalgia noted during the study [17, 18]. Regarding the survival of patients in the two studied groups, there was a significant difference between them. This agrees with Motzkus-Feagans and his colleague [17] and agrees with a study done using the Veteran Affairs Clinical Case Registry [22]. This study described the effect of statins in cirrhotic HCV patients matched 1:5 with statin non-users, finding fewer decompensation episodes and death in statin users. No differences in comorbidities, metabolic conditions, or hepatic function were reported between the groups. The positive effect of statins in cirrhosis decompensation and mortality persisted at 10 years after adjustment for age, FIB-4 index score, serum level of albumin, model for end-stage liver disease (MELD), and CTP scores [22]. In our study, no significant difference was observed between the two groups as regards variceal rebleeding. This also agrees with the finding of Motzkus-Feagans et al., who proved that rebleeding rates were not different between the treatment and the control [17].

Regarding survival in CTP score A and B patients, there was a significant difference between the two studied groups. At the same time, there was an increased survival in group II patients compared to group I. The same finding was conveyed by Motzkus-Feagans and his colleague, who reported an increased survival in decompensated cirrhotic patients who received simvastatin after variceal bleeding [17]. Similarly, Pollo-Flores and colleagues reported the same findings after evaluating statin use in cirrhotic patients to look for increased mortality or decompensation with a mean follow-up of 36 months, including most cirrhotic patients at an early stage (CTP score A) [23]. They show that statin use was associated with lower mortality and fewer hepatic decompensation episodes in multivariate analysis.

More prolonged administration of simvastatin treatment than placebo for severe PHT was assessed in a blinded randomized controlled trial. Three months of 40 mg simvastatin in 24 patients, most CTP A and B nearly two-thirds with use of NSBB and medium/ large esophageal varices including 30% with previous variceal bleeding, showed a significant reduction in HVPG with greater effect in patients with previous variceal bleeding and medium/large esophageal varices. Again, no significant increase in adverse events from the use of simvastatin was reported [23]. Regarding survival in Child C patients, no significant difference was observed between the two studied groups, which matches the published data in this regard [17].

The current study has some limitations, such as the relatively small sample size, which could be attributed to our narrow inclusion criteria and the long-term follow-up required for the participants. Repeating the experiment with a larger sized sample could confirm our findings.

Conclusions

Adding simvastatin to the standard therapy in secondary prevention of variceal bleeding could be associated with survival benefits in patients with Child A and B cirrhosis, while it was incapable of reducing rebleeding. Further studies are required to confirm this survival benefit.

Abbreviations

CTP score: Child-turcotte-pugh score; GOVs: Gastroesophageal varices; HCV: Hepatitis C virus; HBV: Hepatitis B virus; MELD: Model for end-stage liver disease; NSBB: Non-selective β-blockers; PHT: Portal hypertension

Acknowledgements

None

Authors' contributions

The study was designed by HE, HA, and EST. AA and DNE collected the study data and oversaw the participant visits. MEK and RE provided regulatory oversight. DNE, RE, and MEK wrote the first draft of the article. All authors contributed to the reviewing and editing of the article and approved the final version. Article preparation was done by all study authors, and the decision to submit the article for publication was made by all the study authors.

Declarations

Ethics approval and consent to participate

All procedures performed in this study involving human participants were following the ethical standards of the institutional and/or national research committee and with the 1964 Helsinki Declaration and its later amendments or comparable ethical standards. The study was approved by the Research Ethics Committee (REC) for human subject research at the National Liver Institute in 2017. Informed consent was obtained from all individual participants included in the study.

Competing interests

The authors declare that they have no competing interests.

Author details

[1]Hepatology and Gastroenterology Department, National Liver Institute, Menoufia University, Menoufia, Egypt. [2]Tanta Fever Hospital, Tanta, Gharbiah, Egypt. [3]Tropical Medicine Department, Faculty of Medicine, Minia University, Minya, Egypt. [4]Endemic Medicine Department, Faculty of Medicine, Helwan University, Ain Helwan, Cairo 11795, Egypt.

References

1. Bosch J, Abraldes JG, Berzigotti A, García-Pagan JC (2009) The clinical use of HVPG measurements in chronic liver disease. Nat Rev Gastroenterol Hepatol. 6(10):573–582. https://doi.org/10.1038/nrgastro.2009.149

2. Bosch J, Abraldes JG, Groszmann R (2003) Current management of portal hypertension. J Hepatol. 38(Suppl 1):S54–S68. https://doi.org/10.1016/S0168-8278(02)00430-0
3. Vargas V, Rimola A, Casanovas T, Castells L, Navasa M, Baliellas C, Bilbao I, Visa J, Jaurrieta E, Margarit C (2003) Applicability of liver transplantation in Catalonia at the end of the millennium. A prospective study of adult patient selection for liver transplantation. Transpl Int. 16(4):270–275. https://doi.org/10.1111/j.1432-2277.2003.tb00298.x
4. Failli P, DeFranco RM, Caligiuri A et al (2000) Nitrovasodilators inhibit platelet-derived growth factor-induced proliferation and migration of activated human hepatic stellate cells. Gastroenterology. 119(2):479–492. https://doi.org/10.1053/gast.2000.9354
5. García-Calderó H, Rodríguez-Vilarrupla A, Gracia-Sancho J, Diví M, Laviña B, Bosch J, García-Pagán JC (2011) Tempol administration, a superoxide dismutase mimetic, reduces hepatic vascular resistance and portal pressure in cirrhotic rats. J Hepatol. 54(4):660–665. https://doi.org/10.1016/j.jhep.2010.07.034
6. Morales-Ruiz M (2003) Cejudo-martín P, Fernández-Varo G, et al. Transduction of the liver with activated Akt normalizes portal pressure in cirrhotic rats. Gastroenterology. 125(2):522–531. https://doi.org/10.1016/S0016-5085(03)00909-0
7. de Franchis R (2005) Evolving consensus in portal hypertension report of the Baveno IV Consensus Workshop on methodology of diagnosis and therapy in portal hypertension. J Hepatol. 43(1):167–176. https://doi.org/10.1016/j.jhep.2005.05.009
8. Blum A, Shamburek R (2009) The pleiotropic effects of statins on endothelial function, vascular inflammation, immunomodulation and thrombogenesis. Atherosclerosis. 203(2):325–330. https://doi.org/10.1016/j.atherosclerosis.2008.08.022
9. Trebicka J, Hennenberg M, Laleman W, Shelest N, Biecker E, Schepke M, Nevens F, Sauerbruch T, Heller J (2007) Atorvastatin lowers portal pressure in cirrhotic rats by inhibition of RhoA/Rho-kinase and activation of endothelial nitric oxide synthase. Hepatology. 46(1):242–253. https://doi.org/10.1002/hep.21673
10. Violi F, Calvieri C, Ferro D, Pignatelli P (2013) Statins as antithrombotic drugs. Circulation. 127(2):251–257. https://doi.org/10.1161/CIRCULATIONAHA.112.145334
11. Zafra C, Abraldes JG, Turnes J, Berzigotti A, Fernández M, García-Pagán JC, Rodés J, Bosch J (2004) Simvastatin enhances hepatic nitric oxide production and decreases the hepatic vascular tone in patients with cirrhosis. Gastroenterology. 126(3):749–755. https://doi.org/10.1053/j.gastro.2003.12.007
12. Garcia-Pagan J-C, Villanueva C, Albillos A, Banares R, Morillas R, Abraldes JG, Bosch J, on behalf of the Spanish Variceal Bleeding Study Group (2009) Nadolol plus isosorbide mononitrate alone or associated with band ligation in the prevention of recurrent bleeding: a multicentre randomised controlled trial. Gut. 58(8):1144–1150. https://doi.org/10.1136/gut.2008.171207
13. Sauerbruch T, Mengel M, Dollinger M et al (2015) Prevention of rebleeding from esophageal varices in patients with cirrhosis receiving small-diameter stents versus hemodynamically controlled medical therapy. Gastroenterology 149(3):660–8. e1
14. Abraldes JG, Bureau C, Stefanescu H, Augustin S, Ney M, Blasco H, Procopet B, Bosch J, Genesca J, Berzigotti A, for the Anticipate Investigators (2016) Noninvasive tools and risk of clinically significant portal hypertension and varices in compensated cirrhosis: the "Anticipate" study. Hepatology. 64(6):2173–2184. https://doi.org/10.1002/hep.28824
15. Singh S, Singh PP, Singh AG, Murad MH, Sanchez W (2013) Statins are associated with a reduced risk of hepatocellular cancer: a systematic review and meta-analysis. Gastroenterology. 144(2):323–332. https://doi.org/10.1053/j.gastro.2012.10.005
16. Elwan N, Salah R, Hamisa M et al (2018) Evaluation of portal pressure by Doppler ultrasound in patients with cirrhosis before and after simvastatin administration–a randomized controlled trial. F1000Research. 7:256. https://doi.org/10.12688/f1000research.13915.1
17. Motzkus-Feagans C, Pakyz A, Ratliff S et al (2013) Statin use and infections in Veterans with cirrhosis. Aliment Pharmacol Ther. 38(6):611–618. https://doi.org/10.1111/apt.12430
18. Schuppan D, Afdhal NH (2008) Liver cirrhosis. Lancet. 371(9615):838–851. https://doi.org/10.1016/S0140-6736(08)60383-9
19. Bays H, Cohen DE, Chalasani N, Harrison SA (2014) An assessment by the statin liver safety task force: 2014 update. J Clin Lipidol. 8(3):S47–S57. https://doi.org/10.1016/j.jacl.2014.02.011
20. Russo MW, Hoofnagle JH, Gu J, Fontana RJ, Barnhart H, Kleiner DE, Chalasani N, Bonkovsky HL (2014) Spectrum of statin hepatotoxicity: experience of the drug-induced liver injury network. Hepatology. 60(2):679–686. https://doi.org/10.1002/hep.27157
21. Mohanty A, Tate JP, Garcia-Tsao G (2016) Statins are associated with a decreased risk of decompensation and death in veterans with hepatitis C–related compensated cirrhosis. Gastroenterology 150(2):430–40. e1
22. Kumar S, Grace ND, Qamar AA (2014) Statin use in patients with cirrhosis: a retrospective cohort study. Dig Dis Sci. 59(8):1958–1965. https://doi.org/10.1007/s10620-014-3179-2
23. Pollo-Flores P, Soldan M, Santos UC, Kunz DG, Mattos DE, da Silva AC, Marchiori RC, Rezende GFM (2015) Three months of simvastatin therapy vs. placebo for severe portal hypertension in cirrhosis: a randomized controlled trial. Dig Liver Dis. 47(11):957–963. https://doi.org/10.1016/j.dld.2015.07.156

13

Validity of serum leukotriene B4 as a marker of decompensated liver cirrhosis in chronic HCV patients: leukotriene B4 in decompensated liver cirrhosis

Ayman El-Shayeb[1], Sawsan El-Mallah[1], Akram Deghady[2], Samar El-Hewely[1] and Doaa Elwazzan[1*]

Abstract

Background: Liver cirrhosis is divided into two stages: compensated stage and another advanced stage which includes both decompensated cirrhosis and acute-on-chronic liver failure. The immune system is of major importance in cirrhosis pathophysiology. Sustained bacterial translocation from the intestine to systemic circulation causes a chronic systemic inflammatory syndrome. Inflammatory markers are emerging in the scope of cirrhosis and its complications due to their deleterious effects on disease progression and prognosis. The aim of the study was to assess the value of leukotriene B4 (LTB4) as a marker of decompensated cirrhosis and to evaluate its relation to disease progression and complications.

Results: The current study was conducted on 80 candidates in the Alexandria Main University Hospital, Tropical Medicine Department; they were categorized into three groups: group I ($n = 30$) compensated cirrhotic patients, group II ($n = 30$) decompensated cirrhotic patients, and group III ($n = 20$) apparently healthy individuals. Serum LTB4 was measured by ELISA. LTB4 showed statistically significant higher values in the decompensated group than the compensated group ($p = 0.007$) and the control group ($p = 0.002$). However, there was no statistically significant difference between the compensated group and the controls ($p = 0.510$). LTB4 correlated positively with the Child-Pugh score ($p = 0.003$). Moreover, it correlated positively with the MELD-Na score ($p = 0.012$). There was a significant correlation between the degree of ascites and serum LTB4 ($p < 0.001$). However, there was no significant correlation between hepatic encephalopathy and LTB4 ($P > 0.204$).

Conclusion: Serum LTB4 could be used as a sensitive biomarker of decompensation in cirrhotic patients.

Keywords: Hepatitis C virus, Liver cirrhosis, Bacterial translocation, Leukotriene B4

Background

Chronic HCV infection is often asymptomatic and ultimately leads to cirrhosis [1]. The clinical course of cirrhosis is divided into two stages: compensated and decompensated [2]. Progression of a compensated stage to a decompensated one has a significantly negative effect on the prognosis and is related to an abrupt decrease in survival probability to less than 3–5 years [3].

Our concepts on the pathophysiology of cirrhosis progression have undergone major changes and the axis formed by the bowel, liver, and immune system became of major importance [4]. Sustained bacterial translocation from the intestinal lumen to the systemic circulation and organs triggers the innate immune system and results in a chronic systemic inflammatory syndrome which may be a mechanism for decompensation and multiorgan dysfunction [5].

*Correspondence: d.elwazzan@gmail.com
[1] Tropical Medicine Department, Faculty of Medicine, Alexandria University, Alexandria, Egypt
Full list of author information is available at the end of the article

LTB4 is a pro-inflammatory compound that displays strong chemoattractant properties. Increased LTB4 has been found in lots of inflammatory and allergic diseases and levels correlate with disease activity in some of these [6]. However, leukotriene B4 role in decompensated cirrhosis has not been studied in depth.

Aim of the work

The aim of this study was to assess the value of LTB4 as a marker of decompensated cirrhosis and to study its relation to complications and disease progression.

Subjects

This study was conducted on 80 candidates in the Alexandria Main University Hospital, Tropical Medicine Department; subjects were divided into three groups: group I ($n = 30$) compensated cirrhotic patients, group II ($n = 30$) decompensated cirrhotic patients, and group III ($n = 20$) apparently healthy individuals. The age of the candidates ranged between 21 and 79 years old.

Exclusion criteria

Patients with concurrent allergic diseases, diabetes mellitus, obesity, malignancies, and history of anti-inflammatory and immunosuppressive drugs were excluded from the study.

Methods

All patients were subjected to thorough history taking and proper clinical examination. Laboratory investigations included complete blood count, liver function tests, renal function tests, erythrocyte sedimentation rate and C reactive protein (CRP), viral hepatitis markers B and C, polymerase chain reaction test for HCV RNA, and serum alpha-fetoprotein. Triceps fold thickness and basal metabolic index were estimated in addition to Child-Pugh classification and MELD score calculation. Serum LTB4 was measured by the ELISA kit named Human Leukotriene B4 (LTB4) ELISA kit. Ultrasound abdomen and triphasic CT scan were done for patients with ultrasound positive focal hepatic lesions.

Data were analyzed using the IBM SPSS software package version 20.0. The used statistical tests were chi-square test, Monte Carlo correction, Student's t test, F-test (ANOVA), Mann-Whitney test, Kruskal-Wallis test, and Spearman's coefficient. Receiver operating characteristic curve (ROC (was generated by plotting sensitivity (TP) on Y-axis versus 1-specificity (FP) on X-axis at different cutoff values. The area under the ROC curve denotes the diagnostic performance of the test. Area more than 50% gives acceptable performance and area about 100% is the best performance for the test.

Ethical approval

The ethical committee of the Faculty of Medicine, Alexandria University, approved this study. Written informed consent was obtained from all patients.

Results

This study was conducted on 80 candidates in the Alexandria Main University Hospital, Tropical Medicine Department; subjects were divided into three groups.

Regarding their demographic data, see Table 1.

Group I included 30 compensated cirrhotic patients. They were 63.3% males and 36.7% females. Their mean age was 48.0 ± 11.06 years old. All the patients were HCV positive.

Group II included 30 decompensated cirrhotic patients. They were 50% females and 50% males. Their mean age was 55.47 ± 12.62 years old. All the patients were HCV positive.

Group III control group included 20 apparently healthy individuals. They were 35.0% males and 65% females. Their mean age was 55.47 ± 12.62 years old.

Regarding LTB4 results, in the control group, it ranged 6.21–47.45 ng/L with a mean of 19.83 ± 13.17 ng/L. In compensated cirrhosis group, it ranged 9.11–58.73 ng/L with a mean of 9.11–58.73 ng/L. On the other hand, LTB4 in the decompensated cirrhosis group ranged between 13.62 and 346.1 ng/L with a mean of 47.34 ± 65.18 ng/L. LTB4 showed a statistically significantly higher value in the decompensated cirrhosis group than the compensated cirrhosis group ($p = 0.007$) and the control group ($p = 0.002$). However, there was no statistically significant difference between the compensated cirrhosis group and the control groups with $p = 0.510$ (Table 1, Fig. 1). Going through lab results (Table 1), bilirubin was statistically significantly higher in group II than group I ($p < 0.001$). Albumin was statistically significantly lower in group II than group I ($p < 0.001$). INR was statistically significantly higher in group II than group I ($p < 0.001$).

In the current work, we assessed serum creatinine and serum sodium in the studied groups. Creatinine was statistically significantly higher in group II than group I with ($p = 0.007$). There was a positive correlation between serum level of creatinine and LTB4 where $p = 0.035$. As regards serum sodium, it was statistically significantly lower in group II than group I and III ($p = 0.001$); however, there was no statistically significant difference between group I and III ($p = 0.798$). There was a statistically significant correlation between serum level of sodium and LTB4 where $p = 0.040$. LTB4 showed higher values in patients with lower sodium levels.

Regarding serum CRP, it was statistically significantly higher in the patients than in the control group.

Table 1 Comparison between the three studied groups ($n = 80$) according to demographic data and other different parameters

	Group I ($n = 30$)	Group II ($n = 30$)	Group III ($n = 20$)	Test of Sig.	*P*
Gender					
Male	19	15	7	$\chi^2 = 3.886$	0.143
Female	11	15	13		
Age (years)					
Min-Max	28.0–70.0	36.0–79.0	21.0–45.0	$F = 39.150$*	<0.001*
Mean ± SD	48.0 ± 11.06	55.47±12.62	28.60±5.36		
Median (IQR)	45.50(39.0–57.0)	54.0(45.0–67.0)	28.0(25.50–31.0)		
Degree of ascites					
Mild	-	9	-	30	-
Moderate	-	9	-	30	
Massive	-	12	-	40	
Hepatic encephalopathy	-	17	-	$\chi^2 = 23.721$*	<0.001*
Total bilirubin (mg/dl)					
Min.-Max.	0.20–1.40	0.50–9.0	0.80–1.20	$H = 29.980$*	<0.001*
Serum albumin (g/dl)					
Min.-Max.	3.50–4.30	1.60–3.0	4.0–5.50	$F = 245.85$*	<0.001*
INR					
Min.-Max.	0.80–1.50	1.10–2.50	0.90–1.40	$F = 45.043$*	<0.001*
CRP					
Min.-Max.	10.0–18.0	24.0–50.0	1.0–5.0	$H = 69.618$*	<0.001*
Child-Pugh Classification					
A	30	0	NA	$\chi^2 = 60.00$*	<0.001*
B	0	15			
C	0	15			
MELD/Na score					
Min-Max	6.0–18.0	10.0–30.0	NA	$t = 10.592$*	<0.001*
Mean ± SD	10.43 ± 3.07	20.23 ± 4.03			
Median (IQR)	10.0 (9.0–12.0)	20.0 (18.0–22.0)			
Serum Leukotriene B4 (ng/L)					
Min.-Max	9.11–58.73	13.62–346.1	6.21–47.45	$H = 11.517$*	0.003*
Mean ± SD	21.12 ± 11.0	47.34 ± 65.18	19.83 ± 13.17		
Median (IQR)	17.90(12.63–28.69)	24.27(19.59–39.35)	13.11(9.13–27.23)		

Group I: Compensated liver cirrhosis due to chronic HCV infection

Group II: Decompensated liver cirrhosis due to chronic HCV infection

Group III: Healthy controls

INR International normalization ratio, *CRP* C-reactive protein, χ^2 Chi-square test, *H* Kruskal-Wallis test, pairwise comparison bet. the 2 groups were done using post hoc test (Dunn's for multiple comparisons test), *F* ANOVA test, pairwise comparison bet. the 2 groups were done using post hoc test (Tukey), *t* Student's *t* test, *p p* value for comparing between the studied groups

*Statistically significant at $p \leq 0.05$

Moreover, it was statistically significantly higher in group II than group I ($p = 0.001$). There was a statistically significant positive correlation between CRP and LTB4 ($p < 0.006$) (Table 1, Fig. 2).

All patients in the decompensated cirrhosis group were suffering from different degrees of ascites. Twelve out of thirty patients presented with a massive degree of ascites. The rest of the patients, half of them, had moderate ascites and the other half had a mild degree of ascites assessed by ultrasound (Table 1). The relation between LTB4 and degree of ascites was assessed and results showed a positive correlation between LTB4 and the degree of ascites ($p < 0.001$). Serum LTB4 levels in patients with massive ascites ranged 32.39–346.1 ng/L. It was lower in patients with moderate ascites ranging 20.54–27.81 ng/L. The lowest values were in patients with a mild degree of ascites ranging 13.62–19.88 ng/L.

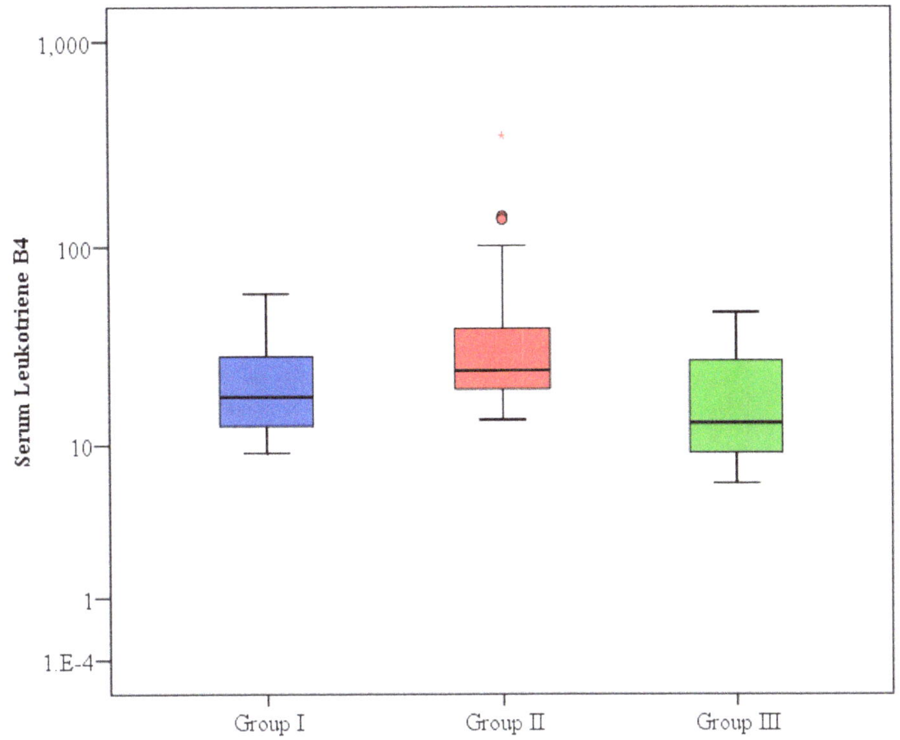

Fig. 1 Comparison between the three studied groups ($n = 80$) according to serum LTB4

Seventeen out of thirty decompensated patients were suffering from hepatic encephalopathy (Table 1). In these patients, LTB4 ranged 13.62–346.1 ng/L compared to patients without hepatic encephalopathy where LTB4 ranged 9.11–140.8 ng/L. There was no significant correlation between hepatic encephalopathy and LTB4 ($p > 0.204$).

As regards the Child-Pugh classification, in group I, all patients were Child A class. Group II included 15 patients with Child score B and 15 patients with Child score C (Table 1). There was a statistically significant difference between groups I and II ($p < 0.001$). The Child classification showed a statistically significant correlation with LTB4 ($p = 0.003$) (Fig. 3).

MELD/Na score calculation was done; it ranged 6.0–18.0 in the compensated cirrhosis group. On the other hand, MELD/Na score ranged 10.0–30 in the decompensated group (Table 1). It was statistically significantly higher in decompensated cirrhosis group than in compensated group ($p < 0.001$). The relation between LTB4 and Meld/Na score showed a statistically significant correlation ($p < 0.012$) (Fig. 4).

ROC curve was done to estimate the cutoff point of LTB4 to discriminate compensated cirrhosis from decompensated cirrhosis. The ROC curve for Serum LTB4 was significant (p 0.002*) and showed that the cutoff level of LTB4 discriminating decompensated patients from compensated patients was >16.2 ng/L, with a sensitivity of 93.33%, specificity of 43.33%, positive predictive value of 62.2%, and negative predictive value of 86.7% with a diagnostic accuracy of 66.7%. (Table 2, Fig. 5)

Discussion

There is now much evidence that inflammatory mediators have direct deleterious effects in the pathophysiology of liver cirrhosis and its complications [7]. Several studies have shown several circulatory chemokines involved in leukocyte migration and chemotaxis to be increased in decompensated cirrhotic patients, which correlated with survival [8].

Leukotrienes are potent biological mediators implicated in lots of disease processes. LTB4 is a pro-inflammatory compound that displays strong chemoattractant properties. Increased LTB4 has been found in lots of inflammatory and allergic diseases and levels correlate with disease activity in some of these [9].

In the current study, serum LTB4 value was elevated with worsening severity of liver disease measured by Child-Pugh classification and MELD/Na score. LTB4 was significantly higher in decompensated cirrhosis group

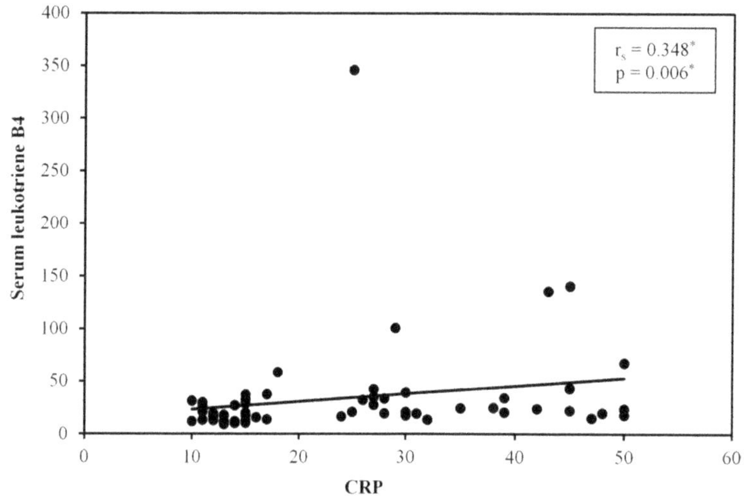

Fig. 2 Correlation between serum leukotriene B4 and CRP in total cases ($n = 60$)

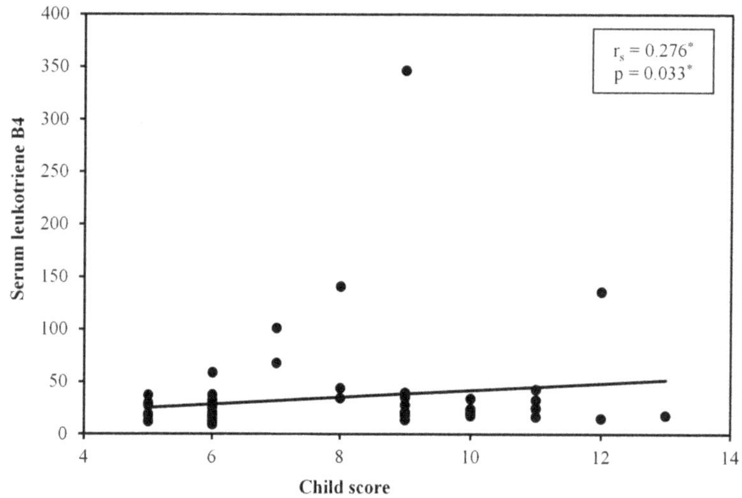

Fig. 3 Correlation between LTB4 and Child Score in cirrhotic patients ($n = 60$)

than the compensated group and controls ($p = 0.003$). However, there was no significant difference between compensated cirrhosis group and controls ($p = 0.510$). LTB4 showed a statistically significant correlation with Child class ($p = 0.003$). Moreover, LTB4 values showed a significant positive correlation with MELD/Na score ($p = 0.012$). This proves the idea of systemic inflammation in cirrhosis which may be a mechanism for decompensation and multiorgan dysfunction.

Our results showed that LTB4 cutoff value to discriminate compensated cirrhosis from decompensated cirrhosis was >16.2 ng/L with a sensitivity of 93.33% and specificity of 43.33%.

In addition to our study, Becares et al. study [10], quantified serum LTB4 in a cohort of 26 patients with cirrhosis divided into 3 groups: group I healthy volunteers ($n = 5$), group II decompensated stable patients ($n = 11$), and group III ACLF ($n = 10$). Becares et al. study [10] concluded that ACLF patients display significantly higher neutrophil recruitment to a site of inflammation than healthy volunteers in addition to increased plasma levels of the chemotactic LTB4 according to cirrhosis disease severity which was compatible with our findings.

Another study discussing the value of LTB4 in chronic liver disease is Asano et al.'s study [11], which measured LTB4 using peripheral blood mononuclear cells (PBMC)

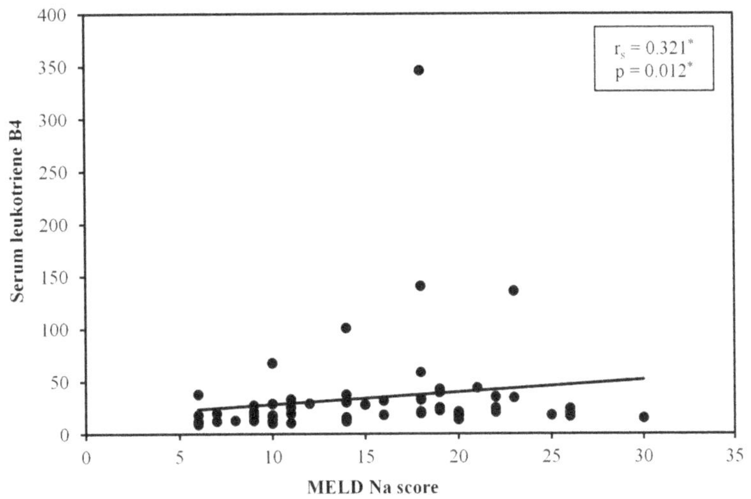

Fig. 4 Correlation between LTB4 and MELD/Na score in cirrhotic patients ($n = 60$)

Table 2 Agreement (sensitivity, specificity) for LTB4 to diagnose decompensated cirrhosis group ($n = 30$) from compensated cirrhosis group ($n = 30$)

	AUC	*P*	95% C.I	Cut off[a]	Sensitivity %	Specificity %	PPV %	NPV %	Accuracy of the test %
Serum leukotriene B4	0.728	0.002*	0.601–0.855	>16.2	93.33	43.33	62.2	86.7	66.7

AUC Area under a curve, *p value* Probability value, *CI* Confidence Intervals, *NPV* Negative predictive value, *PPV* Positive predictive value

*Statistically significant at $p \leq 0.05$

[a] Cutoff was chosen according to the Youden index

in patients with fulminant hepatitis (FH) and other liver diseases. The production rate of LTB4 was elevated in 16 of 17 FH patients. However, in discordance to our study, LTB4 was below the detectable level in patients with chronic hepatitis. Asano et al. concluded that enhanced LTB4 production may indicate the primed state of PBMC and their role in the development of massive liver necrosis and of other organ failures in FH.

Serum sodium was measured and results showed statistically lower values in Child B and C than Child A patients ($p < 0.001$) and controls ($p < 0.001$); however, there was no statistically significant difference between group I and III ($p = 0.798$). This was in agreement with James et al.'s study [12], who evaluated serum sodium among 97 decompensated patients, 42 had serum sodium levels ≥136 mEq/L, while 32 had serum sodium levels between 131 and 135 mEq/L and 23 patients had serum sodium level ≤130 mEq/L. Serum sodium levels were associated strongly with the severity of liver disease as assessed by Child-Pugh and MELD score. Patients with serum sodium levels ≤130 mEq/L had increased mortality (30.4% with $p = 0.002$). In our study, serum sodium showed a significant negative correlation with LTB4 ($p = 0.040^*$).

Regarding CRP, it was statistically significantly higher in Child B and C patients ($p < 0.001$) than Child A patients. This was compatible to Lai et al.'s study [13] where patients with class B and C scores showed the highest level of high-sensitivity C-reactive protein when compared with class A patients or healthy subjects. Lai et al. [13] aimed to assess the association of liver cirrhosis with increased inflammatory responses and the relation between CRP and the severity of the liver disease. In our study, LTB4 correlated positively with CRP values with $p = 0.006$.

LTB4 correlated positively with the degree of ascites (mild – moderate – massive) with $p < 0.001$. LTB4 relation to ascites was studied in Ouwendijk et al. study [14]; they collected ascitic fluid from six patients with liver cirrhosis and isolated macrophages that were labeled with 14C-arachidonic acid. After stimulation of these cells, the main substances formed were LTB4 and LTC4. This suggests that human peritoneal macrophages are capable of producing LTs and prostaglandins. Moreover, it supports the idea that the production of these substances might play a role in some of the complications of patients with liver cirrhosis and ascites.

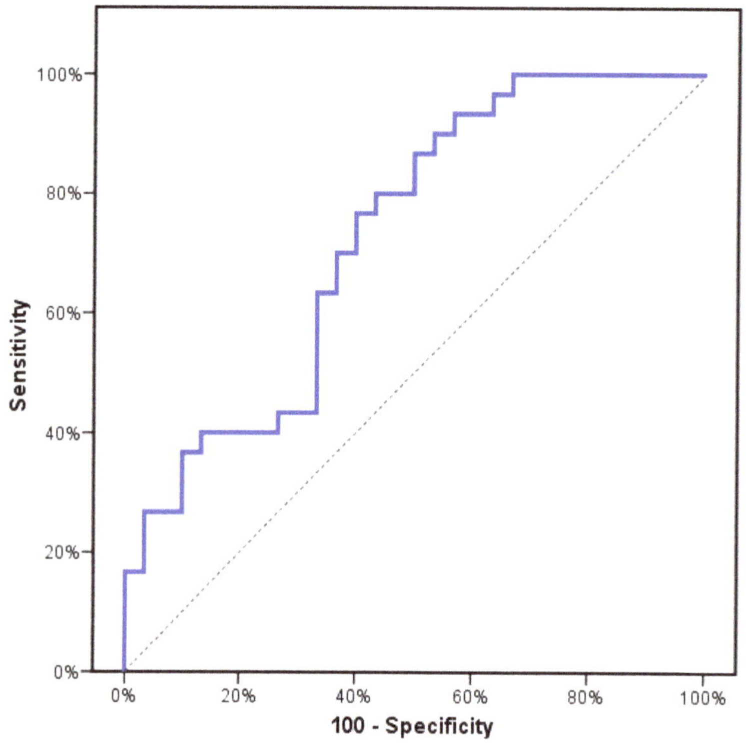

Fig. 5 ROC curve for LTB4 to discriminate compensated cirrhosis patients ($n = 30$) from decompensated cirrhosis patients ($n = 30$)

Other leukotrienes studied in cirrhosis and its related complications are cysteinyl leukotrienes and their metabolite leukotriene E4 (LTE4). According to Moore et al.'s study [15], urinary LTE4 was elevated in patients with HRS compared with normal controls and with renal failure alone. Urinary LTE4 was also elevated in subjects with decompensated liver disease; it showed high results in cirrhosis with ascites and even higher results in severe hepatocellular dysfunction; however, it was normal in compensated liver disease. They concluded that LTE4 production is increased in HRS and that this may be one of the factors involved in its pathogenesis.

Conclusions

Serum LTB4 could be used as a sensitive biomarker of decompensation in cirrhotic patients. Furthermore, the significant correlation of serum LTB4 with Child-Pugh class, MELD/Na score, and CRP could suggest that it can be used as a tool to follow up the clinical outcomes of patients with liver cirrhosis and prioritize listing for liver transplantation.

Abbreviations

LTB4: Leukotriene B4; MELD: Model for end-stage liver disease; HCV: Hepatitis C virus; CRP: C-reactive protein; ACLF: Acute on chronic liver failure; PBMC: Peripheral blood mononuclear cells; LTE4: Leukotriene E4.

Acknowledgements

The authors would like to thank all patients for their participation in this research.

Authors' contributions

AE initiated the project, designed the study, and was responsible for the concept. SE shared in the literature review, data collection, and writing the manuscript. AD did all the laboratory work. DE shared in manuscript writing, study design, analysis of the results, and final revision of the manuscript. All authors provided critical feedback and helped shape and revise the research, the analysis, and the manuscript. All authors have read and approved the manuscript.

Declarations

Ethics approval and consent to participate

The ethical committee of the Faculty of Medicine, Alexandria University, approved this study. Written informed consent was obtained from both patients and the control. Committee reference No.: 0106135. Date: 24 September 2019. IRB No.: 00012098. FWA No.: 00018699.

Competing interests

The authors declare that they have no competing interests.

Author details

[1]Tropical Medicine Department, Faculty of Medicine, Alexandria University, Alexandria, Egypt. [2]Clinical Pathology Department, Faculty of Medicine, Alexandria University, Alexandria, Egypt.

References

1. Gill K, Ghazinian H, Manch R, Gish R (2016) Hepatitis C virus as a systemic disease: reaching beyond the liver. Hepatol Int 10(3):415–423
2. Crismale JF, Friedman SL (2020) Acute liver injury and decompensated cirrhosis. Med Clin North Am 104(4):647–662
3. D'Amico G, Morabito A, D'Amico M, Pasta L, Malizia G, Rebora P, Valsecchi MG (2018) Clinical states of cirrhosis and competing risks. J Hepatol 68(3):563–576
4. Tawfik N, El-Gendy N, Elhassan HAE, Ebrihem E, Saleh RA (2019) Inflammatory biomarkers as prognostic indicators for liver cirrhosis. Al-Azhar Assiut Med J 17(1):68–74
5. European Association for the Study of the Liver (EASL) (2018) EASL Clinical Practice Guidelines for the management of patients with decompensated cirrhosis. J Hepatol 69(2):406–460
6. Yokomizo T (2011) Leukotriene B4 receptors: novel roles in immunological regulations. Adv Enzyme Regul 51(1):59–64
7. Kalogeris T, Baines CP, Krenz M, Korthuis RJ (2012) Cell biology of ischemia/reperfusion injury. Int Rev Cell Mol Biol 298:229–317
8. Dirchwolf M, Podhorzer A, Marino M, Shulman C, Cartier M, Zunino M et al (2015) Immune dysfunction in cirrhosis: distinct cytokines phenotypes according to cirrhosis severity. Cytokine 77:14–25
9. Primdahl KG, Tungen JE, Aursnes M, Hansen TV, Vik A (2015) An efficient total synthesis of leukotriene B4. Org Biomol Chem 13(19):5412–5417
10. Becares N, Maini A, Colas R, Dalli J, Gilroy D, O'Brien A (2019) FRI-109-Increased plasma leukotriene B4 in decompensated cirrhosis associates with disease progression and leads to increased skin window neutrophil infiltration. J Hepatol 70:e435
11. Asano F, Moriwaki H, Shiratori Y, Shimazaki M, Sakai T, Koshino Y et al (1993) Enhanced production of leukotriene B4 by peripheral blood mononuclear cells in patients with fulminant hepatitis. J Gastroenterol Hepatol 8(3):228–231
12. James P, Vajaravelu S, Radhakrishnan A (2016) Study of serum sodium levels in decompensated chronic liver disease. Glob J Res Anal 5(10):77–82
13. Lai C-Y, Cheng S-B, Lee T-Y, Liu H-T, Huang S-C, Huang Y-C (2018) Possible synergistic effects of glutathione and C-reactive protein in the progression of liver cirrhosis. Nutrients 10(6):678
14. Ouwendijk RJ, Zijlstra FJ, Wilson JH, Vincent JE, Bonta IL (1985) Production of leukotrienes and prostaglandins by human ascites cells. Eur J Clin Invest 15(6):327–331
15. Moore KP, Taylor GW, Maltby NH, Siegers D, Fuller RW, Dollery CT, Williams R (1990) Increased production of cysteinyl leukotrienes in hepatorenal syndrome. J Hepatol 11(2):263–271

14

Serum Beclin 1 and autophagy-related protein-5 and the risk of hepatocellular carcinoma among cirrhotic hepatitis C patients

Ayman El Shayeb[1], Akram Deghedy[2], Essam Saeed Bedewy[1], Sahar Badawy[1*] and Nermeen Abdeen[1]

Abstract

Background: The most common primary liver cancer in adults is hepatocellular carcinoma (HCC) which is commonly presented with a poor prognosis. Therefore, it is important to explore effective biomarkers and therapeutic targets for HCC patients. Autophagy is involved in the development and prevention of cancer. Mammalian Beclin-1 is needed for an autophagic vesicle in HCC. Autophagy-related protein-5 (ATG5) is an important molecule involved in cell death during autophagy. The objective is to investigate serum ATG 5 and Beclin 1 levels in HCV-induced liver cirrhosis with and without HCC. The study was conducted on 80 individuals classified into 3 groups:

Group 1: 30 patients with HCV-induced liver cirrhosis without HCC.
Group 2: 30 patients with HCV-induced liver cirrhosis with HCC.
Group 3: 20 healthy subjects (control group).

Results: Serum ATG 5 was significantly lower in HCC than liver cirrhosis patients. Serum Beclin 1 was significantly higher in HCC than liver cirrhosis patients. A cutoff value of < 95.7 and > 5.3 of serum ATG5 and Beclin 1 could be suggested for diagnosis of HCC among patients with HCV-related cirrhosis.

Conclusion: Serum Beclin 1 and ATG 5 could be used as a novel diagnostic marker for HCC. Moreover, scoring of serum BECLIN 1, ATG 5, and cachexia might be a future promising tool to predict the risk of HCC development.

Keywords: Liver cirrhosis, Hepatocellular carcinoma, Hepatitis C virus, Serum Beclin 1, Serum ATG5

Background

Hepatocellular carcinoma (HCC) is the fifth most common cancer and the second most common cause of cancer-related death worldwide accounting for 7% of all cancers [1]. The most frequent risk factor for HCC is cirrhosis. All causes of cirrhosis can be complicated by HCC, but the risk increased in patients with viral hepatitis. Moreover, around one-third of cirrhotic patients will develop HCC during lifetime [2]. The autophagic response is deregulated in chronic liver conditions which can develop HCC [3].

Autophagy has a pro-survival function during HCC. Increased autophagy flux was detected in advanced cases of HCC and an increased autophagy response was found to be associated with malignant development and poor prognosis of HCC [4, 5]. Autophagy helps HCC invasion by having effect on the epithelial–mesenchymal transition [6]. It explains why HCC develops in cirrhotic liver rather than in normal liver.

BECLIN1 is a dual function molecule which acts as a tumor suppressor and autophagy regulator [7]. Mice with alteration of BECLIN1 showed a decreased

*Correspondence: saharbadawy70@gmail.com
[1] Tropical Medicine Department, Faculty of Medicine, Alexandria University, Alexandria, Egypt
Full list of author information is available at the end of the article

autophagy activity and the formation of malignant lesions like HCC [8].

Autophagy-related protein-5 (ATG5) can control autophagy. Calpain 1 is a calcium-dependent non-lysosomal cysteine protease that digests ATG5 [9]. Low intracellular calcium levels decrease the cleavage activity of Calpain 1, increase the level of ATG5 and ATG12-ATG5 and increase autophagy [10]. MicroRNA (miR181a) interacts with a miRNA response element in the 3′ untranslated region (UTR) of *ATG5*, which inhibits its transcription. Increased expression of miR181a decreases *ATG5* mRNA and protein levels, resulting in autophagy inhibition [11].

The aim of the work is to evaluate the level of serum Beclin1 and serum ATG5 among cirrhotic hepatitis C virus patients with and without hepatocellular carcinoma.

Subjects

This study was conducted on 80 individuals admitted to the Tropical Medicine Department of Alexandria Main University Hospital during the period from October 2018 to January 2020 who were divided into 3 groups:

Group 1: 30 patients with HCV-induced liver cirrhosis without HCC
Group 2: 30 patients with HCV-induced liver cirrhosis with HCC
Group 3: 20 healthy subjects of matched age and sex as control

Informed consent was taken from every participant in this study.

Exclusion criteria

Patients with chronic HBV infection, any other identifiable cause of chronic hepatitis other than HCV, and patients with any suspected malignancies other than HCC, diabetes mellitus, chronic kidney disease, coronary disease, organ transplantation, and autoimmune hepatitis were excluded.

Methods

All participants were subjected to a detailed history taking and clinical assessment. The presence or absence of cirrhosis and HCC existence were documented by an ultrasound followed by a triphasic CT for those who had suspected focal hepatic lesions.

Serum AFP [12], Beclin 1 [13], and ATG 5 [14] levels were measured by using an enzyme linked immunosorbent assay (ELISA) according to the manufacturer's instructions.

Statistical analysis of the data [15]

Data were fed to the computer and analyzed using IBM SPSS software package version 20.0 [16]. Qualitative data were described using number and percent. Quantitative data were described using range (minimum and maximum), mean, standard deviation, and median. Comparison between the three studied groups regarding categorical variables was tested using Chi-square test.

For normally distributed data, comparison between the three studied groups was analyzed, *F*-test (ANOVA) to be used and post hoc test (Scheffe). For abnormally distributed data, comparison between two independent population were done using Mann–Whitney test while Kruskal–Wallis test was used to compare between the three studied groups and pair wise comparison was assessed using Mann–Whitney test. Correlations between two quantitative variables were assessed using Spearman coefficient.

Receiver operating characteristic curve (ROC) was plotted to analyze a recommended cutoff for the 3 markers; the area under the ROC curve denotes the diagnostic performance of the test. Multivariate logistic regression was performed.

Results

Table 1 lists the demographic data between liver cirrhosis, HCC patients, and control group as regards age, sex, MELD score, Child–Pugh score, and BCLC.

In cirrhotic patients, the number of patients with cachexia was 7 out of 30 with 23.3%. In HCC patients, the number of patients with cachexia was 17 out of 30 with 56.7%. There was higher statistical significance of cachexia in patients with HCC than patients with liver cirrhosis (p value < 0.001) as shown in Table 2.

In HCC patients, 15 patients preseAls with portal vein thrombosis (PV). As regards multicentricity, there were 20 patients that presented with multiple lesions of HCC lesions, while 10 patients presented with single lesion as shown Table 3.

Serum alpha-fetoprotein was significantly higher in HCC patients than cirrhotic patients and control group (p 0.025, $p < 0.001$*). Also, there was statistically significant difference between cirrhosis and control group (p value 0.001) as shown in Table 4.

Serum ATG 5 was significantly lower in patients with HCC than in patients with cirrhosis and control group (p value 0.022, p value 0.001). But there was no statistically significant difference between patients with cirrhosis than control individuals (p value 0.258) as shown in Table 5.

Serum Beclin 1 was significantly higher in HCC patients than cirrhotic patients and control group (p

Table 1 Comparison between the three studied groups according to different parameters

	Cirrhotic (n = 30)	HCC (n = 30)	Control (n = 20)	Test of Sig	p
Sex					
Male	15 (50%)	19 (63.3%)	10 (50%)	χ^2 = 1.347	0.510
Female	15 (50%)	11 (36.7%)	10 (50%)		
Age (years)					
Mean ± SD	58.1 ± 6.8	55.3 ± 6	54.3 ± 4.6	F = 2.881	0.062
Median (Min. – Max.)	56.5 (48 – 75)	54 (45 – 65)	52.5 (48 – 62)		
MELD					
Mean ± SD	15.1 ± 4.9	18.9 ± 5.3	–	t = 2.879*	0.006*
Median (Min. – Max.)	15 (7 – 24)	19 (10 – 31)	–		
Child Pugh					
A	6 (20%)	3 (10%)	–	χ^2 = 1.344	^{MC}p = 0.539
B	13 (43.3%)	13 (43.3%)	–		
C	11 (36.7%)	14 (46.7%)	–		
Mean ± SD	8.9 ± 2.75	9.5 ± 2.3	–	U = 385.0	0.331
Median (Min. – Max.)	9 (5 – 14)	9 (5 – 14)	–		
BCLC					
A		3			
B		9			
C		4			
D		14			

χ^2: Chi square test; MC: Monte Carlo; F: F for ANOVA test

U: Mann Whitney test; t: Student t-test

H: H for Kruskal Wallis test, Pairwise comparison bet. each 2 groups were done using Post Hoc Test (Dunn's for multiple comparisons test)

p: p value for comparing between the studied groups

*: Statistically significant at p ≤ 0.05

Table 2 Comparison between the three studied groups according to cachexia

Cachexia	Cirrhotic (n = 30)		HCC (n = 30)		Control (n = 20)		χ^2	p
	No	%	No	%	No	%		
No cachexia	23	76.7	13	43.3	20	100.0	19.365*	< 0.001*
Yes	7	23.3	17	56.7	0	0.0		

2 : Chi square test

p: p value for comparing between the three studied groups

*: Statistically significant at p ≤ 0.05

Table 3 Distribution of the studied cases according to CT findings in HCC group (n = 30)

CT findings	No	%
PV Thrombosis	15	50.0
Number of lesions		
Single	10	33.3
Multiple	20	66.7

value < 0.001, *p* value 0.001). But there was no statistically significant difference between patients with cirrhosis than control individuals (*p* value 0.20) as shown in Table 6.

The diagnostic performance, cutoff point, sensitivity, specificity, PPV, NPV, and accuracy for discriminating HCC from liver cirrhosis for ATG5, Becline 1, and AFP were shown in Table 7. Receiver operating characteristic

Table 4 Comparison between the three studied groups according to AFP

AFP (ng/ml)	Cirrhotic (n = 30)	HCC (n = 30)	Control (n = 20)	H	p
Min. – Max	4.0 – 200.0	8.0 – 3200.0	4.0 – 12.0	39.415*	0.001*
Mean ± SD	39.60 ± 47.44	442.4 ± 809.4	7.02 ± 2.33		
Median	15.0	48.50	5.0		
IQR	10.0 – 50.0	14.0 – 800.0	6.0 – 9.0		
Sig. bet. grps	p1 = 0.025*, p2 = 0.510, p3 < 0.001*				

H: H for Kruskal Wallis test, Pairwise comparison bet. each 2 groups were done using Post Hoc Test (Dunn's for multiple comparisons test)

p: p value for comparing between the studied groups

p_1: p value for comparing between Cirrhotic and HCC

p_2: p value for comparing between Cirrhotic and Control

p_3: p value for comparing between HCC and Control

*: Statistically significant at $p \le 0.05$

curves (ROC curves) were done to estimate the cutoff points for ATG5, Becline 1, and AFP for predicting the probability for HCC as shown in Fig. 1.

The diagnostic performance for combined ATG5, Beclin1, and AFP for detection of HCC from cirrhosis was significant, its diagnostic performance was 0.833* ($p < 0.001$*), with sensitivity of 96.7%, specificity of 63.3%, positive predictive value of 72.5%, negative predictive value of 95%, and accuracy of 80% as shown in Table 8.

Cachexia, ATG 5 level, Beclin 1, level, AFP, and Child–Pugh score were entered in a stepwise logistic regression model; the significant variables were cachexia ($P < 0.031$*), ATG 5 ($P < 0.009$*), and Beclin 1 level ($P < 0.018$*); on the other hand, the Child–Pugh score was insignificant in the multivariate analysis ($P = 0.931$) and AFP ($P = 0.620$) as shown in Table 9.

Prognostic fidelity was improved when combining these parameters in a scoring system with ATG 5 < 95.7, Beclin1 > 5.3, and presence of cachexia. Cachexia was

Table 5 Comparison between the three studied groups according to ATG5

ATG5(ng/ml)	Cirrhotic (n = 30)	HCC (n = 30)	Control (n = 20)	H	p
Min. – Max	44.0 – 256.5	11.0 – 149.5	64.40 – 186.6	11.080*	0.004*
Mean ± SD	100.8 ± 50.18	74.08 ± 32.52	109.2 ± 34.60		
Median	98.0	69.50	98.50		
IQR	62.10 – 116.6	49.70 – 95.70	84.95 – 133.60		
Sig. bet. grps	$p_1 = 0.022^*$, $p_2 = 0.258$, $p_3 = 0.001^*$				

H: H for Kruskal Wallis test, Pairwise comparison bet. each 2 groups were done using Post Hoc Test (Dunn's for multiple comparisons test)

p: p value for comparing between the studied groups

p_1: p value for comparing between Cirrhotic and HCC

p_2: p value for comparing between Cirrhotic and Control

p_3: p value for comparing between HCC and Control

*: Statistically significant at $p \le 0.05$

Table 6 Comparison between the three studied groups according to BECLIN1

BECLIN1 (ng/ml)	Cirrhotic (n = 30)	HCC (n = 30)	Control (n = 20)	H	p
Min. – Max	1.20–12.0	3.90 – 19.80	0.70–13.60	22.344*	< 0.001*
Mean ± SD	5.62 ± 2.46	8.65 ± 3.30	4.49 ± 3.06		
Median	5.25	7.90	4.70		
IQR	4.15 – 6.95	6.20 – 10.40	3.10 – 6.60		
Sig. bet. grps	$p_1 < 0.001^*$, $p_2 = 0.200$, $p_3 = 0.001^*$				

H: H for Kruskal Wallis test, Pairwise comparison bet. each 2 groups were done using Post Hoc Test (Dunn's for multiple comparisons test)

p: p value for comparing between the studied groups

p_1: p value for comparing between Cirrhotic and HCC

p_2: p value for comparing between Cirrhotic and Control

p_3: p value for comparing between HCC and Control

*: Statistically significant at $p \le 0.05$

Table 7 Agreement (sensitivity, specificity) for ATG5, BECLIN1 and AFP to diagnose HCC patients from Cirrhotic

	AUC	p	95% C. I		Cut off[#]	Sensitivity	Specificity	PPV	NPV	Accuracy
			LL	UL						
ATG5(ng/ml)	0.670	0.024[*]	0.534	0.806	≤95.7	76.67	53.33	62.2	69.6	65.0
BECLIN1(ng/ml)	0.824	<0.001[*]	0.715	0.933	>5.3	93.33	66.67	73.7	90.9	80.0
AFP(ng/ml)	0.659	0.034[*]	0.521	0.798	>70	26.7	83.3	61.5	54.2	49.3
p value for comparative	ATG5 vs. BECLIN1 Z=1.623, p=0.105									
	ATG5 vs. AFP Z=0.104, p=0.917									
	BECLIN1 vs. AFP Z=1.830, p=0.067									

AUC: Area Under a Curve; p value: Probability value

CI: Confidence Intervals

NPV: Negative predictive value; PPV: Positive predictive value

[*]: Statistically significant at p ≤ 0.05

[#] Cut off was choose according to Youden index

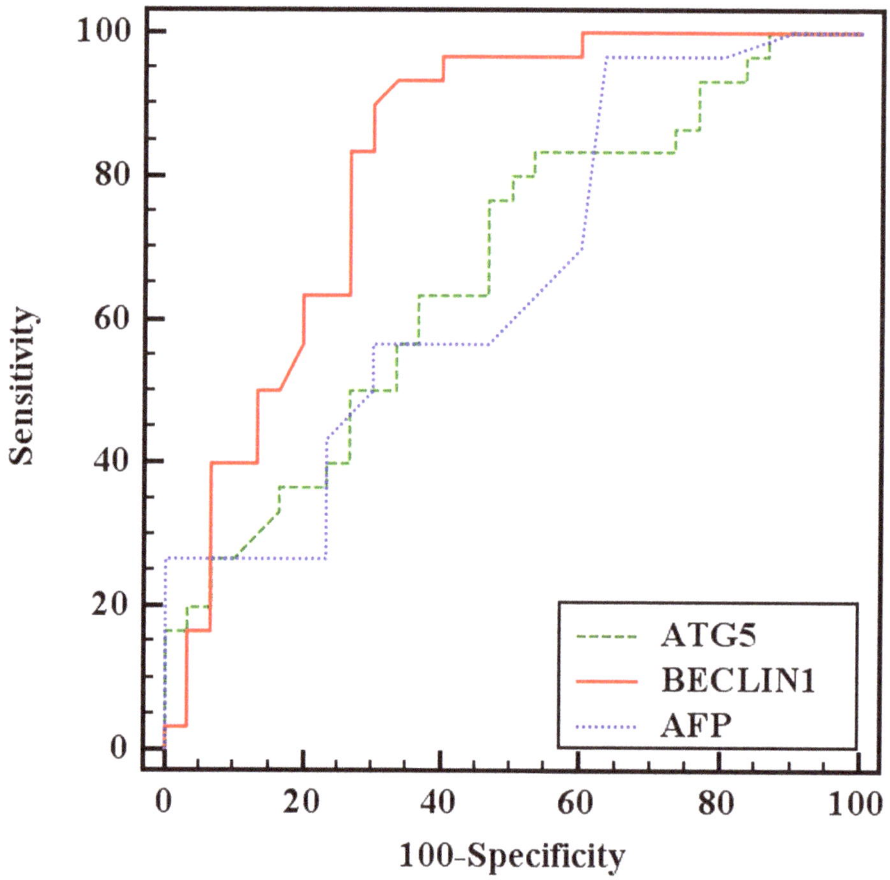

Fig. 1 ROC curve for AFP, ATG5, and BECLIN1 to diagnose HCC patients from cirrhotic patients

assigned 1 point, ATG 5<95.7 was assigned 1 point, and Beclin1>5.3 was given 2. So cachexia, ATG 5, and Beclin1 level were identified as being independently predicting HCC.

The score ranged from 0 to 4 with a cutoff point 2 to predict HCC. At cutoff 2 scoring points, the PPV was 83.3% and NPV was 75.8%, with (sensitivity 70, specificity 94%) as shown in Tables 10 and 11.

Table 8 Agreement (sensitivity, specificity) for Combined AFP, ATG5 and BECLIN1 to diagnose HCC patients from Cirrhotic

Combined	AUC	p	95% C. I		Sensitivity	Specificity	PPV	NPV	Accuracy
			LL	UL					
ATG5 & BECLIN1& AFP	0.833	< 0.001*	0.730	0.937	96.7	63.3	72.5	95.0	80.0

AUC: Area Under a Curve p value: Probability value

CI: Confidence Intervals

NPV: Negative predictive value PPV: Positive predictive value

*: Statistically significant at $p \leq 0.05$

Table 9 Multivariate analysis logistic regression for predict HCC

Parameters	B (weight)	Sig	OR	95% CI	
				LL	UL
Cachexia	1.348	0.031*	3.850	1.128	13.148
ATG5 (ng/ml)	1.288	0.009*	3.619	1.376	9.521
BECLIN.1(ng/ml)	1.70	0.018*	5.460	1.340	22.244
Child class	0.076	0.931	0.926	0.164	5.230
AFP(ng/ml)	-0.475	0.620	0.622	0.095	4.075

Table 10 Cutoff and scoring points for the different parameters

Parameters	Cutoff	Scoring points
Cachexia	-	1
ATG5(ng/dl)	95.7	1
BECLIN.1(ng/dl)	5.3	2

Table 11 Cutoffs, sensitivity and specificity for the total score

Criterion	Sensitivity	Specificity	+PV	-PV
≥0	100.00	0.00	37.5	
>0	80.00	58.00	53.3	82.9
>1	63.33	76.00	61.3	77.6
>2	70.00	94.00	83.3	75.8
>3	30.00	98.00	90.0	70.0
>4	0.00	100.00		62.5

Discussion

Hepatocellular carcinoma (HCC) counts around 90% of primary liver cancers. The poor prognosis of patients with HCC is due to a late diagnosis. Therefore, it is important to detect new biomarkers which can be used as complements or substitutes for AFP in HCC diagnosis and to be a proper tool for assessment of tumor spread and patient prognosis as these markers can be a tool for HCC treatment and outcomes [17, 18].

Autophagy is a degradation of lysosomes which is important for cell survival under starvation, stress, and infection. The mechanism is regenerating of energy from intracellular materials (cytoplasm, organelles, protein aggregates, etc.) to meet energy requirements in low-nutritional conditions [19].

In this study, serum ATG 5 was significantly lower in patients with HCC than in patients with cirrhosis, but there was no statistically significant difference between patients with cirrhosis than control individuals. The ROC curve for ATG5 for detection of HCC from cirrhosis was significant, its diagnostic performance was 0.670* (p < 0.024*), and the cutoff point discriminating HCC from liver cirrhosis was < 95.7 with sensitivity of 76.6%, specificity of 53.33%, positive predictive value of 62.2%, negative predictive value of 69.9%, and accuracy of 65%.

This is in concordance with Yang et al. [20] who found that Atg5 were decreased in human HCC tissue in comparison with control tissue which suggests that autophagy is decreased in HCC. Also, this result is consistent with findings in Takamura et al.'s [21] study that autophagy might be a suppressor mechanism in HCC. Therefore, autophagic deficiency increases tumor growth in HCC.

In this study, serum Beclin 1 was significantly higher in HCC patients than patients with cirrhosis but there was no statistically significant difference between patients with cirrhosis than control individuals (p value < 0.001).

The ROC curve for Beclin 1 for detection of HCC from liver cirrhosis was significant, its diagnostic performance was 0.824 (p < 0.001), and the cutoff point discriminating HCC from cirrhosis was > 5.3 with sensitivity of 93.33, specificity of 66.67%, positive predictive value of 73.3%, negative predictive value of 90.9%, and accuracy of 80%.

In contrast to the results of Qiu et al. [22] that have detected that Beclin1 expression in HCC is significantly lower than that in normal and cirrhotic tissues. They have also shown that Beclin1 expression is correlated with liver cirrhosis and vascular invasion but not with TNM stage, AFP level, number of tumors, and capsule.

In this study, we developed a simple score that consisted of routinely available clinical and laboratory parameters to predict the risk of HCC in patients with HCV-related cirrhosis. This prediction score is accurate. The score ranged from 0 to 4, it is composed of Cachexia which was assigned 1 point since its estimated coefficient in logistic regression model was 1.348, ATG 5 < 95.7 was assigned 1 point as its estimated coefficient I logistic regression model was 1.288, and Beclin 1 > 5.3 was given 2 points for its estimated coefficient in logistic regression model was 1.7.

A cutoff point 2 is used to predict HCC in HCV-related cirrhotic patients. At cutoff value of 2 scoring points, the PPV was 83.3% and NPV was 75.8%. Using a cutoff of 2 points led to false negative results in 4 out of 30 with HCC (sensitivity 70%, specificity 94%).

Compared with current guidelines, the prediction score provides more systematic stratification of HCC risk [23, 24].

The score suggests that patients with cachexia can predict the development of HCC. And this is consistent with Nozoe et al. [25], who used the prognostic nutritional index (PNI) as a prognostic marker in a number of gastrointestinal malignancies, and more recently, in a study by Proctor et al. [26], the PNI was found to affect the prognosis in malignancy regardless of the site of origin.

Also, in this study, assessment of serum marker may have the advantage of being noninvasive rather than other studies in which assessment of Beclin 1 and ATG 5 used the invasive technique by liver biopsy.

Conclusion

Serum Beclin 1 and ATG 5 could be used as a novel diagnostic marker for HCC. Moreover, scoring of serum BECLIN 1, ATG 5, and cachexia might be a future promising tool to predict the risk of HCC development.

Limitation of this study

Small number of patients therefore studying on a large number of patients could be suggested.

Recommendation

Wide sample sizes are suggested to validate this result.

Abbreviations

HCV: Hepatitis C virus; HCC: Hepatocellular carcinoma; ATG 5: Autophagy-related protein 5; BCLC: Barcelona Clinic Liver Cancer.

Acknowledgements

The authors are thankful to the Tropical Medicine Department, Faculty of Medicine, Alexandria University.

Authors' contributions

SB was responsible for the practical section, analysis of data, and manuscript preparation. The authors read and approved the final manuscript.

Declarations

Ethics approval and consent to participate

The Ethical Committee (EC) at our institution approved the study. The EC has FWA since 2010 and operates according to the ICH GCP guidelines and applicable local and institutional regulations and guidelines (serial number of ethical approval 0201134) (FWA no. 00018699 expires January 21, 2026) (IRB no. 00012098 expires June 10, 2022). Patients included in the study signed an informed written consent to participate.

Competing interests

The authors declare that they have no competing interests.

Author details

[1]Tropical Medicine Department, Faculty of Medicine, Alexandria University, Alexandria, Egypt. [2]Clinical Pathology Department, Faculty of Medicine, Alexandria University, Alexandria, Egypt.

References

1. Akinyemiju T, Abera S, Ahmed M, Alam N, Alemayohu MA, Allen C, Al-Raddadi R, Alvis-Guzman N, Amoako Y et al (2017) The burden of primary liver cancer and underlying etiologies from 1990 to 2015 at the global, regional, and national level: results from the Global Burden of Disease Study 2015. JAMA Oncol 3(12):1683–1691
2. Sangiovanni A, Prati GM, Fasani P, Ronchi G, Romeo R, Manini M, Del Ninno E, Morabito A, Colombo M (2006) The natural history of compensated cirrhosis due to hepatitis C virus: A 17-year cohort study of 214 patients. Hepatology 43(6):1303–1310
3. Dash S, Chava S, Chandra PK, Aydin Y, Balart LA, Wu T (2016) Autophagy in hepatocellular carcinomas: from pathophysiology to therapeutic response. Hepat Med 8:9–20
4. Lazova R, Camp RL, Klump V, Siddiqui SF, Amaravadi RK, Pawelek JM (2012) Punctate LC3B expression is a common feature of solid tumors and associated with proliferation, metastasis, and poor outcome. Clin Cancer Res 18(2):370–379
5. Wu DH, Jia CC, Chen J, Lin ZX, Ruan DY, Li X, Lin Q, Min D, Ma XK et al (2014) Autophagic LC3B overexpression correlates with malignant progression and predicts a poor prognosis in hepatocellular carcinoma. Tumour Biol 35(12):12225–12233
6. Li J, Yang B, Zhou Q, Wu Y, Shang D, Guo Y, Song Z, Zheng Q, Xiong J (2013) Autophagy promotes hepatocellular carcinoma cell invasion through activation of epithelial-mesenchymal transition. Carcinogenesis 34(6):1343–1351
7. Liang XH, Yu J, Brown K, Levine B (2001) Beclin 1 contains a leucine-rich nuclear export signal that is required for its autophagy and tumor suppressor function. Cancer Res 61(8):3443–3449
8. Qu X, Yu J, Bhagat G, Furuya N, Hibshoosh H, Troxel A, Rosen J, Eskelinen EL, Mizushima N et al (2003) Promotion of tumorigenesis by heterozygous disruption of the beclin 1 autophagy gene. J Clin Invest 112(12):1809–1820
9. Yousefi S, Perozzo R, Schmid I, Ziemiecki A, Schaffner T, Scapozza L, Brunner T, Simon HU (2006) Calpain-mediated cleavage of Atg5 switches autophagy to apoptosis. Nat Cell Biol 8(10):1124–1132
10. Xia HG, Zhang L, Chen G, Zhang T, Liu J, Jin M, Ma X, Ma D, Yuan J (2010) Control of basal autophagy by calpain1 mediated cleavage of ATG5. Autophagy 6(1):61–66
11. Tekirdag KA, Korkmaz G, Ozturk DG, Agami R, Gozuacik D (2013) MIR181A regulates starvation- and rapamycin-induced autophagy through targeting of ATG5. Autophagy 9(3):374–385
12. Medline plus (2020) Alpha-fetoprotein (AFP) test. https://medlineplus.gov/lab-tests/alpha-fetoprotein-afp-test/. Accessed 28 April 2021.
13. Novus Biologicals (2020) Novus Biologicals. Human Beclin 1 ELISA Kit (Colorimetric). https://www.novusbio.com/products/beclin-1-elisa-kit_nbp2-69959;2020. Accessed 28 April 2021.

14. Cloud-Clone Corp (2020) SEL221Hu 96 tests enzyme-linked immunosorbent assay kit for autophagy related protein 5 (ATG5) organism species: *Homo sapiens* (human) instruction manual. http://www.cloud-clone.com/manual/ELISA-Kit-for-Autophagy-Related-Protein-5-(ATG5)-SEL221Hu.pdf. Accessed 6 March 2020.
15. Kotz S, Balakrishnan N, Read CB, Vidakovic B (2006) Encyclopedia of statistical sciences. 2nd ed. Wiley-Interscience, Hoboken, N.J.
16. Kirkpatrick LA, Feeney BC (2013) A simple guide to IBM SPSS statistics for version 20.0. Student ed. Wadsworth, Cengage Learning, Belmont, Calif.
17. Kim DY, Han KH (2012) Epidemiology and surveillance of hepatocellular carcinoma. Liver Cancer 1(1):2–14
18. Zhu K, Dai Z, Zhou J (2013) Biomarkers for hepatocellular carcinoma: progression in early diagnosis, prognosis, and personalized therapy. Biomark Res 1(1):10
19. He C, Klionsky DJ (2009) Regulation mechanisms and signaling pathways of autophagy. Annu Rev Genet 43:67–93
20. Yang J, He Y, Zhai N, Ding S, Li J, Peng Z (2018) MicroRNA-181a inhibits autophagy by targeting Atg5 in hepatocellular carcinoma. Front Biosci (Landmark Ed) 23:388–396
21. Takamura A, Komatsu M, Hara T, Sakamoto A, Kishi C, Waguri S, Eishi Y, Hino O, Tanaka K et al (2011) Autophagy-deficient mice develop multiple liver tumors. Genes Dev 25(8):795–800
22. Qiu DM, Wang GL, Chen L, Xu YY, He S, Cao XL, Qin J, Zhou JM, Zhang YX et al (2014) The expression of beclin-1, an autophagic gene, in hepatocellular carcinoma associated with clinical pathological and prognostic significance. BMC Cancer 14:327
23. Ueno S, Tanabe G, Sako K, Hiwaki T, Hokotate H, Fukukura Y, Baba Y, Imamura Y, Aikou T (2001) Discrimination value of the new western prognostic system (CLIP score) for hepatocellular carcinoma in 662 Japanese patients. Cancer of the Liver Italian Program. Hepatology 34(3):529–534.
24. Bruix J, Sherman M (2005) Management of hepatocellular carcinoma. Hepatology 42(5):1208–1236
25. Nozoe T, Kohno M, Iguchi T, Mori E, Maeda T, Matsukuma A, Ezaki T (2012) The prognostic nutritional index can be a prognostic indicator in colorectal carcinoma. Surg Today 42(6):532–535
26. Proctor MJ, Morrison DS, Talwar D, Balmer SM, Fletcher CD, O'Reilly DS, Foulis AK, Horgan PG, McMillan DC (2011) A comparison of inflammation-based prognostic scores in patients with cancer. A Glasgow Inflammation Outcome Study. Eur J Cancer 47(17):2633–2641

15

Effect of directly acting anti-viral agents on immunological imprints in chronic HCV-4a patients: interleukin-10 and vascular endothelial growth factor genes expression level

Iman S. Naga[1*], Amel Abdel Fattah Kamel[2], Said Ahmed Ooda[3], Hadeer Muhammad Fath Elbab[2] and Rania Mohamed El-Sharkawy[2]

Abstract

Background: Hepatitis C virus infection is a global health challenge with Egypt being one of the highly affected countries. IL-10 has been suggested as a suitable marker to assess necroinflammation and to monitor the progression of liver damage. Vascular endothelial growth factor (VEGF) is a potent angiogenic factor playing a central role in many physiological as well as pathological processes. Several factors can be predictive of the response to treatment and achievement of SVR; some of which are host-related, and others are virus-related. The gene expression of IL-10 and VEGF have multiple effects for treatment response. The aim of the present work was to study the effect of treatment with directly acting agents (DAA) on the expression of VEGF and IL-10 genes in chronic hepatitis C virus-infected Egyptian genotype-4a patients. Twenty-five HCV subjects where evaluated for IL-10 and VEGF gene expression before and after treatment with DAA.

Results: IL-10 expression was downregulated in 92% of the cases. VEGF expression was heterogeneous showing spreading of values along a wide range with 64% of the cases being downregulated.

Conclusion: DAAs do not completely reverse the immunological imprints established upon chronic HCV infection.

Keywords: HCV, VEGF, IL-10, Gene expression, Genotype-4, DAA

Background

Hepatitis C virus (HCV) infection is a global health challenge with Egypt being one of the highly affected countries [1]. HCV genome exhibits significant genetic variability which leads to its classification into 7 major genotypes and up to 67 different subtypes. This genetic variability affects the response to treatment and the virus capability to escape the immune surveillance [2]. Genotype 4 is the most common genotype in Egypt [3].

In 2018, a meta-analysis for HCV viremic rate among the Egyptian population indicated that HCV prevalence was estimated by 11.9% among the general population; 67% of them are chronically infected and are in need for treatment [4].

Both innate and adaptive immune responses are essential for viral clearance. The innate response is the first line of defense during infection [5]. Cytokines play an important role in viral clearance, inflammation, regeneration, and fibrosis. Interleukin 10 (IL-10) and vascular

* Correspondence: iman.naga@alexu.edu.eg; imannaga80@gmail.com
[1]Department of Microbiology, Medical Research Institute, University of Alexandria, Alexandria, Egypt
Full list of author information is available at the end of the article

endothelial growth factor (VEGF) are key players in the immune response against HCV infection. Both are seen elevated in patients with HCV, cirrhosis, and HCC and their levels are associated with disease progression and prognosis [6]. IL-10 can also be used as a marker to assess necroinflammation and to monitor the progression of liver damage [7]. High levels of IL-10 are associated with Th-2-like response which leads to viral persistence and chronicity. Moreover, IL-10 inhibits Th-1-like response that is responsible for viral clearance after acute infection [8].

The adaptive immune response through CD4+T cells has a central role in induction of anti-viral immune response against viral infection which can be subdivided according to two predominant profiles referred to as T helper 1 (Th1)-like and T helper 2 (Th2)-like responses. Th1-like responses include the secretion of IL-2, TNF-α, and IFN-γ which are required for generation of cytotoxic T lymphocytes and activation of natural killer (NK) cells, while Th2-like responses produce IL-4 and IL-10, which inhibit development of the Th1 response [9]. In early HCV infection, those who clear the infection have significant Th1 responses with high IFN- γ and IL-2, while those who progress to chronicity have a significantly high magnitude of IL-10 and significantly higher ratio of IL-10 to IFN-γ production early in infection and along the course of the disease [10].

VEGF is a potent angiogenic factor playing a central role in many physiological as well as pathological processes. VEGFs exert their effects by activation of different signaling pathways stimulating endothelial cell proliferation and migration and increasing the vascular permeability [11, 12]. It is a powerful mitogen for microvascular and macrovascular endothelial cells. VEGF reduces hepatocellular tight junction (TJ) integrity and hepatocellular polarity through a VEGFR-2 dependent pathway [13]. The increased hepatic angiogenesis in chronic HCV could provide the molecular basis for liver carcinogenesis and contribute to the increased risk of HCC in patients with cirrhosis on top of HCV [14].

"The goal of treatment of HCV-infected persons is to reduce mortality and liver-related health adverse consequences, including end-stage liver disease and hepatocellular carcinoma, by the achievement of virologic cure as evidenced by a sustained virologic response." as recommended by the EASL-IDSA. The introduction of the directly acting anti-viral agents (DAAs) in the treatment of chronic HCV infections has led to dramatic improvement in outcome of HCV-infected patients [15].

The present work aimed to study the effect of treatment with directly acting agents (DAA) on the expression of VEGF and interleukin-10 genes in chronic HCV-infected patients in Alexandria, Egypt.

Methods

After the approval of the Ethical Committee of the Medical Research Institute, 25 chronic HCV genotype-4-infected patients were selected from the Department of Experimental and Clinical Internal Medicine, Medical Research Institute, Alexandria University. An informed consent was taken from each patient. The 25 HCV-positive patients were assessed before and after the end of DAA treatment. Exclusion criteria included co-infection with HBV infection, co-morbidities with renal or cardiac diseases, having any malignancies, and any immunological disorders.

The 25 HCV-positive patients were diagnosed by positive anti-HCV test result and confirmed by measuring the viral load by real-time polymerase chain reaction (PCR). The patients received sofosbuvir/ledipasvir once daily for 12 weeks. Virological response was assessed at the end of treatment. In this prospective study, the following was performed for all patients:

Complete physical examination

Abdominal examination for signs of hepatic failure as ascites. Abdominal ultrasound to confirm the presence or absence of cirrhosis and any liver mass if present and Child-Pugh classification [16].

Blood sampling

Sampling was performed at baseline and at the end of treatment. Ten milliliters of venous blood was withdrawn from each patient and divided into different vacutainers for molecular studies, coagulation studies, and complete blood count. Sera was separated for the determination of the concentrations of serum levels of albumin [17], total and direct bilirubin [18], and serum activities of the enzymes alanine and aspartate aminotransferases using fully automated chemistry analyzer Beckman AU400 [19, 20]. Also, plasma prothrombin activity (PT) was done [21].

Determination of HCV viral load

Viral RNA was extracted from patients' sera using QIAamp viral RNA mini spin Kit (Qiagen®) according to manufacturer's instructions. The extracted viral RNA was used as a template for HCV viral load determination before initiation of treatment and 12 weeks after treatment using Artus HCV QS-RGQ-PCR Kit (Qiagen®) and real-time PCR machine MX3000 TM (Stratagene) according to manufacturer's instructions [22].

Determination of HCV genotype

HCV genotype via amplification, sequencing, and nucleotide blasting of NS5b domain. Briefly, cDNA strand was synthesized from HCV RNA using RevertAid First Strand cDNA Synthesis Kit (Thermo Scientific) using random hexamer primers provided with the kit. NS5b domain was amplified using nested PCR primers JA 230 CTACCATCATGGCTAA(A/G)AA(C/T)GAGGT JA 233 ATGATGTTATGAGCTCCA(A/G)GTC(A/G)TA JA 231 TATGA(C/T)ACCCGCTG(C/T)TTTGAC 50 JA 232 CCTGGTCATAGCCTCCGTGAA. The PCR reaction was performed in 25 μl final reaction containing 2× DreamTaq green PCR master mix (Thermo Scientific, USA) and 5 μM of each primer and 1 μl of cDNA or first amplification. The thermal cycling consisted of 35 cycles of denaturation at 95 °C for 30 s, annealing at 50 °C for 30 s and extension at 72 °C for 30 s, and preceded by 1 cycle of initial denaturation at 95 °C for 5 min and followed by 1 cycle of final extension at 72 °C for 5 min. The same reaction was used for the second amplification (nested) in 50 μL final reaction volume containing 1 μL of the first amplification product as a template. The purified NS5b PCR products were sequenced using the BigDye Terminator V 3.1 Cycle Sequencing Kit (Applied Biosystems) on the automated sequencer ABI prism 310 genetic analyzers (Applied Biosystems). For determination of HCV genotypes and subtypes, NS5b sequencing results were analyzed using a HCV BLAST free online tool from HCV sequence database (https://hcv.lanl.gov/content/sequence/BASIC_BLAST/basic_blast.html).

IL-10 and VEGF relative gene expression:

Peripheral blood mononuclear cells (PBMC) were isolated from anticoagulated blood by Ficoll-Paque™ method then total RNA was purified from mononuclear cells using Qiagen RNeasy Mini Kit Spin Technology according to manufacturer's instructions. The concentration of RNA was determined using Nano Drop Thermo Spectrophotometry (Thermo Scientific) by measuring the absorbance at 260 nm A260. The purity of RNA was assessed using ratio A260/A280 ratio. Ratio between 1.7 and 1.9 was considered acceptable. Reverse transcription of 1 ug of RNA and effective genomic DNA elimination was performed by the Quantitect Reverse Transcription kit according to manufacturer's instructions then quantification of IL-10, VEGF, and GAPDH genes was performed using SBR-green real-time PCR. QuantiTect Primer Assays (Qiagen®) was used for accurate real-time quantification of target RNA. The reaction was performed in 20 μl final volume containing 10 μl Quantitect sybr green PCR Master Mix, 2 μl Quantitect primer assay, and 2.5 μl template cDNA on real-time PCR machine MX3000 TM (Stratagene). The reaction took place under the following thermal profile: initial incubation at 50 °C for 15 min to activate the DNA polymerase. This was followed by 45 cycles of 3 PCR-step amplification, denaturation at 94 °C for 15 s, followed by annealing at 57 °C for IL-10 and 60 °C for VEGF for 30 s, and followed by extension at 72 °C for 30 s, with real-time fluorescence detection.

Calculation of relative gene expression

Relative expression of target genes (IL-10, VEGF) was calculated using the comparative CT method ($2^{-\Delta\Delta CT}$ method) [23]. CT values of the target genes were normalized against the CT value of housekeeping gene (GAPDH). The fold changes after treatment was compared to the control group (before treatment) which was set to 1 [24].

Calculation of platelet ratio index (APRI) and fibrosis- (FIB-) 4 scores

Platelet ratio index (APRI) and fibrosis- (FIB-) 4 indexes were calculated using simple mathematical formulas as follows [25]:

$$\text{APRI} : (\text{AST [level]}/\text{AST[upper limit of normal]}/\text{platelet count } [109/\text{L}]) \times 100$$

For APRI, cut-off value of < 0.5 rules out fibrosis while ≥ 1 was assigned for marked fibrosis and ≥2 for cirrhosis.

$$\text{FIB–4} : \text{age [years]} \times (\text{AST [U/L] platelets} \times 109/\text{L}] \times \text{ALT}1/2\ [\text{U/L}]).$$

For FIB-4, a cut-off value of < 1.45 rules out advanced fibrosis while ≥ 3.25 was assigned for marked fibrosis.

Statistical analysis

Data were fed to the computer and analyzed using IBM SPSS software package version 20.0. (Armonk, NY: IBM Corp.). Qualitative data were described using number and percent. The Kolmogorov-Smirnov test was used to verify the normality of distribution. Quantitative data were described using range (minimum and maximum), mean, standard deviation, and median. Significance of the obtained results was judged at the 5% level. The Student *t* test was used for normally distributed quantitative variables to compare between two studied groups while Mann-Whitney test was used for abnormally distributed quantitative variables. Correlations between quantitative continuous variables parameters were evaluated by linear regression with analysis of Pearson's coefficients.

Results

A total of 25 HCV genotype-4-infected patients were enrolled in the present study; all of which (100%) were treatment-naïve cases. Females represented 52% (13/25) while males were 48% (12/25) and their ages ranged from 17 to 65 years.

There is a statistically significant difference between the ALT and AST activity as well as prothrombin activity (INR) before and after treatment in the studied cases

(p = 0.0003, p = 0.0001, p = 0.022, respectively). There is no correlation between the viral load and ALT and AST activity, albumin, bilirubin level (total and direct), or the studied hematological parameters before treatment (Table 1).

Child-Pugh score, APRI, and FIB-4 were calculated for all cases enrolled in the present study before treatment to estimate the severity of liver injury and the majority of the patients were categorized as Child-Pugh class (A) 88% (22/25), while class (B) were 12% (3/25), and none were classified as class (C). Additionally, APRI and FIB-4 were calculated for all cases in the present study as a non-invasive marker for assessment of hepatic fibrosis or cirrhosis before and after treatment. Before treatment, APRI ranged from 0.108 to 2.43 with a mean of 0.87 while FIB-4 ranged from 0.27 to 6.49 with a mean of 2.20. After treatment, APRI ranged from 0.214to 0.987 with a mean of 0.44 while FIB-4 ranged from 0.27 to 4.88 with a mean of 1.60. The difference between the APRI and FIB-4 scores before and after treatment was found statistically significant (p = 0.002, p = 0.048 for APRI and FIB-4, respectively).

Table 1 Hematological, chemical profile, and viral load of HCV patients before and after DAA treatment

	Before treatment	After treatment	*p* value
ALT (U/L)			
Min–max	13–135	4–35	0.0003*
Mean	46.40	21.08	
AST (U/L)			
Min–max	8–124	16–35	0.0001*
Mean	43.96	21.96	
Albumin (g/dl)			
Min–max	2.8–5.2	3.5–4.8	0.3310
Mean	3.98	4.04	
Total bilirubin (mg/dl)			
Min–max	0.3–3.05	0.3–1.2	0.406
Mean	0.73	0.67	
Direct bilirubin (mg/dl)			
Min–max	0.1–2.14	0.1–0.6	0.155
Mean	0.35	0.26	
Platelets count (× 10^3/μl)			
Min–max	40–304	55–266	0.481
Mean	178.08	177.28	
PT (INR)			
Min–max	1–1.9	1–1.2	0.022*
Mean	1.18	1.08	
HCV load (×10^5 IU/L)			
Min–max	0.241–130	Undetectable	–
Mean	13.22		

*Statistically significant at $p \leq 0.05$

The majority of HCV patients (80%) had a viral load ranging between > 10^5–< 10^7 IU/ml. The remaining 20% had a viral load < 10^5. NS5b region was successfully amplified and sequenced in all 25 patients included in this study. The 25 HCV patients involved in this study were genotyped as HCV genotype 4a.

As regards the relative expression of IL-10 (Fig. 1), 92% (23/25) of the cases showed downregulated expression and only 2 (8%) showed upregulated expression. As for the relative expression of VEGF (Figure 2), 64% (16/25) of the cases showed downregulated expression while 36% (9/25) of the cases showed upregulated expression (Table 2).

Correlation between IL-10 expression and the liver functions, hematological parameters, viral load, and calculated fibrosis scores before treatment shows a strong positive correlation with the viral load (r = 0.721, p = 0.0001) while other parameters show no correlation, while correlation between VEGF expression and liver functions, hematological parameters, viral load, and calculated fibrosis scores before treatment shows a positive correlation with AST activity (r = 0.573, p = 0.003) as well as with the viral load (r = 0.488, p = 0.013) while other parameters show no correlation (Table 3).

Correlation between IL-10 and VEGF expression and the liver functions (AST, ALT, bilirubin total and direct, albumin), hematological parameters (platelet count, INR), viral load, and calculated fibrosis scores (APRI and FIB-4) after treatment shows no correlation with any of the mentioned parameters.

Discussion

The use of DAAs for the treatment of viral hepatitis has led to dramatic improvement in outcome of HCV-infected patients. They target 3 main parts of viral particle NS3/4A protease, NS5A, and NS5B RNA-dependent polymerase [26].

In the current study, all HCV patients received sofosbuvir-based regimen for 12 weeks. The results showed that 100% of the cases (25/25) achieved SVR by the end of the treatment course confirmed by an undetectable PCR viral load. This is consistent with other studies that reported high SVR on sofosbuvir-based regimen. El Raziky et al. [27] had presented his results from a phase II open-label study (OSIRIS) conducted in Egypt on 63 patients with/without cirrhosis and has reported 100% SVR-12 for both groups. Similar results were reported by Lawitz et al. (2015) [28], Feld et al. [29], and Gayam et al. (2018) [30].

Although HCV RNA monitoring during HCV treatment has been a standard practice, aminotransferases (ALT and AST) monitoring is also important to assess

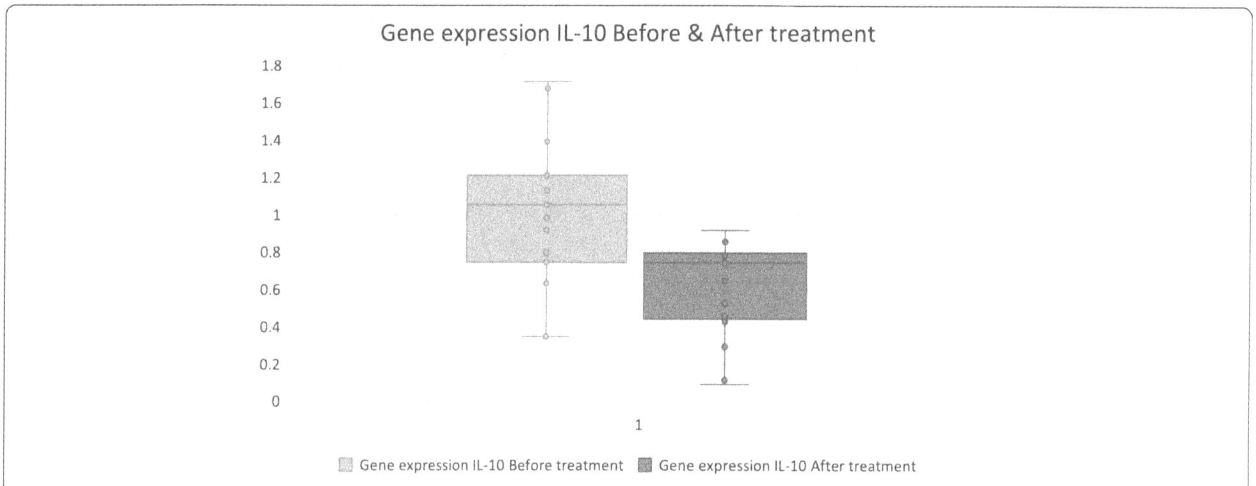

Fig. 1 Box plot showing the expression of IL-10 in HCV patients before and after DAA treatment

improvement of liver injury, drug side effects or interactions, and treatment response. Typically, SVR is accompanied by normalization of ALT, AST which reflects a positive response to therapy and subsequent reduction in risk for progressive cirrhosis and HCC [31]. In the present study, cases showed normalization of the mean of liver enzymes after treatment. There is a statistically significant difference between the ALT and AST activity before and after treatment. In agreement with these results, Huynh T et al. (2018) [32] assessed the dynamic patterns of both ALT and AST during and after DAA treatment for HCV infection and the study provided evidence that normalization of both ALT and AST is well associated with sustained HCV clearance and could be a potential biochemical marker to assess HCV treatment responses. In addition, some authors [31, 33] concluded that AST and ALT may serve as a more economical predictive factor for viral clearance for SVR.

Chronic HCV-infected patients are at high risk for development of advanced fibrosis as part of the natural course of the disease, 20% of patients will progress to advanced liver disease with cirrhosis or HCC [34]. In the present study, 12% of the cases were categorized by Child-Pugh score as class B while 88% were classified as class A. Before treatment, APRI index had a mean of 0.87 while the FIB-4 had a mean of 2.2. After treatment, APRI index showed a mean of 0.44 while the FIB-4 showed a mean of 1.6. The difference between the APRI score and FIB-4 index before and after treatment was statistically significant.

Bachofner et al. (2017) [35] measured the transient elastography (TE) and calculated the FIB-4 and APRI scores for 549 HCV patients who received a DAA-based treatment and reported that the cases recorded an improvement in liver stiffness recorded by TE and regression of validated fibrosis scores of the FIB-4 and APRI in

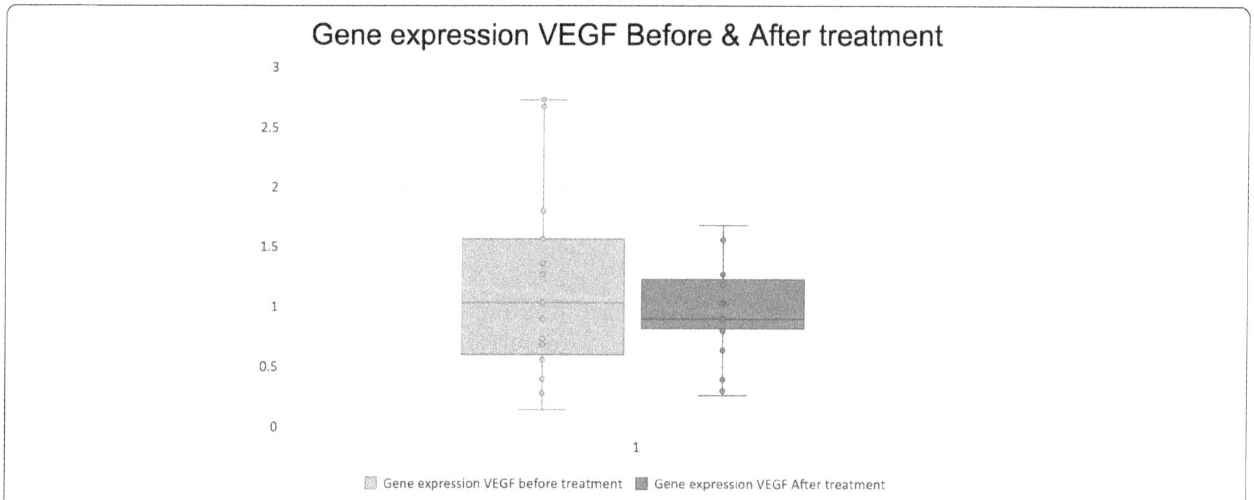

Fig. 2 Box plot showing the expression of VEGF in HCV patients before and after DAA treatment

Table 2 IL-10 and VEGF gene expression among HCV-infected patients

Gene expression	Number	%
IL-10		
< 1	23	92
> 1	2	8
Range	0.093-7.345	
Mean ± SD	1.00 ± 1.50	
VEGF		
< 1	16	64
> 1	9	36
Range	0.258–6.712	
Mean ± SD	1.32 ± 1.35	

concordance with the HCV eradication by DAAs. Additionally, Hengst et al. [36] reported a rapid decline in APRI and FIB-4 scores after treatment coinciding with HCV clearance. Although this study results are in concordance with the previous reported studies but these results raise a question of whether this improvement in liver status reflects a true regression of fibrosis or merely resolution of chronic liver inflammation as the course of improvement is too short for such significant remodeling in liver tissue and such improvement requires long-term follow-up to confirm it.

Several studies addressed the effect of DAAs on the host immune response indicating the reconstitution of innate immunity and downregulation of interferon (IFN) cell signaling after DAA treatment suggesting that the rapid reduction in viremia induced by DAAs may attenuate inflammation with minimizing effects on hepatitis progression [37].

The aim of the present study was to investigate the effect of DAAs on VEGF and IL-10 expression coinciding with the viral clearance. The information on the expression of VEGF and IL-10 mRNA is still incomplete and it has not yet been determined in cases of HCV genotype-4 under DAAs treatment which makes the approach of this study a novel one since other studies used the protein serum level [38, 39].

In the present study, the gene expression of IL-10 in HCV genotype-4 patients before and by the end of treatment with DAAs drugs was measured. IL-10 expression was downregulated in 92% (23/25) of the cases, while 8% (2/25) of the cases were upregulated with a range from 0.093 to 7.345. Despite of the apparent differences in expression levels within the studied group, the majority of the cases showed IL-10 down expression after DAA treatment coinciding with the viral clearance which can be explained by improvement of the inflammatory process ongoing with the persistent HCV infection and normalization of the liver functions. As for 2 cases who showed upregulation of IL-10 expression, they had the highest viral load of all the studied cases which may explain the delay in normalization of the immune response due the possible larger burden of the high viral load on the immune system of these 2 cases.

In this study, the data was grouped according to viral and host factors that influence or reflect progression of the disease, i.e., HCV RNA load, ALT, AST, and the stage of fibrosis. Before treatment, IL-10 showed a positive correlation with the HCV viral load which coincides with the previously mentioned reports linking high HCV replication with upregulation of IL-10 explained by inhibition effector T cell responses.

Several studies investigated the hypothesis that DAAs may modify the inflammatory pattern along the course of treatment. Saraiva et al. (2018) [40]; studied the dynamics of 30 different circulating cytokines and growth factors in HCV patients before DAA therapy initiation

Table 3 Correlation between IL-10 and VEGF gene expression with other studied variables before and after DAA treatment

	IL10 gene expression				VEGF gene expression			
	Before treatment		After treatment		Before treatment		After treatment	
	Pearson correlation	*p* value	Pearson correlation	*p* value	Pearson correlation	*p* value	Pearson correlation	*p* value
ALT	− 0.205	0.325	− 0.128	0.551	0.361	0.076	0.280	0.184
AST	− 0.192	0.358	− 0.172	0.421	**0.573****	**0.003**	0.269	0.204
Albumin	− 0.041	0.846	0.050	0.813	0.060	0.775	− 0.248	0.232
Total bilirubin	0.051	0.809	− 0.237	0.265	− 0.035	0.868	− 0.068	0.754
Direct bilirubin	− 0.004	0.986	− 0.228	0.284	− 0.173	0.409	− 0.227	0.286
PT (INR)	0.005	0.983	0.133	0.525	− 0.032	0.881	− 0.103	0.624
PLT	− 0.158	0.451	− 0.147	0.484	0.110	0.600	0.189	0,365
ASPRI	0.047	0.822	0.114	0.597	0.272	0.189	− 0.061	0.777
FIB-4	0.045	0.829	0.078	0.718	0.134	0.524	− 0.035	0.873

*Statistically significant at $p \leq 0.05$

and after the end of therapy. The study concluded that there was a decrease in IL-10 serum levels in association with viral clearance after DAA therapy suggesting that it could be explained by loss of the suppressive function of regulatory T cells (Treg) which secrets IL-10 and other anti-inflammatory cytokines. Also, Villani et al. [41]; confirmed that DAAs resulted in a very rapid decline in viremia and normalization of ALT in less than 4 weeks; together with remarkable decrease in serum IL-10 coinciding with the viral clearance indicating a systemic inflammatory pattern change occurring in chronic HCV patients with very long lasting inflammation. Moreover, Alhetheel et al. [42] reported that following successful treatment with DAAs, the IL-10 levels declined with a concomitant increase in the serum IL-12 levels.

On the other hand, Hengst et al. [36] study showed that treatment with DAAs showed a dramatic response in clearance of the viral load and normalization of ALT but the studied cytokines (including IL-10) showing a baseline increase in expression although had significantly decreased during and after therapy but they did not completely reach normal values suggesting that the inflammatory changes are not fully reversible upon viral clearance.

These conflicting results in literature could be attributed to the differences in the ability of each patient to trigger an efficient immune response against HCV infection. In addition, age, gender, viral load, and liver disease status are also considered interference factors in HCV infection pathogenesis and response of the immune system to treatment. Also, longer follow-up is required to answer the important question of whether the inflammatory parameters will further decline over time in successfully treated patients with HCV infection and whether long-term restoration of the interferon system is achieved after HCV clearance [43].

In the present study, the hypothesis that DAAs cause an increase in VEGF which may be a risk factor for HCC development was addressed. By evaluating the serum expression of VEGF before and after DAA treatment in our cohort of HCV genotype-4 patients, VEGF expression was heterogeneous showing spreading of values along a wide range showing 64% (16/25) of the cases being downregulated, while 36% (9/25) of the cases were upregulated. This heterogeneity can be explained by variability in the immune response among the studied patients; although all patients were chronically infected with HCV, but they differed in many ways as the duration of illness, clinical stage of the disease, host genetic, and immune background. Moreover, further follow-up for this group was performed clinically by doing ultrasound at least once after end of treatment and none showed any detectable masses through the period of follow-up (6 months). A positive correlation was found between VEGF expression and each of the viral load as well as AST activity.

Up to our knowledge, only a limited number of studies have been performed to investigate effect of DAAs on different cytokines and growth factors but none of these studies has evaluated the expression level in the setting of follow-up study along the course of DAA treatment as the present study. Different researchers investigated the assumption that treatment with DAA increases the risk for occurrence/recurrence of HCC.

Saraiva et al. in 2018 [40] investigated the circulating levels of inflammatory and profibrogenic cytokines (including VEGF) in 88 patients before and after the end of treatment with DAAs. Serum level of VEGF was increased in HCV-infected patients before treatment while there was a significant decrease after anti-viral therapy. The final conclusion of the study suggested that viral control induced by DAA therapy restores inflammatory mediators in association with improvement in liver function. Similarly, Hengst et al. [36] showed that the expression of VEGF was significantly higher in all patients before treatment which normalized by end of treatment.

On the other hand, Debes et al. [44] in 2018 evaluated serum levels of 52 immune mediators (including cytokines, growth factors, and apoptosis markers) before, during, and after DAA treatment. VEGF-A which showed significantly higher serum expression levels before DAA treatment in patients that later developed HCC. These results potentially suggest that immune modulation by DAA probably does not trigger HCC development but rather that the immune background could be already affected before DAA treatment and induced a carcinogenic or pre-carcinogenic activity. Kawaguchi et al. [45] in 2018 reported that VEGF was continuously rising and maintained a high level until 12 weeks after DAA treatment ended in patient that showed rapidly growing HCC after treatment. Villani et al. [41] measured the pattern of change in VEGF which showed a 4-fold increase at week 4 after start of DAA treatment and remained elevated up to the end of treatment. The study concluded that the increase of VEGF and change in the inflammatory pattern may alter the balance between inflammatory and anti-inflammatory processes and modify anti-tumor surveillance in the host.

The increased risk for HCC reported by the previous studies was explained by the fact that DAA-mediated clearance of HCV leads to loss of intrahepatic immune activation by IFN-α which activates immune cells as natural killer cells and macrophages that directly inhibits tumor cell proliferation. Consequently, loss of immune activation of these cells by IFN-α may allow tumor growth [46]. However, there are no robust preclinical studies to support this hypothesis. Additionally, even using the best imaging modality cannot exclude a small HCC mass before treatment with certainty [47].

A moderate positive correlation between IL-10 and VEGF genes was shown in the studied group which was statistically significant. IL-10 and VEGF have some similarities and overlap in various functions as the processes of inflammation and angiogenesis are intimately linked, inflammatory mediators have a significant effect on the process of angiogenesis, and the reverse is also true [48].

Conclusion

DAAs has shown excellent SVR in HCV genotype-4 patients reaching 100% in this study which is associated with improvement in the liver functions and fibrosis scores indicating an improvement in liver inflammation and progression of fibrosis. The relative expression of IL-10 has shown a strong positive correlation with the viral load and data from this study provide evidences that successful viral clearance induced by DAAs leads to the downregulation of IL-10 expression in the majority of cases that could be explained by a possible shift in the pretreatment Th2 dominant immune response to the Th1 response. Despite of the viral clearance, relative expression VEGF was heterogeneous although showed a positive correlation with IL-10 but the upregulation in its expression after treatment in a considerable fraction of patients in this study shows that DAAs do not completely reverse the immunological imprints established upon chronic HCV infection. Another investigation at the SVR or even later may be needed to determine sustained outcome of the DAA therapy on the immunological response of chronic HCV-infected patients.

Abbreviations

HCV: Hepatitis C virus; IL-10: Interleukin-10; VEGF: Vascular epidermal growth factor; HCC: Hepatocellular carcinoma; Th1: T helper 1; Th2: T helper 2; TNF-α: Tumor necrosis factor-alpha; NK cells: Natural killer; DAA: Directly acting agents; PCR: Polymerase chain reaction; PBMC: Peripheral blood mononuclear cells; FIB-4: Fibrosis-4 index; APRI: Platelet ratio index; PKC: Protein kinase C; MAPK: Mitogen activated protein kinase; SVR: Sustained virological response; IFN: Interferon; Treg: Regulatory T cells; TE: Transient elastography; AST: Aspartate transaminase; ALT: Alanine aminotransferase; NS: Non-structural protein

Acknowledgements

Not applicable

Authors' contributions

IN supervised and helped perform all the practical work including determination of HCV viral load, HCV genotyping, and genes expression, as well as writing, revising, and editing the manuscript. AK supervised all the work and helped in data interpretation. SO provided all patients' clinical information and physical examination. HE was performed the practical work. RE supervised all the work. All authors read and approved the final manuscript.

Declarations

Ethics approval and consent to participate

Medical research Institute Ethics Committee IORG#: IORG0008812

The Medical Research Institute–Alexandria University Ethics Committee reviewed the documents for the above-mentioned study. On 8/5/2017, they granted approval for the above mentioned study to be conducted at the Medical Research Institute–Alexandria University.

The ethics committee of the Medical Research Institute–Alexandria University is constituted and operating according to ICH GCP guidelines and applicable local and institutional regulations and guidelines which govern IRB operation. Informed written consent was taken from each patient.

Competing interests

The authors declare that they have no competing interests.

Author details

[1]Department of Microbiology, Medical Research Institute, University of Alexandria, Alexandria, Egypt. [2]Department of Chemical Pathology, Medical Research Institute, University of Alexandria, Alexandria, Egypt. [3]Department of Experimental and Clinical Internal Medicine, Medical Research Institute, University of Alexandria, Alexandria, Egypt.

References

1. Buonfiglioli F, AP CF, Crespi C, Foschi FG, Lenzi M et al (2016) Development of hepatocellular carcinoma in HCV cirrhotic patients treated with direct acting antivirals. Annual Meeting of EASL, Barcelona
2. Elgharably A, Gomaa AI, Crossey MM, Norsworthy PJ, Waked I, Taylor-Robinson SD (2017) Hepatitis C in Egypt - past, present, and future. Int J Gen Med 10:1–6. https://doi.org/10.2147/IJGM.S119301
3. Messina JP, Humphreys I, Flaxman A, Brown A, Cooke GS, Pybus OG, Barnes E (2015) Global distribution and prevalence of hepatitis C virus genotypes. Hepatology. 61(1):77–87. https://doi.org/10.1002/hep.27259
4. Kouyoumjian SP, Chemaitelly H, Abu-Raddad LJ (2018) Characterizing hepatitis C virus epidemiology in Egypt: systematic reviews, meta-analyses, and meta-regressions. Sci Rep 8(1):1661. https://doi.org/10.1038/s41598-017-17936-4
5. Li K, Lemon SM (2013) Innate immune responses in hepatitis C virus infection. Semin Immunopathol 35(1):53–72. https://doi.org/10.1007/s00281-012-0332-x
6. Zekri A-RN, Ashour MSE-D, Hassan A, Alam El-Din HM, El-Shehaby AMR, Abu-Shady MA (2005) Cytokine profile in Egyptian hepatitis C virus genotype-4 in relation to liver disease progression. World J Gastroenterol 11(42):6624–6630. https://doi.org/10.3748/wjg.v11.i42.6624
7. Bruno CM, Valenti M, Bertino G, Ardiri A, Amoroso A, Consolo M, Mazzarino CM, Neri S (2011) Relationship between circulating interleukin-10 and histological features in patients with chronic C hepatitis. Ann Saudi Med 31(4):360–364. https://doi.org/10.4103/0256-4947.83215
8. Wilson EB, Brooks DG (2011) The role of IL-10 in regulating immunity to persistent viral infections. Curr Top Microbiol Immunol 350:39–65. https://doi.org/10.1007/82_2010_96
9. El-Emshaty HM, Nasif WA, Mohamed IE (2015) Serum cytokine of IL-10 and IL-12 in chronic liver disease: the immune and inflammatory response. Dis Markers 2015:707254
10. Ejrnaes M, Filippi CM, Martinic MM, Ling EM, Togher LM, Crotty S, von Herrath MG (2006) Resolution of a chronic viral infection after interleukin-10 receptor blockade. J Exp Med 203(11):2461–2472. https://doi.org/10.1084/jem.20061462
11. Taktak-BenAmar A, Morjen M, Ben Mabrouk H, Abdelmaksoud-Dammak R, Guerfali M, Fourati-Masmoudi N et al (2017) Expression, purification and

functionality of bioactive recombinant human vascular endothelial growth factor VEGF(165) in E. coli. AMB Express 7(1):33
12. Koch S, Claesson-Welsh L (2012) Signal transduction by vascular endothelial growth factor receptors. Cold Spring Harb Perspect Med 2(7):a006502. https://doi.org/10.1101/cshperspect.a006502
13. Mee CJ, Harris HJ, Farquhar MJ, Wilson G, Reynolds G, Davis C, van IJzendoorn SCD, Balfe P, McKeating JA (2009) Polarization restricts hepatitis C virus entry into HepG2 hepatoma cells. J Virol 83(12):6211–6221. https://doi.org/10.1128/JVI.00246-09
14. Llovet JM, Pena CE, Lathia CD, Shan M, Meinhardt G, Bruix J (2012) Plasma biomarkers as predictors of outcome in patients with advanced hepatocellular carcinoma. Clin Cancer Res 18(8):2290–2300. https://doi.org/10.1158/1078-0432.CCR-11-2175
15. Hepatitis C (2018) Guidance 2018 update: AASLD-IDSA recommendations for testing, managing, and treating hepatitis C virus infection. Clin Infect Dis 67(10):1477–1492
16. WHO (2016) WHO guidelines for the screening care and treatment of persons with chronic hepatitis C infection. World Health Organization, Geneva, pp 25–26
17. Doumas BT, Watson WA, Biggs HG (1971) Albumin standards and the measurement of serum albumin with bromcresol green. Clin Chim Acta 31(1):87–96. https://doi.org/10.1016/0009-8981(71)90365-2
18. Jendrassik LGP (1938) Vereinfachte photometrische Methode zur Bestimmung des Bilirubins. Biochem Z 297:81–89
19. Bergmeyer HU, Horder M, Rej R (1986) International Federation of Clinical Chemistry (IFCC) scientific committee, analytical section: approved recommendation (1985) on IFCC methods for the measurement of catalytic concentration of enzymes. Part 3. IFCC method for alanine aminotransferase (L-alanine: 2-oxoglutarate aminotransferase, EC 2.6.1.2). J Clin Chem Clin Biochem 24(7):481–495
20. Rej R (1984) Measurement of aminotransferases: part 1. Aspartate aminotransferase. Crit Rev Clin Lab Sci 21(2):99–186. https://doi.org/10.3109/10408368409167137
21. Lewis SMBB, Bates I (2017) Chapter 16:investigation of haemostsis (CBC, PT, INR). In: Dacie and Lewis practical Haematology, 12th edn. J and Churchil Elsevier Ltd, Philadelphia, pp 389–391
22. Halfon P, Bourlière M, Pénaranda G, Khiri H, Ouzan D (2006) Real-time PCR assays for hepatitis C virus (HCV) RNA quantitation are adequate for clinical management of patients with chronic HCV infection. J Clin Microbiol 44(7):2507–2511. https://doi.org/10.1128/JCM.00163-06
23. Kuang J, Yan X, Genders AJ, Granata C, Bishop DJ (2018) An overview of technical considerations when using quantitative real-time PCR analysis of gene expression in human exercise research. PLoS One 13(5):e0196438 Available from: http://europepmc.org/abstract/MED/29746477. https://doi.org/10.1371/journal.pone.0196438, http://europepmc.org/articles/PMC5944930 http://europepmc.org/articles/PMC5944930?pdf=render
24. Livak KJ, Schmittgen TD (2001) Analysis of relative gene expression data using real-time quantitative PCR and the 2(-Delta Delta C(T)) method. Methods. 25(4):402–408. https://doi.org/10.1006/meth.2001.1262
25. WHO (2018) Guidelines for the Care and Treatment of Persons Diagnosed with Chronic Hepatitis C Virus Infection [Internet] Geneva: WHO
26. Horsley-Silva JL, Vargas HE (2017) New therapies for Hepatitis C virus infection. Gastroenterol Hepatol (N Y) 13(1):22–31
27. El Raziky MGM, Hammad R (2015) Treatment of hepatitis C genotype 4 patients with simeprevir and sofosbuvir: preliminary results from a phase IIa, partially randomised, open-label trial conducted in Egypt (OSIRIS). Hepatology 62(1):145A
28. Lawitz E, Poordad F, Brainard DM, Hyland RH, An D, Dvory-Sobol H, Symonds WT, McHutchison JG, Membreno FE (2015) Sofosbuvir with peginterferon-ribavirin for 12 weeks in previously treated patients with hepatitis C genotype 2 or 3 and cirrhosis. Hepatology. 61(3):769–775. https://doi.org/10.1002/hep.27567
29. Feld JJ, Jacobson IM, Hezode C, Asselah T, Ruane PJ, Gruener N et al (2015) Sofosbuvir and Velpatasvir for HCV genotype 1, 2, 4, 5, and 6 infection. N Engl J Med 373(27):2599–2607. https://doi.org/10.1056/NEJMoa1512610
30. Gayam V, Khalid M, Mandal AK, Hussain MR, Mukhtar O, Gill A, Garlapati P, Shrestha B, Guss D, Sherigar J, Mansour M, Mohanty S (2018) Direct-acting antivirals in chronic hepatitis c genotype 4 infection in community care setting. Gastroenterology Res 11(2):130–137. https://doi.org/10.14740/gr999w
31. Chatterjee M, Anju CP, Biswas L, Anil Kumar V, Gopi Mohan C, Biswas R (2016) Antibiotic resistance in Pseudomonas aeruginosa and alternative therapeutic options. Int J Med Microbiol 306(1):48–58. https://doi.org/10.1016/j.ijmm.2015.11.004
32. Huynh T, Zhang J, Hu KQ (2018) Hepatitis C virus clearance by direct-acting antiviral results in rapid resolution of hepatocytic injury as indicated by both alanine aminotransferase and aspartate aminotransferase normalization. J Clin Transl Hepatol 6(3):258–263. https://doi.org/10.14218/JCTH.2018.00014
33. Khan ST, McGuinty M, Corsi DJ, Cooper CL (2017) Liver enzyme normalization predicts success of Hepatitis C oral direct-acting antiviral treatment. Clin Invest Med 40(2):E73–e80
34. Yen Y-H KF-Y, Kee K-M, Chang K-C, Tsai M-C, Hu T-H et al (2018) APRI and FIB-4 in the evaluation of liver fibrosis in chronic hepatitis C patients stratified by AST level. PLoS One 13(6):e0199760. https://doi.org/10.1371/journal.pone.0199760
35. Bachofner JA, Valli PV, Kroger A, Bergamin I, Kunzler P, Baserga A et al (2017) Direct antiviral agent treatment of chronic hepatitis C results in rapid regression of transient elastography and fibrosis markers fibrosis-4 score and aspartate aminotransferase-platelet ratio index. Liver Int 37(3):369–376. https://doi.org/10.1111/liv.13256
36. Hengst J, Falk CS, Schlaphoff V, Deterding K, Manns MP, Cornberg M, Wedemeyer H (2016) Direct-acting antiviral-induced hepatitis c virus clearance does not completely restore the altered cytokine and chemokine milieu in patients with chronic hepatitis C. J Infect Dis 214(12):1965–1974. https://doi.org/10.1093/infdis/jiw457
37. Meissner EG, Lee YJ, Osinusi A, Sims Z, Qin J, Sturdevant D, McHutchison J, Subramanian M, Sampson M, Naggie S, Patel K, Remaley AT, Masur H, Kottilil S (2015) Effect of sofosbuvir and ribavirin treatment on peripheral and hepatic lipid metabolism in chronic hepatitis C virus, genotype 1-infected patients. Hepatology. 61(3):790–801. https://doi.org/10.1002/hep.27424
38. Othman MS, Aref AM, Mohamed AA, Ibrahim WA (2013) Serum levels of interleukin-6 and interleukin-10 as biomarkers for hepatocellular carcinoma in Egyptian patients. ISRN Hepatol 2013:412317
39. Yoneda S, Umemura T, Katsuyama Y, Kamijo A, Joshita S, Komatsu M, Ichijo T, Matsumoto A, Yoshizawa K, Ota M, Tanaka E, the Nagano Interferon Treatment Research Group (2011) Association of serum cytokine levels with treatment response to pegylated interferon and ribavirin therapy in genotype 1 chronic hepatitis C patients. J Infect Dis 203(8):1087–1095. https://doi.org/10.1093/infdis/jiq165
40. Saraiva GN, do Rosario NF, Medeiros T, Leite PEC, Lacerda GS, de Andrade TG et al (2018) Restoring inflammatory mediator balance after Sofosbuvir-induced viral clearance in patients with chronic Hepatitis C. Mediat Inflamm 2018:8578051
41. Villani R, Facciorusso A, Bellanti F, Tamborra R, Piscazzi A, Landriscina M, Vendemiale G, Serviddio G (2016) DAAs rapidly reduce inflammation but increase serum VEGF level: a rationale for tumor risk during anti-HCV treatment. PLoS One 11(12):e0167934. https://doi.org/10.1371/journal.pone.0167934
42. Alhetheel A, Albarrag A, Shakoor Z, Alswat K, Abdo A, Al-Hamoudi W (2016) Assessment of pro-inflammatory cytokines in sera of patients with hepatitis C virus infection before and after anti-viral therapy. J Infect Dev Ctries 10(10):1093–1098. https://doi.org/10.3855/jidc.7595
43. Carlin AF, Aristizabal P, Song Q, Wang H, Paulson MS, Stamm LM, Schooley RT, Wyles DL (2015) Temporal dynamics of inflammatory cytokines/chemokines during sofosbuvir and ribavirin therapy for genotype 2 and 3 hepatitis C infection. Hepatology. 62(4):1047–1058. https://doi.org/10.1002/hep.27971
44. Debes JD, van Tilborg M, Groothuismink ZMA, Hansen BE, Schulze Zur Wiesch J, von Felden J et al (2018) Levels of cytokines in serum associate with development of hepatocellular carcinoma in patients with HCV infection treated with direct-acting antivirals. Gastroenterology 154(3):515–7.e3
45. Kawaguchi T, Ide T, Koga H, Kondo R, Miyajima I, Arinaga-Hino T, Kuwahara R, Amano K, Niizeki T, Nakano M, Kuromatsu R, Torimura T (2018) Rapidly growing hepatocellular carcinoma after direct-acting antiviral treatment of chronic hepatitis C. Clin J Gastroenterol 11(1):69–74. https://doi.org/10.1007/s12328-017-0789-1
46. Serti E, Chepa-Lotrea X, Kim YJ, Keane M, Fryzek N, Liang TJ et al (2015) Successful interferon-free therapy of chronic hepatitis C virus infection normalizes natural killer cell function. Gastroenterology 149(1):190–200.e2
47. Faillaci F, Marzi L, Critelli R, Milosa F, Schepis F, Turola E, Andreani S, Vandelli G, Bernabucci V, Lei B, D'Ambrosio F, Bristot L, Cavalletto L, Chemello L, Sighinolfi P, Manni P, Maiorana A, Caporali C, Bianchini M, Marsico M, Turco

L, de Maria N, del Buono M, Todesca P, di Lena L, Romagnoli D, Magistri P, di Benedetto F, Bruno S, Taliani G, Giannelli G, Martinez-Chantar ML, Villa E (2018) Liver angiopoietin-2 is a key predictor of de novo or recurrent hepatocellular cancer after hepatitis C virus direct-acting antivirals. Hepatology. 68(3):1010–1024. https://doi.org/10.1002/hep.29911

48. Park MS, Kim S, Patel J, Hajdu CH, Do RK, Mannelli L et al (2012) Hepatocellular carcinoma: detection with diffusion-weighted versus contrast-enhanced magnetic resonance imaging in pretransplant patients. Hepatology. 56(1):140–148. https://doi.org/10.1002/hep.25681

16

Safety and efficacy of direct-acting antiviral drugs in the treatment of chronic hepatitis C virus infection in patients with thalassemia: a prospective study

Elsayed Ghoneem[1], Ahmed Saleh[1*], Shahira Aly El-Etreby[1], Metwaly Ibrahim Mortada[2], Mayada A. Ghannam[2], Shaimaa El-Ashwah[3] and Noha Eisa[3]

Abstract

Background: Hepatitis C virus (HCV) infection is a major cause of liver-related morbidity and mortality among thalassemic patients. Direct-acting antiviral agents (DAAs) are highly effective and well-tolerated by chronic HCV patients.

Results: The mean age of our patients was 29 years. Sustained virologic response (SVR) at 12 and 24 weeks was achieved in all patients (100%). The most common side effects were fatigue (18%), anemia (13.63%), and headache (4.5%). There was no statistically significant difference in the hemoglobin level before and after treatment ($p = 0.48$). There was a significant improvement in serum bilirubin and mean ALT levels after treatment compared to baseline data ($p < 0.0005$ each).

Conclusions: DAAs, namely, sofosbuvir plus daclatasvir or sofosbuvir plus ledipasvir, are effective and well-tolerated regimens in thalassemic patients with chronic HCV.

Keywords: Thalassemia, Chronic hepatitis C, Direct-acting antiviral drugs (DAAs), Sustained virologic response (SVR), Post-transfusion hepatitis (PTH)

Background

Viral hepatitis, mainly the hepatitis C virus, is one of the common causes of post-transfusion hepatitis (PTH) in patients who need multiple blood transfusions [1]. Thalassemia is a hereditary disorder characterized by the synthesis of abnormal hemoglobin (genetic deficiency in the synthesis of beta-globin chains), resulting in hemolysis and anemia. Patients with β thalassemia major (BTM) usually require repeated blood transfusion, which keeps them at high-risk of HCV infection [2]. In spite of improvements in the screening of blood products in the last decades to minimize the risk of transmission of blood-borne diseases, viral hepatitis, especially HCV, remains an important problem in patients with β thalassemia [3, 4]. Post-transfusion HCV infection leads to chronic hepatitis with hepatocellular necrosis, fibrosis, and cirrhosis in patients with thalassemia with higher morbidity and mortality [5].

Chronic HCV infection (CHC) treatment in β thalassemia patients was challenging in the interferon (IFN)-based therapy era not only because of its modest efficacy [6–10] but also due to unfavorable safety and tolerability profiles, as it was necessary to be combined with ribavirin (RBV) considering subsequent hemolysis and increased need for blood transfusions, and, thereby, increased risk of iron overload [11].

With the introduction of the new IFN plus RBV free regimens in 2014, the management of all patients with

* Correspondence: drahmedsaleh1981@gmail.com
[1]Department of Internal Medicine, Hepatology & Gastroenterology Unit, Faculty of Medicine, Mansoura University, Mansoura, Egypt
Full list of author information is available at the end of the article

chronic HCV infection, including those with β thalassemia, has dramatically improved. These drugs are direct-acting antivirals (DAAs) that act by targeting specific steps in the HCV life cycle and are used in combinations to treat CHC. In Egypt, depending on the genotype and the drug availability, the available DAAs combinations are the co-formulation of sofosbuvir (SOF) with ledipasvir (LDV) (one tablet of 400/90 mg once daily) and SOF plus daclatasvir (DCV) (in two tablets of 400/60 mg/day once daily). They are nucleotide analog NS5B polymerase inhibitor/NS5A inhibitor. According to guidelines, β thalassemia patients should be treated with IFN- and RBV-free regimens [12].

Different DAAs regimens have been reported to be safe and effective in the treatment of CHC patients in clinical practice [12]. Our thalassemia patients were followed up in a hematology clinic at Oncology Center, Mansoura University (OCMU). Such patients who are also infected with HCV could be a target population for "HCV micro-elimination" on the road toward global HCV elimination in our country.

Methods

Patients

This is a prospective study that included 88 treatment naïve patients with chronic HCV genotype 4 infection and beta-thalassemia major from attendees of Hematology Clinic at Oncology Center, Mansoura University, from January to December 2017. All included patients were transfusion-dependent and were using iron chelation therapy. Only four patients had concomitant hepatitis B virus (HBV) coinfection.

Inclusion criteria for DAAs

Patients of both genders included for DAAs therapy in the current study were diagnosed with Thalassemia major and were on regular transfusion and iron chelation therapy, aged 12 years and above, naïve chronic hepatitis C genotype 4 infection with detectable HCV-RNA by RT-PCR. No additional drugs were used.

Exclusion criteria

Patients were excluded from the study if they were infected with other HCV genotypes, had concomitant HIV infection, or had presence of liver cell failure.

Diagnosis of HCV and genotyping

Chronic HCV infection was diagnosed by positive RT-PCR RNA HCV with or without abnormal liver function tests and the presence of stigmata of chronic liver disease (flapping tremors, ascites, edema lower limb, and hepatic encephalopathy). HCV RNA was quantified by real-time PCR assay (COBAS AmpliPrep/COBAS TaqMan 48, Roche Molecular Diagnostics). The HCV genotype was detected by Versant HCV genotype 2.0 assays (LiPA-Siemens, Erlangen, Germany).

Laboratory assessment

The laboratory tests done included complete blood counts, liver enzymes (ALT, AST), serum bilirubin, serum creatinine, α fetoprotein, and INR. The liver fibrosis stage was assessed by a non-invasive tool known as the FIB-4 score [13].

Treatment protocols

At the Virology unit, Specialized Medical Hospital, Mansoura University, Egypt, all patients were evaluated for anti-HCV treatment. Two DAA regimens were used according to the guidelines of the National Committee for Control of Viral Hepatitis (NCCVH) in Egypt. We treated the patients with the following combinations: SOF(400 mg daily) plus DCV(60 mg daily) for the older age group and LDV(90 mg daily)-SOF in the younger age group (12–18 years) for 12 weeks. Only four patients were coinfected with HBV (diagnosed by the presence of detectable HBV DNA by PCR and all of them were HBeAg positive) and treated using LDV/SOF and lamivudine.

Endpoints of the treatment

The primary endpoint was assessed by the achievement of SVR at 12 weeks and at 24 weeks. The secondary endpoint was assessed by the recording of adverse events, increased transfusion requirements, or stoppage of treatment. All patients were on regular transfusion, and the median packed red blood cell units transfused was a unit per 21 days.

Patients' follow up

Clinical and laboratory data were recorded at baseline and at 4, 8, 12, and 24 weeks of therapy.

Statistical analysis

Data were entered and statistically analyzed using the Statistical Package for Social Sciences (SPSS) version 17. Quantitative data were described as means (standard deviations) or medians (interquartile ranges), as appropriate. Comparisons between the different groups were performed using the Wilcoxon rank-sum test for variables that were not normally distributed. Qualitative data were presented as numbers and percentages and compared by using the chi-square test. A P value of less than 0.05 was considered statistically significant.

Results

Demographic and clinicolaboratory data

Table 1 shows the demographic, baseline clinical, and laboratory parameters for a total of 88 thalassemic

Table 1 Demographic, basal clinical and laboratory parameters

Variables	No (%) or median (IQR)
Male gender	44 (50%)
Age (years)	29 (12–36)
Subjects with comorbidities	28 (31.82%)
Hypertension	8 (13.63%)
Osteoporosis	12 (13.63%)
HBV	4 (4.54%)
Drug users	4 (4.54%)
Splenectomy	88 (100%)
Iron chelation agent	
Deferiprone	28 (31.82)
Deferasirox	60 (68.18)
Hemoglobin (g/dl)	8.25 (7.3–9)
Platelet count (×10^9/L)	543 (430–632)
WBCs (× 10^9/L)	27.3 (18.3–50)
AST (IU/L)	71.50 (47–82.30)
ALT (IU/L)	54.45 (28–74)
S. bilirubin (mg/dl)	2.9 (2.5–4)
Direct bilirubin (mg/dl)	0.6 (0.5–0.98)
Albumin (g/dl)	4 (3.8–4.8)
INR	1.2 (1.1–1.3)
S. creatinine (mg/dl)	0.65 (0.6–0.8)
Ferritin (ng/mL)	2500 (1800–4000)
PCR HCV RNA (IU/ml)	941757 (187771–1400000)
FIB-4 score	0.52 (0.47–0.73)

patients with chronic HCV. The median age of our patients was 29 years and males represented 50% of our study participants. Hypertension was found in 13.63% of cases, osteoporosis in 13.63% of cases, and HBV in four cases. All patients were splenectomized. The median hemoglobin level, platelet count, and white blood cell counts were 8.25 gm/dl, 543 × 10^9/L, and 27.3 × 10^9/L respectively. The median AST, ALT, and serum bilirubin levels were 71.5 IU/L, 54,45 IU/L, and 2.9 mg/dl respectively. Serum ferritin levels were elevated with a median level of 2500 ng/ml. The median PCR for HCV RNA was 941757 IU/ml, with a median FIB-4 score of 0.52.

Efficacy of treatment

All patients were treatment naïve. Overall, 64 (72.72%) patients were treated with a SOF plus DCV, and 24 (27.27%) patients received SOF plus LDV for 12 weeks. All patients achieved SVR at 12 weeks and 24 weeks. There was a significant improvement in the mean ALT values after treatment compared to baseline (42.45 ± 18.56 IU/L vs 57.29 ± 35.07 IU/L, $p < 0.0005$, Fig. 1). Also, there was a statistically significant decrease in serum bilirubin level after treatment ($p < 0.0005$, Fig. 2). There was no statistically significant difference in the hemoglobin level (Fig. 3), platelet count, and WBCs count before and after DAAs (the p values were 0.613, 0.092, and 0.284, respectively) (Table 2). Twelve patients reported increased blood transfusion requirements, although no significant difference was noticed between the mean HB level before and after DAAs.

Safety of the treatment

No major side effects were reported and no patients discontinued the treatment. Only one case required treatment discontinuation (median time of 2 weeks) due to acute kidney injury after the prolonged use of NSAIDs

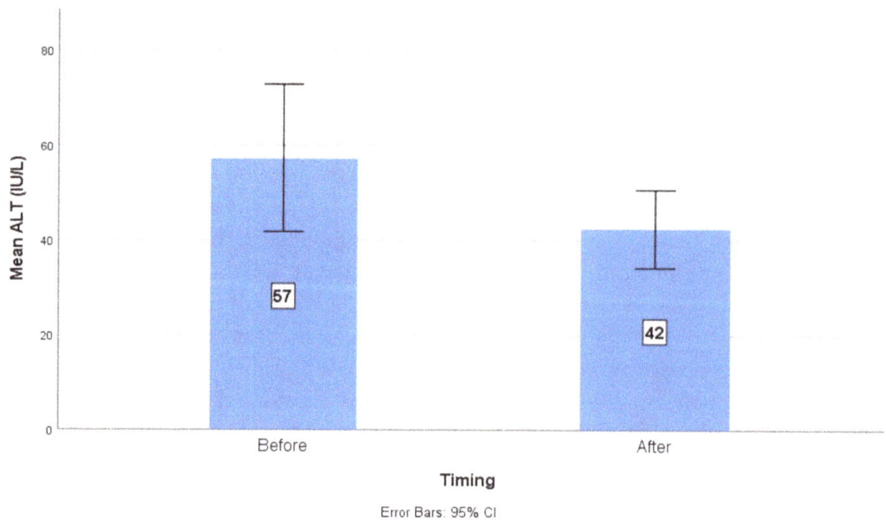

Fig. 1 ALT before and after treatment

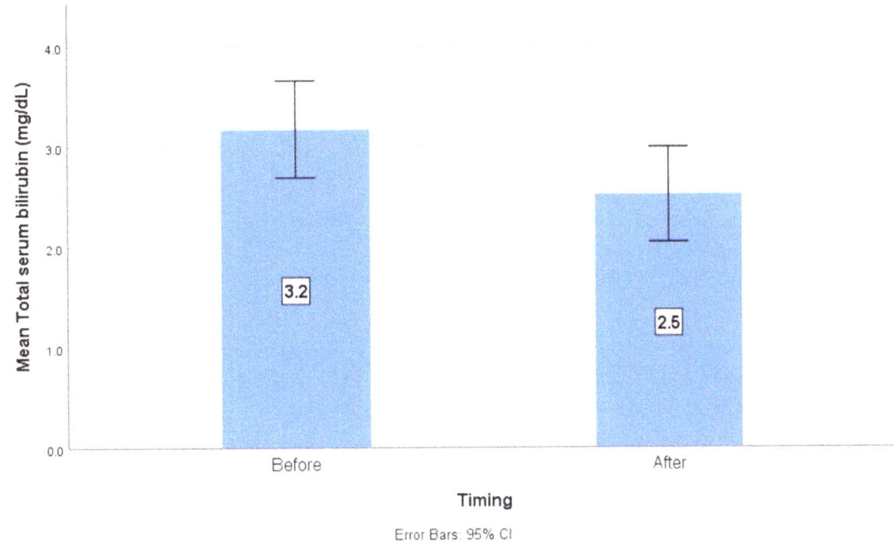

Fig. 2 Serum level of bilirubin before and after treatment

and resumed DAAs after the decline of creatinine to the normal level. Twenty (22.72%) patients complained of mild symptoms. The most common side effects were fatigue (18%), anemia (13.63%), requiring blood transfusion (12 patients) in patients receiving SOF plus DCV, and, lastly, headache (4.5%). These side effects were more frequent among patients receiving SOF plus DCV, than in patients receiving SOF plus LDV; however, this difference in frequency was not statistically significant (60% vs. 40%, $p = 0.58$).

Discussion

HCV infection is considered a major clinical burden in β thalassemia patients. The prevalence of HCV is much higher among patients with beta-thalassemia, as these patients constitute a 4 high-risk group. A systematic review based on the literature database showed that the anti-HCV antibody among β thalassemia patients has been estimated at 18%, 45%, 63%, and 69% in Iran, Pakistan, Saudi Arabia, and Egypt, respectively [14]. Approximately 70–80% of those patients will progress to CHC and up to 20% will go on to cirrhosis [15]. It is also known that HCV infection is a risk factor for HCC, which has been considered as the second common cause of mortality in this population [16].

Herein, our study provides further proof that oral DAAs are highly effective and tolerable by β thalassemia patients with CHC. All enrolled patients achieved SVR

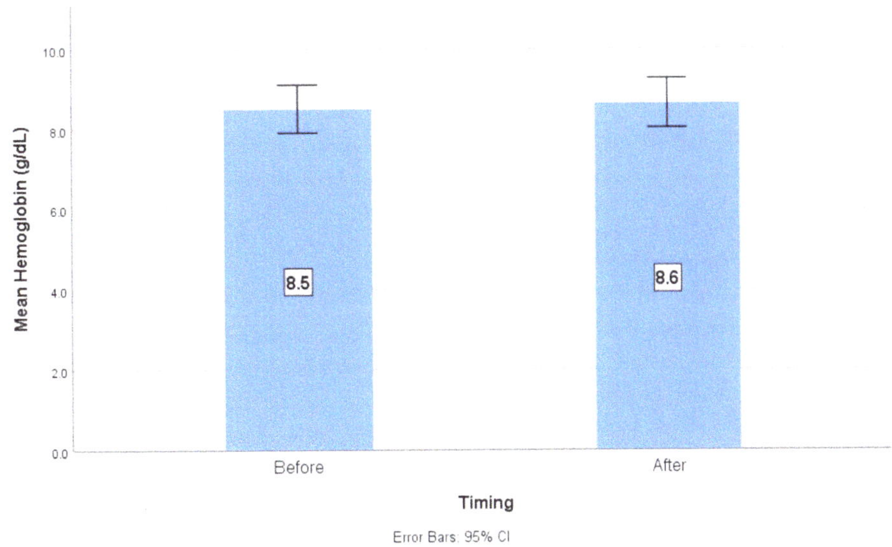

Fig. 3 Hemoglobin level before and after treatment

Table 2 Laboratory parameters before and after treatment with DAAs

Parameter	Before	After	Statistic	*P* value
ALT(IU/ml)	57.29 ± 35.07	42.4545 ± 18.56	3.569	0.0005
S. bilirubin (mg/dL)	3.17 ± 1.08	2.51 ± 1.06	4.800	0.0005
Hemoglobin (g/dL)	8.5 ± 1.34	8.64 ± 1.38	− 0.513	0.613
Platelets count (× 10^9/L)	513.18 ± 160.47	460.14 ± 186.81	1.764	0.092
WBCs (×10^9/L)	27.30 (18.27–51)	20.50 (12.15–49)	− 1.072	0.284

Data presented as mean ± SD except WBCs presented as median (IQR). For WBCs, data were not normally distributed (Shapiro test, $p < 0.05$) with the presence of significant outliers. Accordingly, Wilcoxon test was conducted. Paired samples t test was used for other parameters as the data were normally distributed

at 12 weeks and at 24 weeks. Compared to the Italian cohort [17] and the Greek cohort [18], SVR was achieved in most of the patients (98% and 90%, respectively). Both studies included 57.1% vs. 78.7% and previously treated patients 42.9% vs. 75%. The achievement of 100% SVR in our study could be explained by the fact that all enrolled patients were treatment naïve and had no cirrhosis as the median FIB-4 score was 0.52. However, those patients should be monitored for the possibility of reinfection.

Hezode et al. [19] published a trial using a fixed combination of elbasvir and grazoprevir in patients with congenital blood disorders and CHC, including β thalassemic patients. Forty β thalassemia major patients received treatment for 12 weeks, and SVR was achieved in 97.6% of them. This study showed that treatment was well-tolerated by the patients, and hemoglobin levels were not affected by treatment. The most frequently reported side effects in this study were, e.g., headache, fatigue, nausea, and asthenia. However, this combination is not currently available in Egypt.

Also, in a case series of four β thalassemia patients with CHC associated with advanced hepatic fibrosis, treated with the LDV/SOF combination for 12 weeks, all patients achieved SVR with accepted drug safety and tolerability. The only reported adverse events were mild asthenia and headache. There were no changes in chelation therapy or transfusion requirements during the treatment period. Similar results were presented by Mangia et al. [20, 21].

In the present study, there were no major adverse events, and no discontinuation of treatment was reported. Only one case required temporary treatment discontinuation due to acute kidney injury after the prolonged use of NSAIDs then resumed DAAs after the decline of serum creatinine to the normal value. Mild symptoms occurred in approximately 22.72% of the patients. The most common side effects were fatigue (18%), anemia (13.63%), and headache (4.5%). This is in accordance with the published data from certain clinical trials [18, 22]. These side effects were more common among patients receiving SOF plus DCV than in patients receiving SOF plus LDV; however, this difference in the rates of occurrence of side effects was not statistically significant (p = 0.58). Also, no drug-drug interactions were observed.

There was a significant improvement of mean ALT values and a significant decrease in serum bilirubin after treatment. On the other hand, no statistically significant difference in the hemoglobin level, platelet count, and WBCs count were found before and after DAAs. Only 12 patients had increased blood transfusion requirements, despite a non-significant difference being noticed between the mean HB level before and after DAAs. The dose and type of iron-chelating therapy did not require any modifications during the treatment course.

A high hepatic iron concentration was proposed as a negative predictor of response to DAAs in different ethnic populations. There was no consensus on whether iron accumulation in the sinusoidal cells or hepatocytes and portal track macrophages was more significant for poor response to treatment [23].

Assessment of hepatic iron concentration was limited and mainly based on serum ferritin levels and non-invasive techniques without liver histology and the data of post-treatment assessment of hepatic iron overload were not obtainable during the study. So, we need further studies with larger samples and newer DAA combinations.

Conclusion

Direct-acting antiviral drugs (sofosbuvir plus daclatasvir or sofosbuvir plus ledipasvir) are safe, effective, and well-tolerated regimens for thalassemic patients with chronic HCV.

Abbreviations

HCV: Hepatitis C virus; DAAs: Direct-acting antivirals agents; SVR: Sustained virologic response; PTH: Post-transfusion hepatitis; BTM: β thalassemia major; CHC: Chronic HCV infection; IFN: Interferon; RBV: Ribavirin; SOF: Sofosbuvir; LDV: Ledipasvir; DCV: Daclatasvir; OCMU: Oncology Center, Mansoura University; HBV: Hepatitis B virus; AST: Aspartate aminotransferase; ALT: Alanine aminotransferase; NCCVH: National Committee for Control of Viral Hepatitis; HB: Haemogloin

Acknowledgements

We are thankful to our colleagues in the hepato-gastroenterology and hematology departments, Mansoura University. We are also thankful for our patients for their contribution and trust.

Authors' contributions

The protocol of the study, study design, methodology, follow-up of the patients, collection of the data, data analysis, and writing—original draft preparation: SEA, NE, and EG. Lab investigation: MM and MG. Writing—review and editing: EG. Supervision: SEE and AS. All authors have read and approved the manuscript.

Declarations

Ethics and approval consent to participate

The study has been approved by the ethics committee of our university (Mansoura Faculty of Medicine, Mansoura University, Institutional Review Board Code No R/17.12.71) and has been performed following the ethical standards as laid down in the 1964 Declaration of Helsinki and its later amendments or comparable ethical standards. Informed written consents approved by ethical committee of Mansoura Faculty of Medicine were obtained from all individual participants or their legal guardians if under 16 years.

Competing interests

The authors declare that they have no conflict of interest.

Author details

[1]Department of Internal Medicine, Hepatology & Gastroenterology Unit, Faculty of Medicine, Mansoura University, Mansoura, Egypt. [2]Department of Clinical Pathology, Hematology Unit, Faculty of Medicine, Mansoura University, Mansoura, Egypt. [3]Department of Clinical Hematology, Oncology Center Mansoura University (OCMU), Faculty of Medicine, Mansoura University, Mansoura, Egypt.

References

1. Viral Hepatitis Prevention Board (1995) Hepatitis A, B and C: Defining workers at risk. Viral Hepat 3 Google Scholar
2. Agarwal M, Malkan G, Bhave A, Vishwanathan C, Billa V, Dube S et al (1993) Antibody to hepatitis-C virus in multi-transfused thalassaemics--Indian experience. J Assoc Physicians India 41:195–197 [PubMed] [Google Scholar]
3. Ocak S, Kaya H, Cetin M, Gali E, Ozturk M (2006) Sero-prevalence of hepatitis B and hepatitis C in patients with thalassemia and sickle cell anemia in a long-term follow-up. Arch Med Res 37:895–898 [PubMed] [Google Scholar]
4. Prati D, Maggioni M, Milani S, Cerino M, Cianciulli P, Coggi G et al (2004) Clinical and histological characterization of liver disease in patients with transfusion-dependent beta-thalassemia. A multicenter study of 117 cases. Haematologica 89:1179–1186 [PubMed] [Google Scholar]
5. Angelucci E, Pilo F (2008) Treatment of hepatitis C in patients with thalassemia. Haematologica 93:1121–1123 [PubMed] [Google Scholar]
6. Casu S, Balestrieri C, Figorilli F, Onali S, Serra G, Chessa L, Lai ME (2014) P1155 safety and efficacy of PEG IFnA 2a and ribavirin for treatment of hepatitis C in sardinian adult patients with thalassemia major, a single centre real life experience. J Hepat. 60(1):468. https://doi.org/10.1016/s0168-8278(14)61315-5
7. Paschos P, Vlachaki E, Pasvanti C, Sinakos E, Kalpaka A, Klonizakis P, Perifanis V (2011) Safety and efficacy of combination therapy with pegylated interferon alpha-2a and ribavirin in treating patients with chronic hepatitis C and beta-thalassaemia major: a Greek single-center experience. Acta Haematol. **126**(4):231–233. https://doi.org/10.1159/000330516
8. Harmatz P, Jonas MM, Kwiatkowski JL, Wright EC, Fischer R, Vichinsky E, Giardina PJ, Neufeld EJ, Porter J, Olivieri N, for the Thalassemia Clinical Research Network (2008) Safety and efficacy of pegylated interferon alpha 2a and ribavirin for the treatment of hepatitis C in patients with thalassemia. Haematologica. 93(8):1247–1251. https://doi.org/10.3324/haematol.12352
9. Inati A, Taher A, Ghorra S, Koussa S, Taha M, Aoun E, Sharara AI (2005) Efficacy and tolerability of peginterferon alpha-2a with or without ribavirin in thalassaemia major patients with chronic hepatitis C virus infection. Br J Haematol. 130(4):644–646. https://doi.org/10.1111/j.1365-2141.2005.05645.x
10. Kamal SM, Fouly AH, Mohamed MK, Hochnikos BW, Lamont FT, Gohary IS, Koziel MJ, Afdhal NH, Sayed M, Rasenack JW (2006) 585 Peginterferon alpha 2b therapy with and without ribavirin in patients with thalassemia, a randomized study. J Hepatol. 44:217. https://doi.org/10.1016/s0168-8278(06)80585-4
11. Iavian SM, Tabatabaei SV. Treatment of chronic hepatitis C in polytransfused thalassaemic patients: a meta-analysis. J Viral Hepat. 2010; 17(4):236-244. doi: https://doi.org/10.1111/j.1365-2893.2009.01170.x.
12. European Association for the Study of the Liver (2018) Electronic address EEE. EASL recommendations on treatment of hepatitis C. J Hepatol http://doi.org/10.1016/j
13. Vallet-Pichard A, Mallet V, Nalpas B, Verkarre V, Nalpas A, Dhalluin-Venier V, Fontaine H, Pol S (2007) FIB-4: an inexpensive and accurate marker of fibrosis in HCV infection. comparison with liver biopsy and fibrotest. Hepatology 46(1):32–36. https://doi.org/10.1002/hep.21669
14. Alavian S, Tabatabaei S, Lankarani K (2010) Epidemiology of HCV Infection among Thalassemia Patients in Eastern Mediterranean Countries: a Quantitative Review of Literature. Iran. Red. Crescent. Med. 12(4):365–376
15. Minola E, Prati D, Suter F, Maggiolo F, Caprioli F, Sonzogni A, Fraquelli M, Paggi S, Conte D (2002) Age at infection affects the long term outcome of transfusion associated chronic hepatitis C. Blood. 99(12):4588–4591. https://doi.org/10.1182/blood-2001-12-0192
16. Voskaridou E, Ladis V, Kattamis A, Hassapopoulou E, Economou M, Kourakli A et al (2012) A national registry of haemoglobinopathies in Greece: deducted demographics, trends in mortality and affected births. Ann Hematol. 91(9):1451–1458. https://doi.org/10.1007/s00277-012-1465-7
17. Onali S, Maida I, Balestrieri C, Arcadu F, Urru E, Porcu D, Serra G, Flore G, Dore E, Satta C, Paolo Bitti P, Grazia Sanna M, Serusi L, Casale M, Conti M, Loi M, Figorilli F, Cristina Pasetto M, Babudieri S, Chessa L (2018) Safety and efficacy of direct-acting antivirals in transfusion-dependent thalassemic patients with chronic hepatitis C. Hepat Mon. 18(1):e61453. https://doi.org/10.5812/hepatmon.61453
18. Sinakos E, Kountouras D, Koskinas J, Zachou K, Karatapanis S, Triantos C, Vassiliadis T., Goulis I., Kourakli A., Vlachaki E., Toli B., Tampaki M., Arvaniti P., Tsiaoussis G., Bellou A., Kattamis A., Maragkos K., Petropoulou F., Dalekos G. N., Akriviadis E., Papatheodoridis G.V. Treatment of chronic hepatitis C with direct-acting antivirals in patients with beta thalassaemia major and advanced liver disease. Br J Haematol. 2017; 178(1):130-136. doi: https://doi.org/10.1111/bjh.14640. [PubMed: 28439915].
19. Hezode C, Colombo M, Bourliere M, Spengler U, Ben-Ari Z, Strasser SI, et al. Elbasvir, grazoprevir for patients with hepatitis c virus infection and inherited blood disorders: a phase III study. Hepatology. 2017; 66(3):736-745. doi: https://doi.org/10.1002/hep.29139. [PubMed: 28256747].
20. Biliotti E, Palazzo D, Serani M, Silvestri AM, Volpicelli L, Esvan R, Franchi C, Spaziante M, Sorrentino F, Taliani G Interferon free antiviral treatment of chronic hepatitis C in patients affected by beta-thalassemia major. Ann Hematol. 2017; 96(6):1043-1045. doi: https://doi.org/10.1007/s00277-017-2986-x. [PubMed: 28378040].
21. Mangia A, Sarli R, Gamberini R, Piga A, Cenderello G, Piazzolla V, Santoro R, Caruso V, Quarta A, Ganga R, Copetti M, Forni G (2017) Randomised clinical trial: sofosbuvir and ledipasvir in patients with transfusion dependent thalassaemia and HCV genotype 1 or 4 infection. Aliment Pharmacol Ther. 46(4):424–431. https://doi.org/10.1111/apt.14197
22. European Association for the Study of the Liver. Electronic address EEE (2017) EASL recommendations on treatment of hepatitis C 2016. J Hepatol. 66(1):153–194. https://doi.org/10.1016/j.jhep.2016.09.001
23. Ikura Y, Morimoto H, Johmura H, Fukui M, Sakurai M (1996) Relationship between hepatic iron deposits and response to interferon in chronic hepatitis C. Am. J. Gastroenterol. 91(7):1367–1373

17

Assessment of serum Resistin in detecting Insulin Resistance and their impact on response to direct acting antiviral in chronic viral hepatitis C patients

Amira Isaac, Khaled Hamdy Abd El-Mageed, Hany Haroun Kaisar, Hany Samir Rasmy, Ramy Samir Abd Elhamid Ghait, Ibrahim Magdy Ibrahim* and George Safwat Riad

Abstract

Background: Chronic hepatitis C (CHC) virus is associated with insulin resistance and diabetes which have been linked to progressive liver fibrosis and sustained virologic response (SVR) to antiviral treatment. Resistin is a polypeptide hormone belonging to adipokines that may contribute to the development of obesity, insulin resistance, and metabolic syndrome. Also, the link between resistin and insulin resistance in patients with chronic hepatitis C and the effect of new direct acting antivirals on them seems unclear at present. The aim of this study is to evaluate the role of Resistin in detecting Insulin Resistance and their impact on response to direct acting antiviral in chronic hepatitis C patients.

Results: The Study was prospective Cohort clinical study, in Hepatology outpatient clinic at Ain Shams University Hospitals .This study was performed on 40 Egyptian patients who have Chronic viral hepatitis C, divided into 3 groups: GROUP I includes: 20 patients with Chronic viral hepatitis C on Sofosbovir- Daclatasvir before start of treatment and Sustained viral response after 12 weeks [SVR 12]. GROUP II includes: 20 patients with Chronic viral hepatitis C and non-responders before start of 2nd line of treatment and SVR 12. GROUP III includes: 10 subjects not infected with HCV as control group. The following investigations were done: body mass index calculation, Laboratory investigations including CBC, complete hepatic function tests, FIB-4 calculation, fasting serum insulin, HOMA-IR and serum Resistin level at baseline and re-assessed 12 weeks post end of treatment. Fasting serum Insulin, HOMA-IR and Resistin level were statistically significant higher in both naïve & relapser chronic HCV infected patients than in control group (*p* value <0.001). SVR 12 weeks post treatment was achieved in all 40 patients received new direct acting antivirals with a Significant reduction in Fasting serum Insulin, HOMA-IR and Resistin level at SVR 12 week (*p* value 0,001, <0.001, <0.001) respectively. Significant positive correlation was found between Resistin level and HOMA-IR in both naïve and relapse chronic HCV patients. Calculation of FIB-4 among patients showed significant higher FIB-4 in naïve patients than relapser (*p* value 0,002). Serum Resistin at a cut off value >1800 ng/ml had 38.89 % sensitivity, 86.36 % specificity, 70 % PPV, 63.3 % NPV (with an overall accuracy of 57.1 %) in predicting absence of liver cirrhosis based on FIB-4. And at a cutoff value ≥2400 ng/ml had 93.55% sensitivity, 33.3% specificity, 82.9% positive predictive value, and 60% negative predictive value with an overall accuracy of 62.4% in prediction of significant insulin resistance among chronic HCV patients.

* Correspondence: markmaccar@yahoo.com
Internal Medicine Department, Hepatology and Gastroenterology Department, Faculty of medicine, Ain Shams University, Cairo, Egypt

Conclusion: Serum Resistin level was significantly up regulated in patients with chronic HCV, with significant reduction in its level after achievement of SVR. Resistin has the potential to be a biomarker for screening of insulin resistance among chronic HCV patients.

Keywords: Resistin, Chronic hepatitis C, Insulin resistance, Direct acting antiviral

Background

Hepatitis C virus infection a leading cause of liver cirrhosis that has a significant global impact, where it infects about 71 million in 2015 with highest prevalence in the Eastern Mediterranean and European regions, According to WHO. In Egypt it is 10% prevalent before the National Campaign done in 2018-2019 [1].

The direct-acting antivirals (DAAs) have become the new gold standard of HCV treatment. DAAs are safe and highly effective and achieve a sustained virologic response (SVR) in 90-98% of cases [2].

Experimental and clinical evidences demonstrated that HCV core protein plays a pathogenic role in the development of insulin resistance. Epidemiological studies show that the prevalence of insulin resistance and type 2 diabetes in HCV-infected patients is significantly higher than that observed in hepatitis B virus infection and in the general population. It has been reported that the risk of developing type 2 diabetes mellitus is 11 times higher in patients with HCV infection, in which there is a direct correlation between viremia and insulin resistance levels and the development of type 2 diabetes [3].

Furthermore, insulin resistance in HCV patients is strictly correlated with metabolic syndrome, and it is a determinant for increased vessel wall stiffness. Thus, clearance of HCV could improve insulin resistance related cardiovascular events [4].

Resistin is an adipocyte derived hormone with 12.5 kDa that forms multimeric complexes characterized by the presence of cysteine residues. It is involved in the regulation of glucose homeostasis, inflammation, and adipogenesis and thus influences the development of insulin resistance, obesity, and type 2 diabetes [5].

The resistin expression in the human liver is increased in various liver diseases and the positive correlation between resistin and inflammation and hepatic fibrosis, which suggests the involvement of this adipokine in the pathophysiology of liver fibrosis, has been demonstrated in alcoholic hepatitis and NAFLD [5].

Given the postulate of direct involvement of resistin expression on insulin resistance and their relation to HCV infection, the main aim of this study is to evaluate the role of resistin in detecting Insulin Resistance and their impact on response to Direct acting antiviral in chronic hepatitis C patients.

Methods

This study was conducted on 40 Egyptian > 18 years old, chronic HCV infected patients eligible for antiviral treatment with DAAs, agreeable to regular follow up, recruited from National Committee for Control of Viral Hepatitis (NCCVH) regional center in Ain Shams university hospital during the period from February 2019 to February 2020, and 10 healthy volunteers (non diabetic, non obese) as a control group after approval of the Ain Shams University ethics committee was granted, and informed consents were taken from all patients.

They were divided into three groups, GROUP I (Case group) twenty chronic HCV patients as evident by positive HCV Ab (at least six months duration) and detectable quantitative HCV RNA were subjected to treatment by Sofosbovir 400mg+ Daclatasvir 60mg & GROUP II includes: twenty patients with Chronic HCV and non-responders before start of 2nd line of treatment by Sofosbovir 400mg+ Daclactasvir 60mg+ Ribavirin 1000-1200mg or Sofosbovir 400mg+ Ombitasvir, Paritaprevir & Ritonavir + Ribavirin 1000-1200mg as per the Egyptian NCCVH protocol and accordingly administered an appropriate, personally tailored, DAA regimen for 3 months during the course of this study [6] & GROUP III including 10 subjects not infected with HCV as control group.

All female patients were neither pregnant nor lactating throughout the course of this study. Patients with concomitant HBV or HIV infection, hepatocellular carcinoma, patients with other causes of chronic liver diseases such as autoimmune hepatitis and hemochromatosis, History of alcohol abuse, Diabetes mellitus, intake of certain Medications such as biguanides and thiazolidinediones, renal impairment, and those who refused to be entitled in the study were excluded from the study.

All patients were subjected to the following:

1. Full history taking and clinical examination.
2. Laboratory investigations including:

- Complete blood count
- Liver function tests including serum alanine aminotransferase & aspartate aminotransferase, total & direct bilirubin, serum albumin, Prothrombin time and INR.
- HBsAg – HCVAb - HIVAb.

- Hepatitis C virus RNA levels evaluated by real-time polymerase chain reaction (PCR)
- Serum Alpha fetoprotein.
- Serum creatinine.
- Fasting blood glucose
- HbA1C (BioSystems S.A. Costa Brava, 30.08030 Barcelona (Spain), colorimetric method)
- Fasting Insulin hormone level: Normal values: 0.7-9 μU/ml. (Or mU/L),
- Calculating HOMA-IR.

HOMA was used to evaluate IR and β-cell function by the following formulas: HOMA-IR = ([glycemia (mg/dL) × insulinemia (μU/mL)]/405). ***Normal values:*** (0.5–1.4(, Above 1.9 indicates early insulin resistance. Above 2.9 indicates significant insulin resistance [7].

- Serum Resistin: (measured by ELISA kits, Bioassay Technology Laboratory) normal range of 0.02-6 ng/ml (20-6000 ng/L) was assessed for all patients included in the study, For group I and II, resistin was assessed before starting antiviral treatment (baseline) and three months after end of treatment (SVR)
- FIB-4 index: the fibrosis-4 score at a cut off value of 1.45 (FIB-4 <1.45 had a negative predictive value of 90%of advanced fibrosis. The **FIB-4** index is calculated using the **formula**: **FIB-4** = Age (years)×AST (U/L)/[PLT(10^9/L)×ALT$^{1/2}$ (U/L)] [8].
- Radiological examination: Abdominal ultrasonography

Statistical analysis

The collected data were coded, tabulated, and statistically analyzed using IBM SPSS statistics (Statistical Package for Social Sciences) software version 20. Quantitative data were expressed as mean ±SD (standard deviation) for normally distributed data.

In quantitative data, Independent t-test was used to compare two independent groups with normally distributed data and paired t-test in cases of two dependent groups with normally distributed data. Analysis of variance (ANOVA) was used to compare more than two independent groups with normally distributed data, followed by post hoc test to compare between each two groups. Tukey's test was used as a single-step multiple comparison procedure and statistical test to find means that are significantly different from each other. In qualitative data, inferential analyses for independent variables were done using Chi Square (X^2) test for differences between proportions.

Correlations were done using Pearson correlation coefficient test. The receiver operating characteristic (ROC) curve was constructed to obtain the most sensitive and specific cutoff values for different parameters, *P* value less than 0.05 was sufficient enough to show the statistical significance.

Results

Group I included 20 naive chronic HCV patients, comprising 9 (45%) males and 11 (55%) females, with a mean age of 45.15 ± 14.68 years, Group II included 20 relapser chronic HCV patients, comprising 13 (65%) males and 7 (35%) females, with a mean age of 40.15 ± 14 years, whereas group III included 10 healthy participants who served as a control group, comprising eight (80%) males and two (20%) females, with a mean age of 38.9 ± 13.78 years. The statistical differences between groups regarding age and sex were insignificant (*P*>0.05).

Concerning laboratory findings, naïve chronic HCV patients had statistically significant lower level of hemoglobin and platelets than relapser chronic HCV patients (P<0.001), while INR level was significantly higher among naïve chronic HCV patients (*P*=0.008). (The statistical differences between both studied groups regarding liver function tests were shown in the Table 1

Pretreatment fasting insulin level & HOMA-IR was statistically significantly higher in naive chronic HCV patients than in Relapser HCV patients (*P*<0.001) Table 2.

Regarding pretreatment serum resistin level, it was dramatically higher among both naïve and relapser chronic HCV patients in comparison to control group (*P*<0.001) Table 2.

On applying FIB-4 scoring among naïve chronic HCV patients, 7 (35%) patients had FIB-4 < 1.45 indicating absence of cirrhosis, while 13 (65%) patients had FIB-4 of 1.45-3.25 so they were deemed inconclusive, while among relapser chronic HCV patients, 15 (75%) patients had FIB-4< 1.45 indicating absence of cirrhosis, and 5 (25%) patients had FIB-4 of 1.45-3.25 so they were deemed inconclusive.

All patients among naive and relapser chronic HCV received new direct-acting antiviral drugs for 12 weeks and were reassessed 12 weeks after the end of treatment, where they all achieved undetectable serum HCV RNA concentrations (SVR 12 weeks).The statistical differences between pretreatment and 12 weeks after the end of treatment regarding CBC, liver function tests and FIB-4 are insignificant statistically Table 3.

After achieving SVR, a statistically significant improvement in fasting insulin and HOMA-IR was noticed among both naïve and relapser chronic HCV patients (*P*<0.001). Notably, there was also a statistically significant reduction in serum resistin level (1715 ± 514.80 versus 835.5 ± 668.07) for naïve patients and (1735 ± 707.86 versus 929.5 ± 619.98) for relapser group (*P*<0.001) Table 4.

Table 1 Comparison between the 3 groups regarding demographic and laboratory findings

Baseline parameter	Naive group (*n*=20)	Relapser group (*n*=20)	Control group (*n*=10)		
	Mean ± SD	Mean ± SD	Mean ± SD	F	*p*-value
Age (years)	50.150 ± 14.684	43.150 ± 14.050	41.900 ± 13.788	1.649	0.203
BMI(kg/m^2)	28.895 ± 4.75	25.695±5.18	23.590±4.12	2.216	0.12
AST (IU/L)	39.750 ± 17.302	34.150 ± 19.288	29 .100 ± 10.785	0.768	0.469
ALT (IU/L)	39.200 ± 18.574	40.500 ± 40.565	38.000 ± 14.142	0.026	0.974
Albumin (g/dl)	3.605 ± 0.373	3.775 ± 0.236	3.730 ± 0.306	1.559	0.221
Total bilirubin (mg/dl)	0.925 ± 0.510	0.840 ± 0.357	0.910 ± 0.341	0.221	0.802
INR	1.173 ± 0.208	1.015 ± 0.158	1.002 ± 0.097	5.418	0.008*
Hemoglobin(g/dL)	10.450 ± 0.774	13.110 ± 1.922	12.320 ± 1.062	18.722	<0.001*
TLC(×10^3/μL)	7.005 ± 2.173	6.470 ± 2.682	8.590 ± 2.456	2.538	0.090
Platelets(×10^3/μL)	139.800 ± 57.430	216.600 ± 65.303	289.500 ± 63.400	20.654	<0.001*
HbA1C	6.1 ± 0.3	6 ± 0.5	5.9 ± 0.4	2.443	0.091
Total Cholesterol (mg/dL)	186 ± 20	178 ± 25	159 ± 22	1.54	0.22
LDL (mg/dL)	90 ± 19	84 ± 21	79 ± 27	8.441	0.061
Triglycerides (mg/dL)	132 ± 30	147 ± 24	121 ± 29	10.45	0.07

This table shows no statistical significant difference between the three groups as regards the demographic and laboratory findings of the patients except Hemoglobin and platelets with *p* value <0.001* and INR with *p* value <0.008

For naïve chronic HCV patients' group, there was a positive correlation between baseline *HOMA-IR* and serum resistin level (*P*<0.001), also among relapse group a positive correlation between baseline HOMA-IR and serum resistin level (*P*<0.001) was noticed Table 5.

Notably among naïve chronic HCV patients baseline serum *resistin* level was positively correlated with baseline fasting blood sugar, fasting insulin, HOMA-IR (*P*<0.001, *P*<0.001, *P*<0.027 respectively), while among relapsers it was positively correlated with fasting insulin and HOMA-IR (*P*<0.001, *P*<0.02 respectively) Table 6.

The receiver operating characteristic curve analysis of serum resistin for prediction of absence of liver cirrhosis based on FIB-4 scoring showed the following: fasting serum resistin level at a cutoff value greater than 1800 ng/ml had 38.89% sensitivity, 86.36% specificity, 70% positive predictive value, and 63.3% negative predictive value with an overall accuracy of 57.1% (as shown in figures file, Fig. 1).

The receiver operating characteristic curve analysis of serum resistin for prediction of significant insulin resistance among chronic HCV patients showed the following: fasting serum resistin level at a cutoff value greater than 2400 ng/ml had 93.55% sensitivity, 33.3% specificity, 82.9% positive predictive value, and 60% negative predictive value with an overall accuracy of 62.4% (as shown in figures file, Fig. 2).

Discussion

Chronic HCV infection is the leading cause of hepatocellular carcinoma and the leading indication for liver transplantation in developed countries [9]. Newer combination of DAAs offers cure rates exceeding 90%. However, achieving SVR does not immediately reverse HCV related liver fibrosis or cirrhosis [10].

Table 2 Comparison between the three groups regarding *baseline* Fasting blood sugar, fasting insulin, HOMA-IR and resistin

		Groups			ANOVA		TUKEY'S		Test
		Naïve	Relapser	Control	F	*P*-value	N&R	N&C	R&C
FBS Pre (mg/dl)	Mean ±SD	85 ± 13	83 ± 16	87 ± 13.5	0.16	0.851			
Fasting Insulin Pre (μU/ml)	Mean ±SD	29 ± 7.4	17 ± 5.0	5.9 ± 1.8	59.9	< 0.001	< 0.001	< 0.001	< 0.001
HOMA Pre	Mean ±SD	6.33 ± 2.2	3.5 ± 1.1	1.25 ± 0.4	36.2	< 0.001	< 0.001	< 0.001	0.001
Resistin Pre (ng/L)	Mean ±SD	1715.000 ± 514.807	1735.000 ± 707.869	353.000 ± 85.512	24.209	<0.001	0.99	<0.001	<0.001

This table shows no statistically significant difference between the studied groups before treatment as regard fasting blood sugar. Yet as regard Pre-treatment fasting insulin, HOMA IR & resistin, they were found to be statistically significantly higher in naïve and relapse groups in comparison to control group with *P*-value <0.001, and fasting insulin, HOMA IR were higher in naïve group in comparison to Relapsers with *P*-value <0.001

Table 3 Comparison between baseline and post-treatment different laboratory parameters and FIB-4 in both naive and relapse group of patients

		Naive			Relapser		
		Before ttt	After ttt	*P*-value	Before ttt	After ttt	*P*-value
TLC($\times 10^3/\mu L$)	Mean ±SD	7.005±2.173	6.512±1.99	0.45	6.470±2.682	5.7±2.44	0.48
HB(g/dL)	Mean ±SD	10.450±0.774	10.1± 0.764	0.85	13.110±1.922	11.5±1.877	0.56
PLT($\times 10^3/\mu L$)	Mean ±SD	139.8±57.430	126±55.41	0.51	216.60±65.303	203.5±63.32	0.54
ALT(IU/L)	Mean ±SD	39.200±18.574	40.5± 19.44	0.89	40.50±40.565	41.4± 41.57	0.87
AST(IU/L)	Mean ±SD	39.750± 17.302	40.74 ±17.23	0.92	34.150± 19.288	32.132± 20.22	0.78
Albumin(g/dL)	Mean ±SD	3.605± 0.373	3.51± 0.31	0.83	3.775 ±0.236	3.665± 0.231	0.89
T bilirubin (mg/dL)	Mean ±SD	0.925± 0.510	0.956 ±0.523	0.88	0.840 ±0.357	0.81± 0.345	0.9
INR	Mean ±SD	1.173± 0.208	1.21± 0.213	0.56	1.015 ±0.158	1.055± 0.167	0.7
Fib4	<1.45	7	8	0.41	15	16	0.52
	>1.45	13	12		5	4	

This table shows no statistical significant difference between baseline and post-treatment different laboratory parameters and FIB-4 in both naive and relapse group of patients

In addition to causing liver disease, CHC infection is associated with wide metabolic disarrangements. HCV interacts with lipid metabolism leading to steatosis, causing wide adipocytokine changes and impairs glucose metabolism leading to increased prevalence of insulin resistance and type 2 diabetes [11]. This association is important because the presence of insulin resistance is associated with increased rates of fibrosis [12] and lower rates of rapid and sustained response to antiviral therapy [13].

The mechanism of how metabolic factors influence disease progression is not clearly understood. Adipose tissue secretes bioactive proteins known as adipokines, including leptin, adiponectin, and resistin. These proteins exert different effects on insulin resistance and inflammation [14].

The behavior of circulating resistin during liver disease owing to viral hepatitis is still under investigation. The current study aimed at determining the value of assessment of serum resistin in prediction of insulin resistance among chronic HCV infected patients and their potential prognostic value in CHC patients under new direct-acting antiviral therapy.

On applying a non-invasive scoring to identify liver cirrhosis among the studied patients, pretreatment FIB -4 was statistically significantly higher in naïve group than in relapse group which could be attributed to decline in steatosis index among relapse group as a result

Table 4 Comparison between baseline & post-treatment fasting blood sugar, fasting insulin, HOMA-IR & resistin in *naive* and *relapser* group of patients

			Time		Differences		Paired Test	
			Pre	Post	Mean	SD	t	*P*-value
Naive	FBS (mg/dL)	Mean ±SD	85.350 ± 13.758	76.400 ± 15.551	8.950	6.970	5.743	<0.001*
	Fast Insulin (μU/ml)	Mean ±SD	29.850 ± 7.499	19.150 ± 8.145	10.700	7.263	6.589	<0.001*
	HOMA	Mean ±SD	6.334 ± 2.214	3.645 ± 1.925	2.689	1.477	8.144	<0.001*
	Resistin (ng/L)	Mean ±SD	1715.000 ± 514.807	835.500 ± 668.072	879.500	566.424	6.944	<0.001*
Relapser	FBS (mg/dL)	Mean ±SD	83.800 ± 16.376	74.750 ± 12.422	9.050	8.281	4.887	<0.001*
	Fast Insulin (μU/ml)	Mean ±SD	17.650 ± 5.050	11.250 ± 4.800	6.400	6.992	4.094	<0.001*
	HOMA	Mean ±SD	3.596 ± 1.156	2.012 ± 0.774	1.584	1.495	4.739	<0.001*
	Resistin (ng/L)	Mean ±SD	1735.000 ± 707.869	929.500 ± 619.987	805.500	693.393	5.195	<0.001*

This table shows statistically significant difference between baseline and post-treatment fasting blood sugar, fasting insulin, HOMA-IR, and resistin in naïve and Relapser group of patients being lower post-treatment with *p* value <0.001*

Table 5 Correlation between Pre-treatment HOMA -IR with demographic and laboratory data in *both* Groups of patients

Correlations

	HOMA Pre			
	Naive		Relapser	
	r	*P*-value	r	*P*-value
Age(years)	-0.086	0.717	0.175	0.460
BMI(kg/m^2	-0.097	0.683	0.265	0.258
ALT (IU/L)	0.187	0.431	0.468	0.307
AST(IU/L)	0.004	0.987	-0.416	0.068
Alb(g/dL)	0.095	0.691	-0.227	0.335
Bil(mg/dL)	0.191	0.420	0.107	0.653
Hb(g/dL)	-0.091	0.702	0.130	0.585
TLC(×10^3/µL)	0.244	0.300	0.090	0.705
Plat(×10^3/µL)	-0.093	0.696	-0.013	0.957
INR	0.361	0.118	-0.270	0.251
FBS Pre(mg/dL)	**0.667**	0.001*	0.507	0.075
Fasting Insulin Pre(µU/ml)	**0.856**	<0.001*	**0.794**	<0.001*
Resistin Pre(ng/L)	**0.745**	<0.001*	**0.769**	<0.001*
PCR(IU/mL)	0.014	0.953	-0.061	0.800
AFP(ng/mL)	0.162	0.494	0.070	0.769
FIB4	-0.115	0.629	-0.134	0.573

This table shows a significant positive correlation between Pre-treatment HOMA-IR and Fasting Insulin & Resistin among Naïve & Relapser Patients and FBS among naïve patients with insignificant correlation with all other parameters

Table 6 Correlations between the Resistin Pre-treatment and all other parameters in the study in both groups of patients

Correlations

	Resistin Pre			
	Naive		Relapser	
	r	*P*-value	r	*P*-value
Age(years)	0.224	0.343	-0.109	0.646
BMI(kg/m^2)	0.232	0.325	-0.186	0.432
ALT(IU/L)	-0.207	0.382	0.245	0.298
AST(IU/L)	-0.118	0.621	0.157	0.509
Alb(g/dL)	-0.054	0.822	-0.116	0.627
Bil(mg/dL)	0.232	0.325	-0.039	0.870
Hb(g/dL)	-0.087	0.717	-0.187	0.429
TLC(×10^3/µL)	-0.146	0.538	-0.259	0.271
Plat(×10^3/µL)	0.040	0.866	-0.033	0.889
INR	-0.234	0.321	0.445	0.050
FBS Pre(mg/dL)	**0.695**	<0.001*	0.054	0.822
Fast Insulin Pre(µU/ml)	**0.756**	<0.001*	**0.725**	<0.001*
HOMA	0.494	0.027*	0.510	0.021*
PCR(IU/mL)	-0.026	0.913	-0.047	0.843
AFP(ng/mL)	-0.099	0.677	0.030	0.900
FIB4	0.160	0.499	0.054	0.821

This table shows a significant positive correlation between Pre-treatment Resistin and 'Fasting Insulin and HOMA-IR' among Naïve & Relapser Patient and 'FBS in Naïve patients only' with insignificant correlation with all other parameters

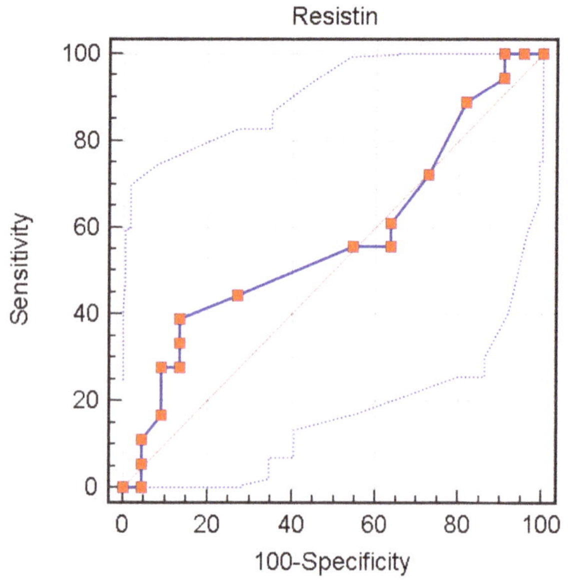

Fig. 1 ROC Curve of serum resistin level in prediction of liver cirrhosis based on FIB4 score in both studied groups of patients

of previous treatment regimen and this was in agreement with Tada et al who stated that viral eradication reduces both liver stiffness and steatosis [15].

In this study, we found that baseline fasting insulin level, HOMA-IR were statistically significantly higher in naïve and relapse chronic HCV patients in comparison to control with P-value <0.001 and these results were in agreement with El Sebaey et al who proved that there is strong link between hepatitis C virus infection and the insulin resistance panel & concluded that Insulin

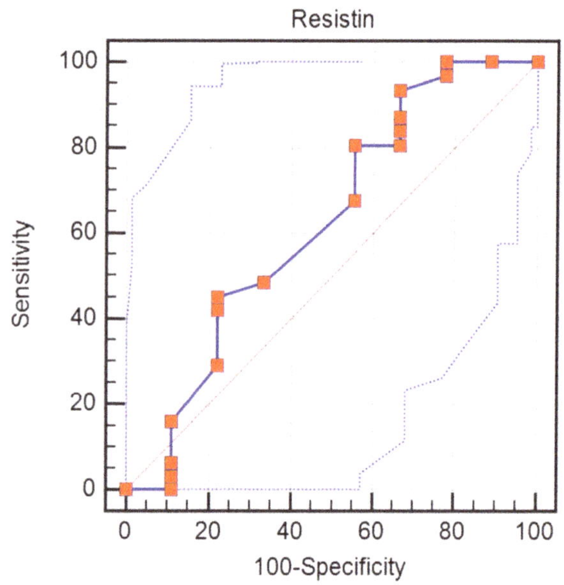

Fig. 2 ROC Curve of serum resistin level in prediction of significant insulin resistance in both studied groups of patients

sensitivity improved markedly in patients who achieved SVR [16].

Also in agreement with Adinolfi et al. who stated that the prevalence of insulin resistance & type 2 diabetes in HCV-infected patients is significantly higher than that observed in hepatitis B virus infection & the general population with a direct correlation between viremia and IR levels and the development of type 2 diabetes [3].

Insulin Resistance in HCV patients has been reported to be mediated by the HCV core protein, which interferes with glucose metabolism and insulin signaling by inhibiting the expression of insulin receptor substrate (IRS)1 and IRS2 [17]. HCV-induced IR in the tissue of HCV-infected patients and animal models has also been indicated to be mediated via several cytokines, including tumor necrosis factor-α [18].

The current study results also showed that there was a statistically significant decline in FBS, Fasting Insulin, HOMA-IR in Both naïve and relapse groups of patients after treatment with DAA in relation to their pre-treatment levels And This goes in agreement with previous data that showed that interferon-based treatment improves insulin resistance and blood glucose levels in patients who clear HCV [19].

Another meta-analysis evaluated data from 8 studies comparing the reduction in IR between SVR and non-SVR groups of HCV patients treated with IFN-based therapy indicated no significant difference in the reduction of IR between the SVR and non-SVR groups. However, patients who achieved SVR had a significantly higher mean reduction in HOMA-IR compared to patients in the non-SVR group [18].

The current study results also showed that pre-treatment serum resistin level was statistically significantly higher in naïve and relapse groups in comparison to control group with a statistically significant decline in its post-treatment level in both groups in relation to pre-treatment level.

Concerning the role of resistin in liver damage associated with viral hepatitis, Resistin expression in human liver was found to be increased in alcoholic liver disease, HCV-induced hepatitis or non-alcoholic steato-hepatitis (NASH). Its expression during liver damage positively correlated with infiltration of inflammatory cells, which represent the principal source of intrahepatic resistin [20].

Regarding this, our results matched with Tiftikci et al. who stated that patients with chronic HCV infection had elevated levels of adipocytokines, such as leptin and resistin, in their sera compared to healthy subjects, although low levels of resistin were associated with the presence of fibrosis in the patient group [21].

Although the possible relationship between resistin and anti-viral treatment has been scarcely studied, Our results go in agreement with Durrazzo et al. who found a significant reduction in resistin levels after anti-viral treatment in a group of CHC patients [22]. On the contrary, the analysis by Lo Iacono et al. found no changes in resistin level in a cluster of chronic HCV patients before and after the anti-viral therapy [23].

Nevertheless, it is yet unclear whether the presence of logistic state stresses the action of resistin as a mediator of IR and moreover its real patho-physiological role is still debated in chronic hepatitis [24].

Resistin may play an important role in the regulation of glucose homeostasis and adipogenesis [25] thereby influencing the development of insulin resistance, type 2 diabetes, and endothelial dysfunction, thrombosis, and angiogenesis [5].

The present study showed that baseline resistin level was found to have significant positive correlation with baseline Fasting insulin in both Naïve and relapser group with r value equal 0.756 and 0.725 with *P*-value <0.001, and with baseline HOMA-IR with r-value 0.877 and 0.789 respectively and *P*-value <0.001. These results agreed with Makni et al who highlighted a significant correlation between resistin and HOMA-IR through Multiple regression models [26].

Possible explanation could be attributed to the important role of resistin in the inflammatory response associated with chronic liver inflammation, such as hepatitis C and NASH [27]. Resistin presents a directed pro-inflammatory activity or mediated by other cytokines such as interleukin (IL)1, IL6 and the TNFα, through nuclear factor-κB pathway. In the course of chronic liver disease, elevated serum levels have been associated with IR, disease progression, severity, clinical complications, and a more severe prognosis [28].

Finally, the present study revealed the best cutoff value of serum resistin in predicting absence of liver cirrhosis based on FIB-4 score among patients with CHC to be greater than 1800 ng/L. This value had 38.89% sensitivity, 86.36% specificity and an overall accuracy of 57.1%.

It also revealed that the best cutoff value of serum resistin in prediction of presence of significant insulin resistance among CHC patients to be greater than 2400ng/L. This value had 93.55% sensitivity, 33.33% specificity and an overall accuracy of 62.4%.

Conclusion

Serum resistin level was significantly upregulated in patients with chronic HCV, with significant reduction in its level after achievement of SVR. Resistin has the potential to be a biomarker for screening of insulin resistance among chronic HCV patients.

Limitation of the study:

- Small number of studied population

Abbreviations

ALT: Alanine Aminotransferase; AST: Aspartate aminotransferase; CHC: Chronic hepatitis C; DAA: Direct acting antiviral; FBS: Fasting Blood sugar; FIB4: Fibrosis 4; HCV: Hepatitis C virus; HOMA-IR: Homeostatic Model Assessment of Insulin Resistance; INR: International Normalized Ratio; IRS: Insulin receptor substrate; IL: interleukin; PCR: Polymerase Chain reaction; SVR: sustained virologic response; TLC: Total leucocytic count

Acknowledgements

The authors express their gratitude to staff members of Internal Medicine Department, Hepatology and Gastroenterology Department, Faculty of medicine, Ain Shams University,
Cairo, Egypt

Authors' contributions

AIS, RSA, KHA had proposed the subject for research and had conducted final revision of gathered data. HSR, GSR had collected the relevant data. IBI, AIS had prepared the manuscript. HHK, RSA had outlined the study design and revised the manuscript. All authors read and approved the final manuscript.

Declarations

Ethics approval and consent to participate

This study was performed according to the ethical standards for human experimentation and in accordance with the ethical principles of the 1975 Declaration of Helsinki. Patients included in this study signed an informed written consent to participate and all the procedures were in accordance with the standards of the Research Ethics Committee (REC) of the Faculty of Medicine, Ain Shams University. (FWA 000017585)

Competing interests

The authors declare that they have no competing interests.

References

1. World Health Organization (WHO) 2017. Global hepatitis report. April. https://www.who.int/hepatitis/publications/global-hepatitis-report2017/en/
2. European Association for the Study of the Liver (EASL) (2017) Recommendations on Treatment of Hepatitis C 2016. J. Hepatol 66:153–194
3. Adinolfi LE, Rinaldi L, Guerrera B et al. (2016). NAFLD and NASH in HCV Infection: prevalence and significance in hepatic and extrahepatic manifestations. Int. J. Mol. Sci; 25: 17(6): 803.
4. Perticone M, Maio R, Tassone EJ, Tripepi G, di Cello S, Miceli S, Caroleo B, Sciacqua A, Licata A, Sesti G, Perticone F (2015) Insulin-resistance HCV infection-related affects vascular stiffness in normotensives. Atherosclerosis 238(1):108–112. https://doi.org/10.1016/j.atherosclerosis.2014.11.025
5. Da Silva TE, Costa-Silva M, Correa CG et al (2018) Clinical Significance of Serum Adiponectin and Resistin Levels in Liver Cirrhosis. Ann hepatol 17(2): 274–285. https://doi.org/10.5604/01.3001.0010.8659
6. El-Akel W, El-Sayed MH, El Kassas M et al (2017) National treatment programme of hepatitis C in Egypt: Hepatitis C virus model of care. J Viral Hepat 24(4):262–267. https://doi.org/10.1111/jvh.12668
7. Singh B, Saxena A (2010) Surrogate markers of insulin resistance: A review. World J Diabetes. 1(2):36–47. https://doi.org/10.4239/wjd.v1.i2.36
8. Sterling RK, Lissen E, Clumeck N, Sola R, Correa MC, Montaner J, S. Sulkowski M, Torriani FJ, Dieterich DT, Thomas DL, Messinger D, Nelson M, APRICOT Clinical Investigators (2006) Development of a simple noninvasive index to predict significant fibrosis in patients with HIV/HCVco-infection. Hepatol 43(6):1317–1325. https://doi.org/10.1002/hep.21178
9. Sebastiani G, Gkouvatsos K, Pantopoulos K (2014) Chronic hepatitis C and liverfibrosis. WorldJ Gastroenterol 20(32):11033–11053. https://doi.org/10.3748/wjg.v20.i32.11033

10. El-Serag HB, Kanwal F, Richardson P et al (2016) Risk of hepatocellular carcinomaafter sustained virological response in veterans with hepatitis C virusinfection. Hepatology 64(1):130–137. https://doi.org/10.1002/hep.28535
11. Eslam M, Khattab MA, Harrison SA (2011) Insulin resistance and hepatitis C: anevolving story. Gut 60(8):1139–1151. https://doi.org/10.1136/gut.2010.228262
12. Moucari R, Asselah T, Cazals-Hatem D et al (2008) Insulin resistance in chronic hepatitis C: association with genotypes 1 and4, serum HCV RNA level, and liver fibrosis. Gastroenterology 134(2):416–423. https://doi.org/10.1053/j.gastro.2007.11.010
13. Khattab M, Eslam M, Sharwae MA, Shatat M, Ali A, Hamdy L (2010) Insulinresistance predicts rapid virologic response to peginterferon/ ribavirin combinationtherapy in hepatitis C genotype 4 patients. Am J Gastroenterol 105(9):1970–1977. https://doi.org/10.1038/ajg.2010.110
14. Shi JP, Fan JG, Wu R, Gao XQ, Zhang L, Wang H, Farrell GC (2008) Prevalenceand risk factors of hepatic steatosis and its impact on liver injury in Chinesepatients with chronic hepatitis B infection. J Gastroenterol Hepatol 23(9):1419–1425. https://doi.org/10.1111/j.1440-1746.2008.05531.x
15. Tada T, Kumada T, Toyoda H, Sone Y, Takeshima K, Ogawa S, Goto T, Wakahata A, Nakashima M, Nakamuta M, Tanaka J (2018) Viraleradication reduces both liver stiffness and steatosis in patients with chronic hepatitis Cvirus infection who received direct-acting anti-viral therapy. Aliment Pharmacol Ther 47(7):1012–1022. https://doi.org/10.1111/apt.14554
16. Alsebaey A, Elhelbawy M, Abdel-Razek W, Hashim M, Elshenawy H, Waked I (2019) HCV treatment with direct acting antivirals improves the insulin sensitivity. Expert Rev Anti Infect Ther 17(9):749–754. https://doi.org/10.1080/14787210.2019.1653184
17. Kralj D, VirovićJukić L, Stojsavljević S et al (2016) Hepatitis C virus, insulin resistance, and steatosis. J Clin TranslHepatol 4:66–75
18. Hu JH, Chang ML, Liu NJ, Yeh CT, Huang TJ (2019) Effect of HCV treatment response on insulin resistance: A systematic review and meta-analysis. Experimental and Therapeutic Medicine 18(5):3568–3578. https://doi.org/10.3892/etm.2019.7995
19. Delgado-Borrego A, Jordan SH, Negre B et al (2010) Halt-C Trial Group. Reduction of insulin resistance with effective clearance of hepatitis C infection: results from the HALT-C trial. Clin. Gastroenterol. Hepatol 8:458–462
20. Bertolani C, Sancho-Bru P, Failli P, Bataller R, Aleffi S, DeFranco R, Mazzinghi B, Romagnani P, Milani S, Ginés P, Colmenero J, Parola M, Gelmini S, Tarquini R, Laffi G, Pinzani M, Marra F (2006) Resistin as an intrahepaticcytokine: over-expression during chronic injury and induction ofproinflammatory actions in hepatic stellate cells. Am J Pathol 169(6):2042–2053. https://doi.org/10.2353/ajpath.2006.060081
21. Tiftikci A, Atug O, Yilmaz Y, Eren F, Ozdemir FT, Yapali S, Ozdogan O, Celikel CA, Imeryuz N, Tozun N (2009) Serum levels of adipokines in patientswith chronic HCV infection: relationship with steatosis and fibrosis. Arch Med Res 40(4):294–298. https://doi.org/10.1016/j.arcmed.2009.04.008
22. Durazzo M, Belci P, Niro G et al (2013) Variations of serum levels of adiponectin and resistin in chronic viral hepatitis. J Endocrinol Invest 36(8): 600–605. https://doi.org/10.3275/8883
23. Lo Iacono O, Venezia G, Petta S et al (2007) The impact of insulin resistance, serum adipocytokines and visceral obesity on steatosis andfibrosis in patients with chronic hepatitis C. Alim PharmacolTher 25(10):1181–1191. https://doi.org/10.1111/j.1365-2036.2007.03309.x
24. Morace C, Spadaro A, Cucunato M, Tortorella V, Consolo P, Luigiano C, Stabile G, Bonfiglio C, Bellerone R, Fortiguerra A, Alibrandi A, Crinò S, Carducci A, Resta ML, Ferraù O, Freni MA (2010) High serum resistin in chronic viral hepatitis is not a marker of metabolic disorder. Hepatogastroenterology 57(102-103):1215–1219
25. Falcao-Pires I, Castro-Chaves P, Miranda-Silva D et al (2012) Physiological, pathological andpotential therapeutic roles of adipokines. *Drug Discov Today* 17(15-16):880–889. https://doi.org/10.1016/j.drudis.2012.04.007
26. Makni E, Moalla W, Benezzeddine-Boussaidi L, Lac G, Tabka Z, Elloumi M (2013) Correlation of Resistin with Inflammatory and Cardiometabolic Markers in Obese Adolescents with and without Metabolic Syndrome. Obes Facts 6(4):393–404. https://doi.org/10.1159/000354574
27. Shen C, Zhao CY, Wang W, Wang YD, Sun H, Cao W, Yu WY, Zhang L, Ji R, Li M, Gao J (2014) The relationship between hepatic resistin overexpression and inflammation in patients with nonalcoholic steatohepatitis. *BMC Gastroenterol* 14(1):39. https://doi.org/10.1186/1471-230X-14-39
28. Yagmur E, Tratwein C, Gressner AM et al (2006) Resistin serum levels are associated with insulin resistance, disease severity, clinical complications and prognosis in patients with chronic liver diseases. Am J Gastroenterol 101(6):1244–1252. https://doi.org/10.1111/j.1572-0241.2006.00543.x

18

Annexin A5 as a marker for hepatocellular carcinoma in cirrhotic hepatitis C virus patients

Waleed Mohamed Serag[1*] and Basem Eysa Elsayed[2]

Abstract

Background: The tumorigenesis and development in a variety of cancers is reportedly encouraged via Annexin A5. The levels of Annexin A5 were tested in patients with or without HCC who were affected by liver cirrhosis. The objective of our study was to detect Annexin A5 levels in such patients in order to assess their function as an HCC marker. The longitudinal study comprised 91 cirrhotic HCV patients with and without HCC, and 20 healthy volunteers in the control group approved by the National Hepatology and Tropical Medicine Research Institute (NHTMRI) between March 2017 and August 2018.The serum levels Annexin A5 were found in all groups with ELISA. ANOVA, Mann-Whitney, and χ^2 tests had been applied.

Results: High scales of Annexin A5 (3.89 + 0.85) were recorded for cirrhosis with HCC, either than cirrhotic patients without HCC (3.06 ± 0.88) (P = 0.041), and either than the control group (0.54 ± 0.11) (P < 0.001).

Conclusion: In HCV cirrhotic patients with and without HCC, AnxA5 can be used as HCC marker.

Keywords: AnxA5 level, HCV, HCC, Cirrhosis

Background

One of the world's most common cancers is hepatocellular carcinomas (HCC). Epidemiologic studies have shown that HCC is the fifth and seventh most diagnosed cancer among men and women and the world's second and sixth cancer cause for death [1]. The main cause of cancer-related death is hepatocellular carcinoma (HCC), which causes about 800,000 deaths worldwide in 2018 [2]. There is a definite need for non-invasive quantifiable biomarkers to classify the early stages of HCC in order to minimize HCC morbidity and mortality [3]. Annexins are water soluble proteins, usually present in many animals, tissues, and cells. These proteins bind calcium and phospholipids and form ion voltage channels which are calcium-dependent. They are inscribed in cell signals, apoptosis, and control of various inflammatory elements, such as cytokines. Annexin A5 (Annex A5) is a member of the 36 kDa molecular weight annexin family which is based on the Ca2+ membrane binding [4]. Inhibition of pro-Inflammatory actions during apoptosis, Annexin-A5 appears to be of significance. Annexin-A5 was suggested to act as an active and selective anti-inflammatory agent to minimize inflammation during apoptosis [5]. The circulating AnxA5 can be emitted from wounded myocardial tissue, vascular endothelial and smooth muscular cells, liver secretary cells, and spleen; once it is in the plasma, it binds to blood cells (platelets and erythrocytes) or to endothelial cells [6] or also can be released from apoptotic particles derived from circulating blood cells, and the level of which has been shown to reflect severity of cell damage [7]. The levels of annexin gene expression inside human organs vary from universal to selective (for example A1, A2, A4, A5, A6, A7, and A11 annexes), including neutrophil annexin A3, placental and skin annexin A8, tongue A9, stomach annexin A10, and small intestine annexin A13 [8]. It is well known that ANXA5 can be liberated from damaged or dying

* Correspondence: waleed.ibrahim@suezuniv.edu.eg
[1]Faculty of Science, Suez University, Suez, Egypt
Full list of author information is available at the end of the article

Table 1 Demographic, clinical, and biochemical properties of all classes

Variables	Cirrhosis with HCC group (*n* = 44)	Cirrhosis without HCC group (*n* = 47)	P1value	Control group (*n* = 20)	*P* value
Age (years)	57.7 ± 5.75	56.8 ± 6.89	0.968 (NS)	54.5(50.5–60.5)	0.337 (NS)
Sex (M/F)	23/21	27/20	0.751 (NS)	10/10	0.587 (NS)
MELD	16.1 ± 4.16	15.1 ± 4.57	0.568 (NS)	–	–
Child–Pugh class (A/B/C)	12/20/12	14/18/14	0.733 (NS)	–	–
ALT (U/L)	51 ± 17.65	53.3 ± 15.94	0.761 (NS)	11.9 ± 3.47	< 0.001* (HS)
AST(U/L)	69 ± 23.39	68.2 ± 19.51	0.944 (NS)	15.4 ± 4.83	< 0.001* (HS)
ALKP (U/L)	107.60 ± 37.05	114.40 ± 41.84	0.068 (NS)	48.6 ± 10.49	< 0.001* (HS)
GGT (mg/dl)	51.09 ± 37.75	48.94 ± 26.37	0.818 (NS)	14.6 ± 4.57	< 0.001* (HS)
INR	1.5 ± 0.47	1.59 ± 0.51	0.542 (NS)	1.005 ± 0.49	< 0.001* (HS)
PT(s)	17.51 ± 4.21	18.62 ± 4.64	0.533 (NS)	13.07 ± 0.18	< 0.001* (HS)
Total bilirubin (mg/dl)	2.55 ± 1.61	2.59 ± 2.01	0.579 (NS)	0.49 ± 0.25	< 0.001* (HS)
Albumin (g/dl)	2.97 ± 0.72	2.54 ± 0.79	0.098 (NS)	4.43 ± 0.59	< 0.001* (HS)
Platelet count (× 10^3/cm^2)	113.04 ± 24.94	111.32 ± 17.63	0.935 (NS)	297.7 ± 17.87	< 0.001* (HS)
APRI score	1.88 ± 0.58	1.93 ± 0.61	0.794 (NS)	0.11 ± 0.03	< 0.001* (HS)
FIB-4 score	5.47 ± 1.04	5.32 ± 1.37	0.709 (NS)	0.57 ± 0.14	< 0.001* (HS)
Annexin A5 (ng/ml)	3.89 ± 0.85	3.06 ± 0.88	0.041 (S)	0.54 ± 0.11	< 0.001* (HS)
AFP (ng/ml)	270 ± 35	98 ± 20	< 0.001* (HS)	5.3 ± 2.9	< 0.001* (HS)

cells not explicitly [9]. In understanding how the presence of HCC can affect the weather equilibrium, it is important to consider the sense in which HCC is present, which is basically often a complication of cirrhosis to the liver [10], with the prevalence of cirrhosis among patients with HCC estimated of 85–95 [11]. By superimposed conditions, like HCC, the rebalanced and unstable hemostasis of hepatic cirrhosis can easily be tipped to thrombotic complications. In non-cirrhotic liver, HCC can develop, according to Kulik L.et al.; in a most recent analysis, the occurrence of HCC without prior cirrhosis is unusual and specifically about 15% of HBV-related cases [12]. The objective of our study was to detect Annexin A5 levels in such patients in order to assess their function as an HCC marker.

Methods

The longitudinal study comprised 44 patients with HCC cirrhosis (23 were male and 21 were female), 47 patients without HCC cirrhosis (27 were male and 20 are female), and 20 control healthy (10 were male and 10 were female) without evidence for the diseases of the liver approved by the National Hepatology and Tropical Medicine Research Institute (NHTMRI) between March 2017 and August 2018. The formal consent was given to all studied citizens. The NHTMRI Ethics Committee has approved this analysis under serial No. 15/2016. The study has been organized in accordance with the Declaration of Research on Human Subject in Helsinki for human subject's research. Both of the patients were diagnosed with hepatic biopsy histology, simple lab changes, and ultrasound from Doppler. The magnitude of liver disease was calculated in accordance with the MELD score and the Child-Pugh classification. Cirrhosis with and without HCC impacted hepatitis C and laboratory and imagery studies based on guidelines for AASLD practice have been clinically conformed. The exclusion criteria were patients of different malignancies that could raise the level of Annexin A5 such as colorectal cancer and pancreatic cancer. The amount of the serum anxA5 was calculated on Stat Fax 4700 Microstrip Reader1 ELISA Microstrip Reader by means of a commercial enzyme immunoassay (SinoGeneClon Biotech Co., Ltd).

Statistical analysis

All statistical analyses were evaluated in SPSS Version 19. Quantitative variables are listed as mean + SD or median, while qualitative variables are listed as frequencies. In order to differentiate the three classes, one way

Table 2 Annexin V level in cirrhotic HCV patients with HCC group

	Cut off	Sens. (%)	Spec. (%)	+PV (%)	−PV (%)	AUC
Serum Annexin A5 level	> 3.2(ng/ml)	80	55.8	43.8	93.5	0.566

Table 3 Annexin V level in cirrhotic HCV patients without HCC group

	Cut off	Sens. (%)	Spec. (%)	+PV (%)	−PV (%)	AUC
Serum Annexin A5 level	≤ 3.1(ng/ml)	50	53.66	13.6	88	0.571

analysis of variance (ANOVA) was used. A non-parametrical analysis was performed by Mann-Whitney, and a parametric student evaluation was performed when a categorical test of χ^2 had been applied. Statistically important was a P value below 0.05.

Results

Ninety-one cirrhotic patients, 44 HCC, and 47 HCC-free were recruited. Twenty healthy people were also hired (control group). Table 1 displays demographic, clinical, and biochemical properties of all classes.

No statistically significant differences in sex, age, albumin, ALKB, ALT, AST, GGT, T-bilirubin, PT, INR, platelet count, APRI score, and FIB-4 score were discovered between cirrhotic group with HCC and cirrhotic group without HCC (Table 1). There were statistically important variations between the two groups regarding AFP ($P < 0.001$) (Table 1). There were statistically relevant differences in Annexin A5 values ($P = 0.041$) between the two groups (Table 1). ROC curve reveals that in the cirrhotic HCC group, Annexin A5 has AUC 0.566 and in the cirrhotic group without HCC has AUC 0.571 (Tables 2 and 3; Figs. 1 and 2).

Discussion

Annexin A5 has been shown to facilitate tumorigenesis and cancers such as hepatocarcinoma, breast, colorectal, pancreas, bladder, and prostate cancer [13, 14]. In most different types of tumors, including liver cancer, ANXA5 exhibits tumor promoter activity. Two-dimension gel electrophoresis was used by Guo et al. to analyze protein expression in five pairs of tumor and tumor thrombal matched samples, which showed an upregulation of ANXA5 in tumor thrombus samples [15]. Sun and others reported that ANXA5 expression was positive for liver cancer progression and metastasis and that ANXA5 promoted cancer through the integrin and mitogen-activated protein kinase-extracellular signal-regulated kinase pathways [16]. Anxa5 could be a predictive biomarker for tumor development, metastasis, and invasion and be of diagnostic, prognostic, and therapeutic significance in cancer [14]. In addition, Sun and Zhuang et al. showed that HCC expression in ANXA5 was higher than normal liver tissue [16, 17]. The findings of the present study indicate, as compared the cirrhotic patients with and without HCC, that the expression of ANXA5 was increased

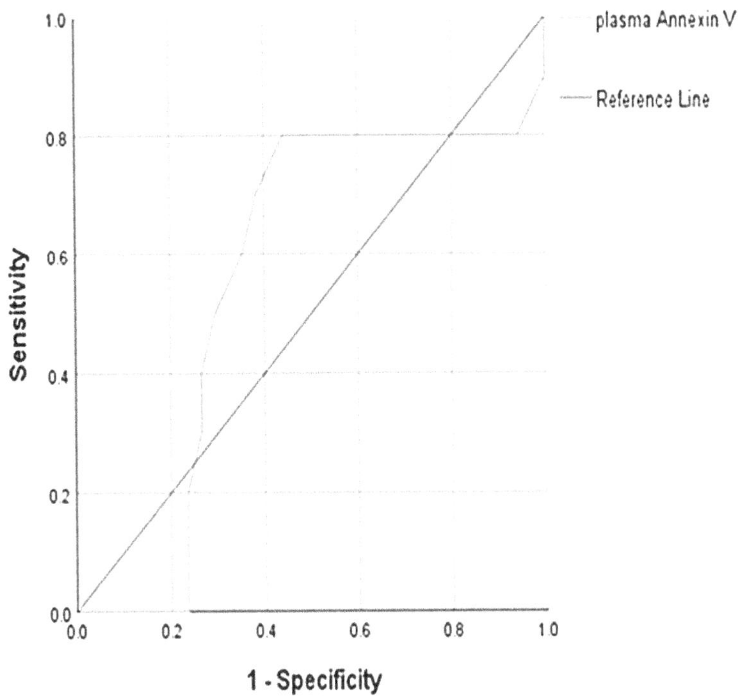

Fig. 1 Serum Annexin A5 ROC curve in HCC group cirrhotic patients

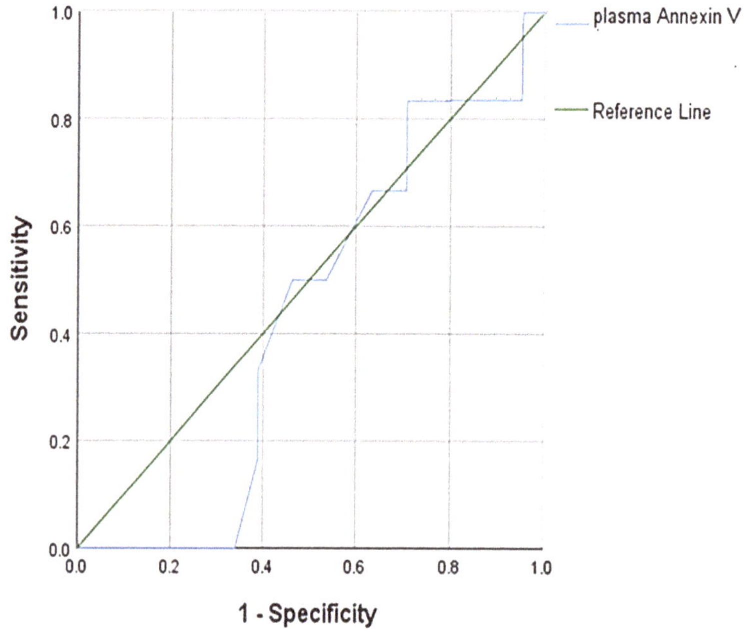

Fig. 2 Serum Annexin A5 ROC curve in cirrhotic patients without HCC

in HCC cirrhotic HCV patients. In addition, the pronounced role of ANXA5 in liver cancer has not been documented to the best of our knowledge. In another review, high ANXA5 expression has been shown to be correlated significantly with poor overall survival [17]. AnxA5 has proved to participate in a wide range of intra- and extracellular processes including blood clotting, signal translation, anti-inflammatory processes, membrane trafficking, and ion channel activity, but it has not yet established the exact biological function of anxA5. However, it is assumed that the biological functions of anxA5 rely primarily on the interaction between them and lipids of the membranes [18], and at least two crucial physiological mechanisms are regulated: the cascade of coagulation, which is known to involve anticoagulant activity, and apoptosis [19]. Various research models have used annexin A5 as a probe to measure apoptosis in vitro and in vivo. A non-invasive imaging protocol using annexin A5 has been developed and applied successfully to measure programmed cell death in patients [20]. In addition, our study match to previous results showing that HCC hepatitis C patients have greater levels of microparticles than HCC-free hepatitis C patients, and these levels of microparticles dynamically alter after surgery [21]. In contrast to healthy controls, the explanation of the presence of microparticles in cirrhotic liver is possibly due to systemic inflammation and liver cell damage [22], asserting microparticulate roles that are included in hepatic fibrosty process in mediation of anti-inflammatory reactions, endothelial damage, and coagulation activation.

Conclusion

In HCC prediction in cirrhotic HCV patients, serum Annexin A5 values were found to be a forecasting factor. Larger scale tests are important to promote the use of an inexpensive and easily accessible Annexin A5 biomarker as HCC marker in HCV cirrhotic patients.

Limitation of study

In our analysis, the sample size of the control group compared to the disease group is relatively small. Finally, it would have been more fitting if the control group number was at least equal to the diseased group.

Recommendation

Wide sample sizes are suggested to validate this result.

Abbreviations

AnxA5: Annexin A5; HCV: Hepatitis C virus; HCC: Hepatocellular carcinoma

Acknowledgements

Great confession of collaboration for all NHTMRI doctors.

Authors' contributions

WS was responsible for the practical section, analysis of data, and manuscript preparation. BE was responsible for the selection and classification of the samples and the manuscript revision. The final manuscript was read and accepted by all contributors.

Declarations

Ethics approval and consent to participate

Informative approval from all study participants, with the number 15/2016 of the National Institute of Hepatology and Tropical Medicine Research, was obtained written and validated by the Ethical Committee.

Competing interests

The authors note that the work reported in this paper was not known for its conflict of financial interests or personal relationships.

Author details

[1]Faculty of Science, Suez University, Suez, Egypt. [2]National Hepatology and Tropical Medicine Research Institute, Cairo, Egypt.

References

1. Jemal A, Bray F, Center MM, Ferlay J, Ward E et al (2011) Global cancer statistics. CA: Cancer J. Clin 61:69–90. https://doi.org/10.3322/caac.201072
2. Bray F, Ferlay J, Soerjomataram I, Siegel RL, Torre LA, Jemal A (2018) Global cancer statistics 2018: GLOBOCAN estimates of incidence and mortality worldwide for 36 cancers in 185 countries. CA: Cancer J. Clin 68(394):424–424. https://doi.org/10.3322/caac.21492
3. Marrero JA, Kulik LM, Sirlin CB, Zhu AX, Finn RS, Abecassis MM, Roberts LR, Heimbach JK (2018) Diagnosis, staging, and management of hepatocellular carcinoma: 2018 practice guidance by the American Association for the Study of Liver Diseases. Hepatology 68:723–750. https://doi.org/10.1002/hep.299132
4. Bouter A, Carmeille R, Gounou C, Bouvet F, Degrelle S et al (2015) Annexin-A5 and cell membrane repair. Placenta 36:S43–SS9. https://doi.org/10.1016/j.placenta.2015.01.193
5. Francesconi L, Ceresér K, Mascarenhas R, Stertz L, Gama C et al (2011) Increased annexin-V and decreased TNF-alpha serum levels in chronic-medicated patients with schizophrenia. Neurosci. Lett. 502:143–146. https://doi.org/10.1016/j.neulet.2011.06.0423
6. Roldán V, Marn F, Pineda J, Marco P, Corral J, Climent V, García A, Martínez JG, Sogorb F (2002) nexina V en pacientes supervivientes de un infarto de miocardio prematuro. Rev Esp Cardiol. 55:1230–1234. https://doi.org/10.1016/S0300-8932(02)76794-812
7. Lai C, Pc C, Wong S, Kw C, Yf C. (2012). Circulating Annexin A5 levels after atrial switch for transposition of the great arteries.
8. Mirsaeidi M, Gidfar S, Vu A, Schraufnagel D (2016) Annexins family: insights into their functions and potential role in pathogenesis of sarcoidosis. J Transl Med 14:1–9. https://doi.org/10.1186/s12967-016-0843-71
9. Kaneko N, Matsuda R, Hosoda S, Kajita T, Ohta Y (1996) Measurement of plasma annexin V by ELISA in the early detection of acute myocardial infarction. Clin. Chim. Acta 251:65–80. https://doi.org/10.1016/0009-8981(96)06294-81
10. Velázquez RF, Rodríguez M, Navascués CA, Linares A, Pérez R et al (2003) Prospective analysis of risk factors for hepatocellular carcinoma in patients with liver cirrhosis. Hepatology 37:520–527. https://doi.org/10.1053/jhep.2003.500933
11. Heimbach JK, Kulik LM, Finn RS, Sirlin CB, Abecassis MM, Roberts LR, Zhu AX, Murad MH, Marrero JA (2018) (2018). AASLD guidelines for the treatment of hepatocellular carcinoma. Hepatology 67:358–380. https://doi.org/10.1002/hep.290861
12. Kulik L, El-Serag HB (2019) Epidemiology and management of hepatocellular carcinoma. Gastroenterology 156:477-91. e1.https://doi.org/10.1053/j.gastro.2018.08.065. 156(2):477–491.e1
13. Wang J, Zhang Y, Liu X, Ma J, Liu P et al (2014) Annexin A5 inhibits diffuse large B-cell lymphoma cell invasion and chemoresistance through phosphatidylinositol 3-kinase signaling. Oncol. Rep. 32:2557–2563. https://doi.org/10.3892/or.2014.35476
14. Peng B, Guo C, Guan H, Liu S, Sun M-Z (2014) Annexin A5 as a potential marker in tumors. Clin. Chim. Acta 427:42–48 https://doi.org/10.1016/j.cca.2013.09.048
15. Guo W-X, Man X-B, Yuan H-X, Shi J, Xue J, Wu MC, Cheng SQ (2007). Proteomic analysis on portal vein tumor thrombus-associated proteins for hepatocellular carcinoma. Zhonghua yi xue za zhi 87:2094-2097. PMID: 17988525, 30
16. Sun X, Liu S, Wang J, Wei B, Guo C, Chen C, Sun MZ et al (2018) Annexin A5 regulates hepatocarcinoma malignancy via CRKI/II-DOCK180-RAC1 integrin and MEK-ERK pathways. Cell Death Dis. 9:1–16. https://doi.org/10.1038/s41419-018-0685-86
17. Zhuang C, Wang P, Sun T, Zheng L, Ming L (2019) Expression levels and prognostic values of annexins in liver cancer. Oncol. Lett. 18:6657–6669 https://doi.org/10.3892/ol.2019.11025
18. Ravassa S, Bennaghmouch A, Kenis H, Lindhout T, Hackeng T, Narula J, Hofstra L, Reutelingsperger C (2005) Annexin A5 down-regulates surface expression of tissue factor a novel mechanism of regulating the membrane receptor repertoir. J. Biol. Chem. 280:6028–6035. https://doi.org/10.1074/jbc.M4117102007
19. Baleva M, Hristova M, Nikolov K (2010) Diagnostic significance of anti-annexin-A5 antibody determination. Open Med. 5:6–11. https://doi.org/10.2478/s11536-009-0132-41
20. Corsten MF, Hofstra L, Narula J, Reutelingsperger CP (2006) Counting heads in the war against cancer: defining the role of annexin A5 imaging in cancer treatment and surveillance. Cancer Res 66(3):1255–1260. https://doi.org/10.1158/0008-5472.CAN-05-3000
21. Brodsky SV, Facciuto ME, Heydt D, Chen J, Islam HK, et al.(2008). Dynamics of circulating microparticles in liver transplant patients. J Gastrointestin Liver Dis 17:261-268. PMID: 18836617
22. Rautou PE, Bresson J, Sainte-Marie Y, Vion AC, Paradis V et al (2012) Abnormal plasma microparticles impair vasoconstrictor responses in patients with cirrhosis. Gastroenterology 143:166–76.e6. https://doi.org/10.1053/j.gastro.2012.03.040

19

Evaluation of mental health and anxiety level among hepatitis C patients during COVID-19 pandemic in Pakistan

Sadia Rafique[1], Muhammad Saleem Khan[1*], Rabia Unar[2], Muhammad Wajid[1], Ahmad Waheed[1] and Ali Umar[1]

Abstract

Background: This study was conducted to check anxiety level and mental stress in the 200 confirmed hepatitis C patients during the COVID-19 pandemic. The Chinese version of the Beck Anxiety Inventory (BAI) score index was used to measure the anxiety level of HCV-positive patients. BAI score index of different demographic factors such as gender, age, occupation, and education of all the sampled population was calculated.

Results: The highest BAI score was recorded in people in the age group of 25–45 years (54.5%). Respondents from public sector employees, own businesses, and postgraduates were highly anxious. A significant difference in BAI score was also recorded between male and female respondents as 33.77% of females were at a severe level of anxiety compared to 17.07% of males. Furthermore, quarantined hepatitis C patients had a significantly higher BAI score (39.5) as compared to non-quarantined patients (27.12), and respondents with HCV infection also had a high BAI score of 37.25 compared to healthy individuals (4.1). Most of the respondents were willing to adopt protective measures against COVID-19.

Conclusion: This study concluded that people with infectious diseases like hepatitis C had high anxiety levels and mental stress in the COVID-19 pandemic and needed psychological aids for better mental health to handle pandemic conditions.

Keywords: Hepatitis C, COVID-19, Anxiety, Mental health, Pakistan

Background

Hepatitis is a serious health concern around the globe and especially in developing countries in Asia [1]. Hepatitis C virus (HCV) is the causative agent of hepatitis C and 3% of the world's population is infected by this virus. Chronic hepatitis C damages hepatic tissues and, in some cases, also develops hepatic carcinoma and hepatic cirrhosis [2].

When a person is infected by HCV, the virus influences the immune system and destroys the recognition and defense system of the host body. Acute or mild infections have less impact on immunology, but if left untreated for a long period of time, the infection can progress to a chronic condition that reduces patients' immunity. These immunosuppressed patients have more chances of developing severe complications in other diseases like COVID-19 than healthier persons [3].

COVID-19 is a pandemic viral infection, caused by a coronavirus (SARS-CoV-2). The outbreak began in Wuhan (China) and spread throughout the world [4]. To date, 151,916,040 people have been infected and 3,190, 948 deaths have been reported globally due to the COVID-19 pandemic [5]. This pandemic also increases anxiety, depression, and restlessness in immune-suppressed individuals such as HCV-infected people.

Psychological problems are often observed in patients suffering from chronic HCV or undergoing HCV treatment such as riboflavin and PegIFNa (pegylated

* Correspondence: SamiiKhan@uo.edu.pk
[1]Department of Zoology, Faculty of Life Sciences, University of Okara, Okara 56130, Pakistan
Full list of author information is available at the end of the article

interferon-alpha). The most frequent and serious side effect of antiviral therapy is depression and poor mental health [6]. Several other factors, such as thinking of being affected by a deadly disease, the negative social impact, and higher complications, are responsible for psychological problems [7]. People are affected very badly in respect of mental health due to the COVID-19 pandemic [8], and this also increases anxiety and stress in HCV patients as recorded in this study. The lockdown situation further increases problems for chronic patients like HCV in terms of availability of medicine and fear of being infected with COVID-19 infection, and this was proved in previous studies by Guerriero et al. [9] that lockdown increases the functional neurological symptoms of mental health disorder by 3.4-fold. Furthermore, similar stressful conditions and anxiety were recorded in individuals that were in direct contact with Ebola-infected individuals (2018) in the Democratic Republic of the Congo and Sierra Leone [10]. Seeing the current situations, this study was designed to find out the anxiety level in HCV-infected individuals.

Methods

Sample population

A cross-sectional study was conducted in different hospitals in Punjab, Pakistan, on a random basis for 4 months. The sample size consisted of 200 HCV-infected patients, who were approached and interviewed in hospitals. Verbal consent was obtained from all individual participants before the interview and the consent was approved by the Ethical Committee, University of Okara (reference number: UO/DOZ/2020/misc.). It was made sure that the ethical standards involving human participants were followed by all means according to the ethical standards of the Ethical Committee, University of Okara, as well as the 1964 Helsinki Declaration and its later amendments or comparable ethical standards.

Assessment of anxiety level

To evaluate the anxiety level, the Chinese version of the Beck Anxiety Inventory (BAI)-based questionnaire was used. This version was used successfully to evaluate the anxiety levels in Chinese populations [11, 12]. The BAI consisted of different questions that describe symptoms of anxiety. Respondents were asked to rate their anxiety level with symptoms on a 4-point Likert type (0–3). The total score ranged between 0 and 63 was used to rate each individual on the anxiety scale [13]. BAI scores were categorized into 4 levels. Normal respondents had scores ranging from 0 to 9, mild or moderate 10–18, moderate to severe 19–29, and severe 30–63 [14].

Statistical analysis

The demographic profile of the sample and BAI scores were characterized by descriptive statistics. Minitab V.17 was used as a statistical tool to analyze the data.

Results

The study population consisted of 200 confirmed HCV-infected patients that regularly visited the hospitals. Out of total respondents, 61.5% (n = 123) were male and 38.5% (n = 77) were female. Most of the respondents (n = 109, 54.5%) were between the ages of 25 and 45. Respondents were of different professions, like labor (maximum, 20.5%) and students (7.5% being minimum). The educational levels of respondents were different from undergraduate (49%), graduate (36.5%), and postgraduate (14.5%) as represented in Table 1.

It was widely assumed that COVID-19 outbreaks cause anxiety and mental stress in the general population. We investigated whether this outbreak also affects patients with compromised immunity, i.e., HCV-infected patients. For this purpose, we recorded the BAI score in HCV patients. There was a significant difference in BAI scores between males and females. A high BAI score was recorded in the age group of 25–45 years, which showed severe anxiety levels in this age group in HCV-infected patients. Furthermore, we also checked whether the demographic characters influence the BAI score or not.

Table 1 Demographic characteristics of HCV-positive participants

Participant characteristics	Respondents	
	N	%
Gender		
Male	123	61.5
Female	77	38.5
Age		
≤ 25 years	11	5.5
25–45 years	109	54.5
> 45 years	80	40
Occupation		
Student	15	7.5
Teachers	36	18
Unemployed	15	7.5
Agriculture	40	20
Own business	20	10
Labor workers	41	20.5
Public sector employee	33	16.5
Education		
Undergraduate	98	49
Graduate	73	36.5
Postgraduate	29	14.5

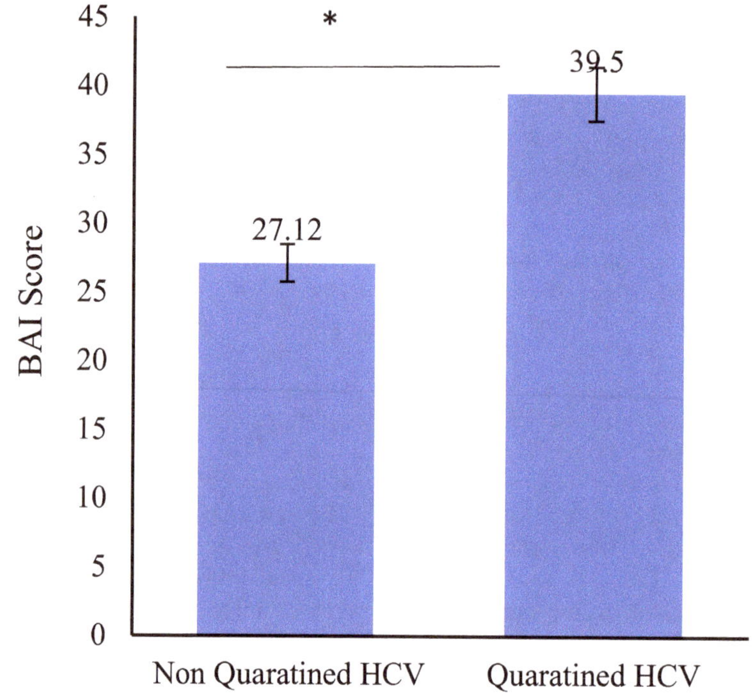

Fig. 1 BAI score of quarantined HCV patients vs non-quarantined HCV patients

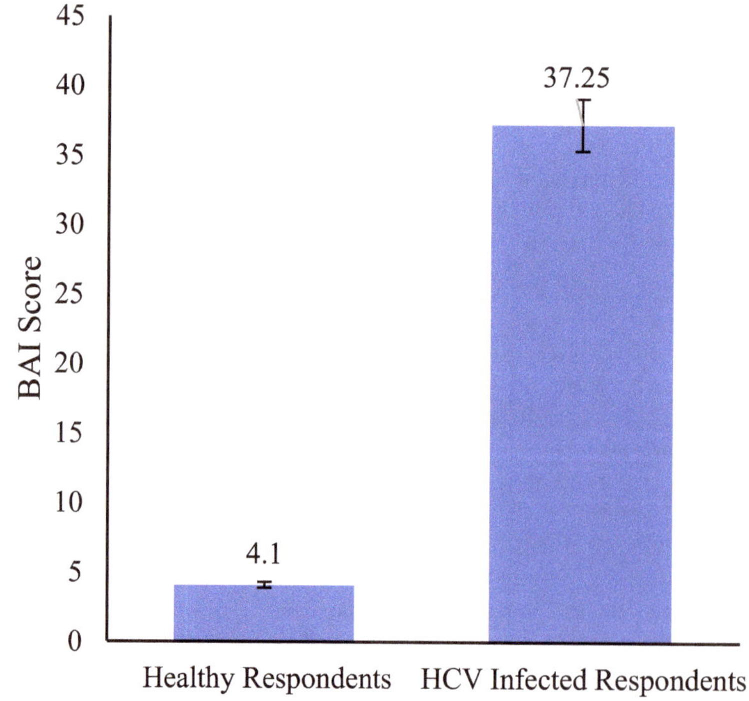

Fig. 2 BAI score of healthy vs HCV-positive patients

Unlike others, a very low level of anxiety was recorded among HCV-infected students as most (80%) of students have BAI level 1.

The quarantined HCV patients had a significantly higher BAI score as compared to non-quarantined HCV patients (Fig. 1), while HCV-positive patients had a highly significant BAI score as compared to healthy individuals (Fig. 2).

Among the professions, the highest percentage of respondents with their business (50%) were at a severe anxiety level (30–63%). The same was in the case of postgraduate patients (Table 2).

The comparison of BAI scores of HCV-positive quarantined and HCV-positive non-quarantined patients showed that quarantined respondents had a significantly higher BAI score compared to non-quarantined patients (Fig. 3).

Table 3 shows that most of the respondents were very conscious of adopting protective measures against being infected by COVID-19. For example, 82.5% of respondents were in the habit of using masks when they went outside their homes. The respondents were using hand sanitizers (47%), and soap (53%) for washing their hands. 82.5% of respondents were frequently washing their hands. 67% of people agreed to quarantine if symptoms of COVID-19 were experienced (Fig. 4).

Discussion

This study aimed to record the anxiety level in HCV-positive respondents in response to the COVID-19 outbreak in the Pakistani population. It was hypothesized that the average BAI score will be higher in HCV patients compared to normal individuals. Our hypothesis was supported by the investigation of [11, 12] as their BAI score of the general population of China in an epidemic-free environment was significantly lower than the sampled population in the present study. Moreover, it was found that hepatitis C patients that were quarantined (n = 32) at the time of sampling had a higher BAI score as compared to patients that were not quarantined. These results support the view that human mental health is significantly affected by communicable diseases [15]. In fact, during the West African Ebola virus disease (EVD) outbreak, healthcare workers confirmed that, in addition to deaths and sadness, mental health services were disrupted due to the intense emotional stress faced

Table 2 BAI score of the HCV-infected respondents classified in various subsamples

Subsamples	BAI score					
	0–9 n (%)	10–18 (%)	19–29 (%)	30–63 (%)	χ^2	P
Gender						
Male (n = 123)	45 (36.59%)	30 (24.39%)	27 (21.95%)	21 (17.07%)	13.070	0.004
Female (n = 77)	13 (16.88%)	16 (20.78%)	22 (28.57%)	26 (33.77%)		
Age						
≤ 25 years (n = 11)	8 (72.73%)	2 (18.18%)	1 (9.09%)	0	13.041	0.042
25–45 years (n = 109)	29 (26.61%)	31 (28.44%)	18 (16.51%)	31 (28.44%)		
> 45 years (n = 80)	31 (38.75%)	21 (26.25%)	14 (17.5%)	14 (17.5%)		
Occupation						
Students (n = 15)	12 (80%)	3 (20%)	0	0	94.589	0.001
Teachers (n = 36)	4 (11.11%)	12 (33.33%)	10 (27.78%)	10 (27.78%)		
Unemployed (n = 15)	2 (13.33%)	3 (20.00%)	8 (53.33%)	2 (13.33%)		
Agriculture (n = 40)	26 (65%)	11 (27.50%)	0	3 (7.50%)		
Own business (n = 20)	2 (10%)	0	8 (40%)	10 (50%)		
Labor workers (n = 41)	12 (29.27%)	12 (29.27%)	14 (34.15%)	3 (7.32%)		
Public sector employee (n = 33)	3 (9.09%)	8 (24.24%)	10 (30.30%)	12 (36.36%)		
Education						
Undergraduate (n = 98)	63 (64.29%)	24 (24.49%)	6 (6.12%)	5 (5.10%)	55.165	0.002
Graduate (n = 73)	34 (46.58%)	3 (4.11%)	24 (32.88%)	12 (16.44%)		
Postgraduate (n = 29)	5 (17.24%)	9 (31.03%)	5 (17.24%)	10 (34.48%)		
Quarantined						
Yes (n = 32)	0	0	11 (33.37%)	21 (66.63%)	45.183	0.004
No (n = 168)	67 (39.88%)	32 (19.04%)	40 (23.81%)	29 (17.26%)		

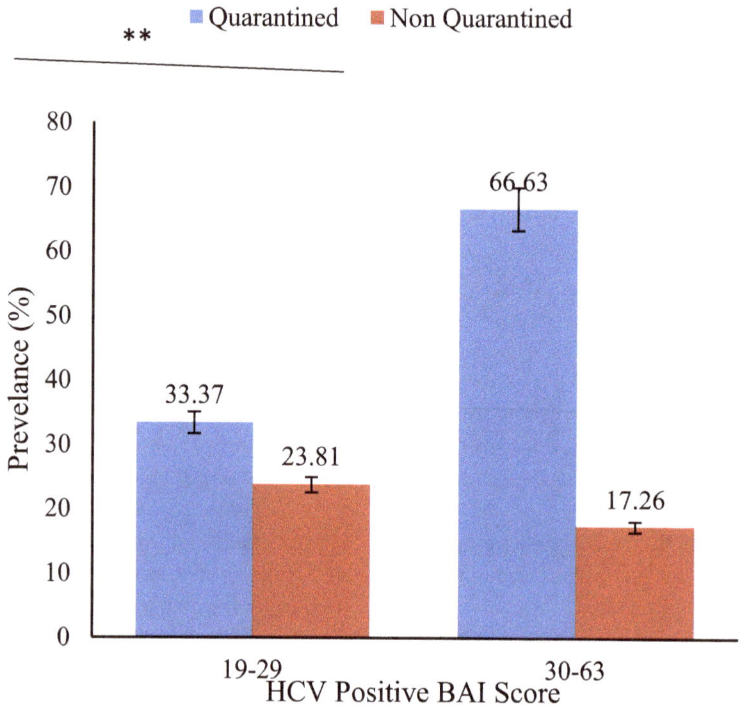

Fig. 3 Prevalence in HCV-positive quarantined vs HCV-positive non-quarantined patients

by patients and their family members, as well as by medical professionals [16].

Out of 200 HCV-positive patients, quarantined (n = 32) patients showed a higher BAI score compared to non-quarantined most probably due to COVID-19 symptoms like sneezing, coughing, difficulty in breathing, malaise, or fever, in the quarantine period, as higher scores of depression subscale as well as Depression, Anxiety and Stress Scale (DASS) were seen in people feeling cold, sore throat, nausea, shortness of breath, and coryza in other studies [17]. Furthermore, the highest BAI score in quarantined patients could be due to viral infection, as found in previous studies, such as the association of neuropsychiatric disease with Borna virus [15], the anxiety experienced by SARS patients [18], and psychological issues such as frustration, depression, fear, anxiety, and suicidal ideation in SARS patients as well [14].

We found a significant difference in the anxiety of females and males, with more anxiety levels in females compared to males. China, Turkey, Italy, and Spain, all have reported similar results [17, 19–21]. A study by Rehman et al. [22] also recorded no significant difference in the anxiety of both sexes in the COVID-19 pandemic. The respondents in the age group of 25–45 years showed higher anxiety levels as compared to the youngsters (≤ 25 years) and older people (> 45 years), and this might be due to 25–45-year-old participants are the backbone of

Table 3 Prevalence of anxiety-related symptoms in HCV-infected respondents regarding COVID-19

Sr #	Parameters	Yes n (%)	No n (%)	Not sure n (%)	χ^2	P
1	Restless due to social distancing?	109 (54.5%)	69 (34.5%)	22 (11%)	56.89	0.05
2	Significant weight loss or gain	69 (34.5%)	117 (58.5%)	14 (7%)	79.69	0.003
3	Insomnia or excessive sleep	69 (34.5%)	124 (62%)	7 (3.50%)	102.79	0.004
4	Repeated thoughts of death?	84 (42%)	105 (52.5%)	11 (5.5%)	73.03	0.013
5	Lacking interest in daily life?	123 (61.5%)	48 (24%)	29 (14.5%)	74.11	0.012
6	Fear leaving house	83 (41.5%)	107 (53.5%)	10 (5%)	76.57	0.001
7	Avoided avail healthcare facilities	116 (58%)	63 (31.5%)	21 (10.5%)	67.99	0.011
8	Limited physical contact	164 (82%)	26 (13%)	10 (5%)	215.08	0.004
9	Avoid watching the news	116 (58%)	74 (37%)	10 (5%)	85.48	0.002

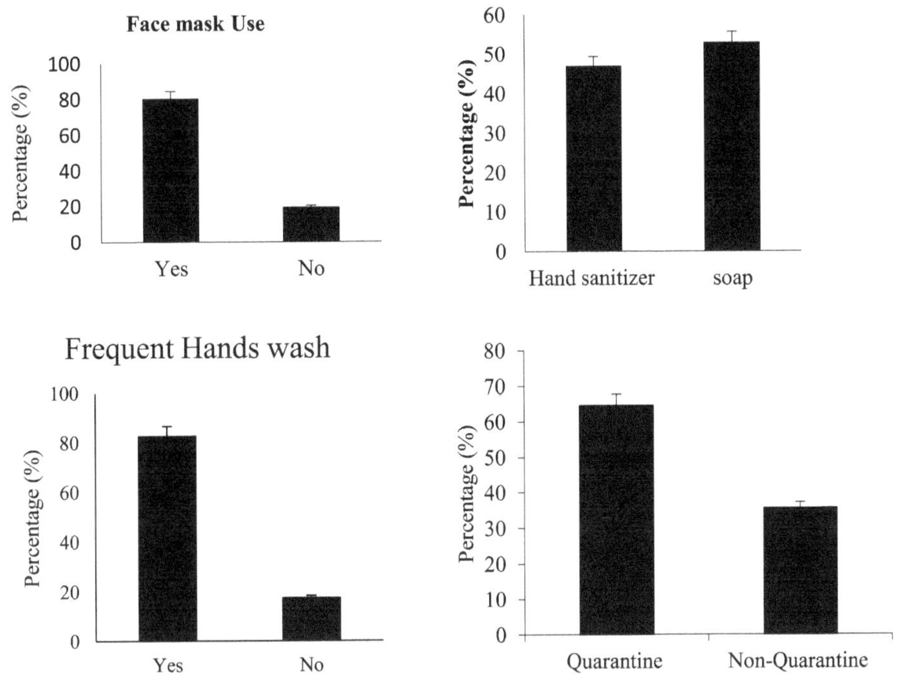

Fig. 4 Percentage proactive measures taken by HCV-infected respondents against COVID-19 infection

their family and they have more burdens of life as well as responsibilities compared to other age groups. Moreover, older people have had more severe anxiety (17.5%) as compared to younger ones. This could be due to a fear of death and dying as a result of an unknown disease. Our study differed in this aspect from Shah et al. [23] and Ozamiz-Etxebarria et al. [24] who found elevated levels of anxiety in age groups 18–24 and 18–26 respectively.

In a comparison based on occupation, those who had owned a business were more anxious (50%) than all other categories, followed by those who worked in the public sector (36.36%). Students found normal (80%) than teachers (11.11%). These outcomes were also opposed to the study of Shah et al. [23] and Cao et al. [25] who found higher levels of anxiety in students, while Rehman et al. [22] found a moderate level of anxiety in students, researchers, and health professionals in India. Furthermore, postgraduates also had anxiety levels (34.48%) followed by graduates (16.44%) and undergraduates (5.10%). This finding contradicted the findings of Zhao et al. [26] who discovered that people in high school or below experienced severe anxiety in China due to COVID-19.

Conclusion

This study concluded that people with infectious diseases such as hepatitis C have higher anxiety levels during COVID-19 pandemic conditions and require adequate psychological aids for better mental health.

Abbreviations

BAI: Beck Anxiety Inventory; SARS-CoV-2: Severe acute respiratory syndrome coronavirus 2; DASS: Depression, Anxiety and Stress Scale; EVD: Ebola virus disease; HCV: Hepatitis C virus; MERS: Middle East respiratory syndrome; SARS: Severe acute respiratory disease

Acknowledgements

The authors are thankful to the Faculty of Zoology and Vice-chancellor, University of Okara, for providing support to complete this research.

Authors' contributions

SR, RU, and MW collected the data. MSK, AW, and AU organized the data, performed the statistical analysis, and prepared the manuscript. All authors read and approved the final manuscript.

Declarations

Ethics approval and consent to participate

All procedures performed in studies involving human participants were in accordance with the ethical standards of the Ethical Committee, University of Okara (reference number: UO/DOZ/2020/misc.), and with the 1964 Helsinki declaration and its later amendments or comparable ethical standards. Verbal consent was obtained from all individual participants included in the study and the consent was approved by the Ethical Committee, University of Okara (reference number: UO/DOZ/2020/misc.).

Competing interests

The authors declare that they have no competing interests.

Author details

[1]Department of Zoology, Faculty of Life Sciences, University of Okara, Okara 56130, Pakistan. [2]Jinnah Post Graduate Medical Center Hospital, Karachi, Pakistan.

References

1. Lu SN, Chen TM, Lee CM, Wang JH, Tung HD, Wu JC (2003) Molecular epidemiological and clinical aspects of hepatitis D virus in a unique triple hepatitis viruses (B, C, D) endemic community in Taiwan. J Med Virol 70(1): 74–80. https://doi.org/10.1002/jmv.10361
2. Mehmood S, Raza H, Abid F, Saeed N, Rehan HM, Javed S, Khan MS (2019) National prevalence rate of hepatitis B and C in Pakistan and its risk factors. J Public Health 28(6):1–14. https://doi.org/10.1007/s10389-019-01081-5
3. Netski DM, Mosbruger T, Depla E, Maertens G, Ray SC, Hamilton RG, Roundtree S, Thomas DL, McKeating J, Cox A (2005) Humoral immune response in acute hepatitis C virus infection. Clin Infect Dis 41(5):667–675. https://doi.org/10.1086/432478
4. Ebrahim SH, Ahmed QA, Gozzer E, Schlagenhauf P, Memish ZA (2020) Covid-19 and community mitigation strategies in a pandemic. British Medical Journal Publishing Group. https://doi.org/10.1136/bmj.m1066
5. Worldometers (2021) COVID-19 coronavirus pandemic. https://www.worldometers.info/coronavirus/.
6. Schaefer M, Capuron L, Friebe A, Diez-Quevedo C, Robaeys G, Neri S, Foster GR, Kautz A, Forton D, Pariante CM (2012) Hepatitis C infection, antiviral treatment and mental health: a European expert consensus statement. J Hepatol 57(6):1379–1390. https://doi.org/10.1016/j.jhep.2012.07.037
7. Fontana RJ, Hussain KB, Schwartz SM, Moyer CA, Su GL, Lok AS (2002) Emotional distress in chronic hepatitis C patients not receiving antiviral therapy. J Hepatol 36(3): 401–407. https://doi.org/10.1016/s0168-8278(01)00280-x
8. Ma K, Zhang Y, Hou T, Wu M, Cai W, Wen T (2020) Investigation of physical and mental health in isolated people during the outbreak of novel coronavirus pneumonia. Chin J Clin Med 27(01):36–40
9. Guerriero RM, Pier DB, De Gusmão CM, Bernson-Leung ME, Maski KP, Urion DK, Waugh JL (2014) Increased pediatric functional neurological symptom disorders after the Boston Marathon bombings: a case series. Pediatr Neurol 51(5):619–623. https://doi.org/10.1016/j.pediatrneurol.2014.07.011
10. Park J-S, Lee E-H, Park N-R, Choi YH (2018) Mental health of nurses working at a government-designated hospital during a MERS-CoV outbreak: a cross-sectional study. Arch Psychiatr Nurs 32(1):2–6. https://doi.org/10.1016/j.apnu.2017.09.006
11. Huang W-L, Chen T-T, Chen I-M, Chang L-R, Lin Y-H, Liao S-C, Gau SS-F (2016) Harm avoidance and persistence are associated with somatoform disorder psychopathology: a study in Taiwan. J Affect Disord 196:83–86. https://doi.org/10.1016/j.jad.2016.02.009
12. Huang W-L, Chen T-T, Chen I-M, Ma H-M, Lee M-T, Liao S-C, Gau S-F (2016) Depression and anxiety among patients with somatoform disorders, panic disorder, and other depressive/anxiety disorders in Taiwan. Psychiatry Res 241:165–171. https://doi.org/10.1016/j.psychres.2016.05.008
13. Beck AT, Epstein N, Brown G, Steer RA (1988) An inventory for measuring clinical anxiety: psychometric properties. J Consult Clin Psychol 56(6):893–897. https://doi.org/10.1037/0022-006x.56.6.893
14. Cheng SK-W, Tsang JS-K, Ku K-H, Wong C-W, Ng Y-K (2004) Psychiatric complications in patients with severe acute respiratory syndrome (SARS) during the acute treatment phase: a series of 10 cases. Br J Psychiatry 184(4):359–360. https://doi.org/10.1192/bjp.184.4.359
15. Tucci V, Moukaddam N, Meadows J, Shah S, Galwankar SC, Kapur GB (2017) The forgotten plague: psychiatric manifestations of Ebola, Zika, and emerging infectious diseases. J Glob Infect Dis 9(4):151–156. https://doi.org/10.4103/jgid.jgid_66_17
16. Reardon S (2015) Ebola's mental-health wounds linger in Africa: health-care workers struggle to help people who have been traumatized by the epidemic. Nature 519(7541):13–15. https://doi.org/10.1038/519013a
17. Wang C, Pan R, Wan X, Tan Y, Xu L, Ho CS, Ho RC (2020) Immediate psychological responses and associated factors during the initial stage of the 2019 coronavirus disease (COVID-19) epidemic among the general population in China. Int J Environ Res Public Health 17(5):1729. https://doi.org/10.3390/ijerph17051729
18. Maunder R, Hunter J, Vincent L, Bennett J, Peladeau N, Leszcz M, Sadavoy J, Verhaeghe LM, Steinberg R, Mazzulli T (2003) The immediate psychological and occupational impact of the 2003 SARS outbreak in a teaching hospital. CMAJ 168(10):1245–1251
19. Özdin S, Bayrak Özdin Ş (2020) Levels and predictors of anxiety, depression and health anxiety during COVID-19 pandemic in Turkish society: the importance of gender. Int J Soc Psychiatry 66(5):504–511. https://doi.org/10.1177/0020764020927051
20. Wang C, Horby PW, Hayden FG, Gao GF (2020) A novel coronavirus outbreak of global health concern. Lancet 395(10223):470–473. https://doi.org/10.1016/S0140-6736(20)30185-9
21. Ozamiz-Etxebarria N, Dosil-Santamaria M, Picaza-Gorrochategui M, Idoiaga-Mondragon N (2020) Niveles de estrés, ansiedad y depresión en la primera fase del brote del COVID-19 en una muestra recogida en el norte de España. Cad Saúde Pública 36(4). https://doi.org/10.1590/0102-311x00054020
22. Rehman U, Shahnawaz MG, Khan NH, Kharshiing KD, Khursheed M, Gupta K, Kashyap D, Uniyal R (2021) Depression, anxiety and stress among Indians in times of Covid-19 lockdown. Community Ment Health J 57(1):42–48. https://doi.org/10.1007/s10597-020-00664-x
23. Shah SMA, Mohammad D, Qureshi MFH, Abbas MZ, Aleem S (2021) Prevalence, psychological responses and associated correlates of depression, anxiety and stress in a global population, during the coronavirus disease (COVID-19) pandemic. Community Ment Health J 57(1):101–110. https://doi.org/10.1007/s10597-020-00728-y
24. Ozamiz-Etxebarria N, Dosil-Santamaria M, Picaza-Gorrochategui M, Idoiaga-Mondragon N (2020) Stress, anxiety, and depression levels in the initial stage of the COVID-19 outbreak in a population sample in the northern Spain. Cad Saude Publica 36(4):e00054020. https://doi.org/10.1590/0102-311X00054020
25. Cao W, Fang Z, Hou G, Han M, Xu X, Dong J, Zheng J (2020) The psychological impact of the COVID-19 epidemic on college students in China. Psychiatry Res 287:112934. https://doi.org/10.1016/j.psychres.2020.112934
26. Zhao H, He X, Fan G, Li L, Huang Q, Qiu Q, Kang Z, Du T, Han L, Ding L (2020) COVID-19 infection outbreak increases anxiety level of general public in China: involved mechanisms and influencing factors. J Affect Disord 276: 446–452. https://doi.org/10.1016/j.jad.2020.07.085

20

Screening for chronic hepatitis C and chronic hepatitis B infections among pregnant females

Rasha Eletreby[1*], Maged Abd Elraouf[2], Ahmed Fouad[1], Mona Nasser[3], Mostafa Al Bassiouni[1], Naglaa Zayed[1], Ayman Yosry[1] and Zeinab Abdellatif[1]

Abstract

Background: In Egypt, an endemic country for both viral hepatitis C and B infections, infection could be more prevalent in pregnant females. This study aimed to assess the prevalence of chronic HCV and HBV in a cohort of pregnant Egyptian females, highlighting the disease burden for better preventive measures and better disease outcome. In this cross-sectional prospective study, 399 pregnant women attending antenatal clinic in a tertiary care center in Egypt were screened for HCV and HBV infection using ELISA testing. Clinical and biochemical characteristics were compared between positive and negative cases.

Results: Mean age was 26.78 years. Prevalence rates of HCV-Ab and HBsAg positivity were 7.02% and 7.52%. Isolated HBcAb positivity was found in only 2 patients (0.5%). All cases were negative for HBsAb. No combined HBV/HCV infection was detected. All positive cases for either HBV or HCV infections did not show any signs of hepatic decompensation. ALT was significantly higher among HBV positive versus negative patients (mean ± SD of 14.2 ± 5.77 IU/L versus 11.95 ± 5.21 IU/L, $p = 0.02$, reference range: 7-56 IU/L), while no significant difference was found between HCV positive and negative cases as regards liver enzymes.

Conclusion: In Egypt, HBV prevalence in pregnant females seems to be higher than general population. This was not evident for HCV infection; however, it is still higher than pooled prevalence rates worldwide. This higher prevalence for both viral infections warrants strict screening programs to prevent vertical transmission and to provide better maternal and fetal outcome.

Keywords: HCV, HBV, Pregnancy, Prevalence rate

Background

Pregnant females represent a vulnerable cohort where infection with either HBV or HCV or both has been linked to adverse pregnancy and birth outcomes, including mother to child transmission (MTCT) [1].

Egypt represents one of the countries with the highest HCV prevalence [2]. Ten percent and 7.0% of the population aged 15-59 years had positive HCV antibody and HCV RNA according to the 2015 Egyptian Health Issues Survey (HIS) [3]. Chronic HCV is the leading cause for end-stage liver disease, hepatocellular carcinoma (HCC), and liver-related mortality in Egypt [4]. Despite shifting to low endemicity area of hepatitis B (HBsAg prevalence < 2%) with the rapid expansion of the coverage of hepatitis B vaccinations following their addition to the national immunization program in the 1990s, HBV still represents disease burden in Egypt [5].

Females represented 55.2% of HCV-infected population in the 2015 HIS. Females aged 15-59 years had HCV antibody and HCV-RNA prevalence of 8.1% and 5.5% respectively and HBcAb, HBsAg prevalence of

* Correspondence: r_m_tawfik@yahoo.com
[1]Endemic Medicine and Hepatogastroentrology Departement, Faculty of Medicine, Cairo University, Cairo, Egypt
Full list of author information is available at the end of the article

13.2% and 1.2% [3]. This infection rate may reflect more prevalent infection among pregnant females.

Women in the child-bearing period can transmit the infection through vertical transmission to their babies. Vertical transmission was a major problem with HBV infection prior to the era of postexposure prophylaxis. Approximately, 85% of infants born to HBsAg and HBeAg positive women acquire HBV infection and about 30% of those born to HBeAg-negative mothers [6]. Vertical transmission is also documented in HCV infection. A meta-analysis revealed a risk of 5.8% for children of HCV antibody, RNA–positive, HIV-negative women, and 10.8% for children of HCV antibody, RNA–positive HIV-positive mothers. This means that more than 1 in every 20 children born to chronically infected mother are HCV infected which is the primary transmission route among children [1]. In Egypt, an endemic country for both viral hepatitis infections, vertical transmission risk may be more prevalent than other regions.

Although females in the reproductive age have a slower rate of disease progression in chronic HCV or HBV than men [7], liver fibrosis rates increase after menopause and become comparable to men [8]. This is principally because postmenopausal women have higher incidence of insulin resistance and metabolic syndrome, and due to loss of protective effects of estrogen [9].

In the current study, we screened a cohort of pregnant Egyptian females for HCV and HBV infections and assessed their liver disease status, clinical and laboratory characteristics with the objective of highlighting the disease burden, and, hence, need for development of guided policies for access to early preventive and therapeutic measures prior to childbearing targeting elimination and better outcomes for both mothers and their children.

Methods

This is a cross-sectional prospective study that included 399 pregnant women attending to obstetric outpatients' clinic, Faculty of Medicine, Cairo University, Cairo, Egypt, in the period from January 2018 till September 2018.

All pregnant women in the first and second trimester of pregnancy who had no history of prior diagnoses or treatment of HCV or HBV were included.

Patients who were included in this study underwent the following:

1. Informed consent: All patients enrolled had signed informed consent including the study procedures. The study was conducted according to Helsinki Declaration [10].
2. Full history taking: including age, sex, residence, presence of hypertension or diabetes, possible risk factors for viral hepatitis acquisition as previous operation or blood transfusion, possible past maternal or fetal complications as history of previous miscarriage, previous preterm labor, still birth or dead fetus, and history of complications during previous pregnancy as postpartum hemorrhage. Past history of chronic liver disease and family history of liver disease.
3. Clinical assessment: with special emphasis on manifestations suggestive of chronic liver disease.
4. Laboratory investigations including: Liver biochemical profile in the form of aspartate aminotransferase (AST), alanine aminotransferase (ALT)
5. Viral hepatitis markers (HBsAg, HBcTotal, HBsAb, HCV Ab) were tested using ELISA technique.

- Prevalence rate of HCV and HBV infections was assessed in the study population with analysis of their demographic and laboratory data.

- Positive cases for HCV and/or HBV infection were counseled. Patients with hepatitis B were managed according to guidelines either during or after pregnancy and were counseled to give their babies hepatitis B immune-globulins at birth and the routine hepatitis B vaccine schedule. Although treatment for hepatitis C was deferred after pregnancy for fear of teratogenicity or adverse pregnancy outcome. They were also counseled to defer treatment after lactation for those who were willing to lactate as direct acting antivirals for HCV treatment are not well studied during lactation.

Statistical analysis

Descriptive statistics were done; categorical variables were presented as frequency (%) and numerical ones as mean (SD) or median (IQR).

Comparison between two groups was done using the Chi-square test or Fischer's exact for categorical variables and the independent samples t test or Mann-Whitney's test as appropriate for numerical variables.

P values <0.05 were deemed significant. STATA 15 was used for the analysis.

Results

Mean age was 26.78 years. Thirty-nine patients (9.77%) were diabetic, 28 patients (7.02%) were hypertensive. In total, 84.96% of participants were in the second trimester. Other demographic and clinical data are shown in Table 1.

Prevalence rates of HCV-Ab and HBsAg positivity were 7.02% and 7.52%. Isolated HBcAb positivity was found in only 2 patients (0.5%). All cases were negative

Table 1 Demographic, risk factors, and clinical data of the study population (number = 399)

		(Number = 399)
Age/years		
Median (IQR)		28 (22-30)
Range		18-37
Residence		
Rural/urban (number %)		219 (54.89%)/180 (45.11%)
DM (number %)		39 (9.77%)
Hypertension (number %)		28 (7.02%)
Trimester of pregnancy (number %)	1st trimester	60 (15.04%)
	2nd trimester	339 (84.96%)
Family history of liver disease (number %)		36 (9.02%)
Blood transfusion (number %)		30 (7.52%)
Previous operations (number %)		47 (11.78%)
History of abortion (number %)		54 (13.53%)
History of preterm labor (number %)		26 (6.52%)
History of stillbirth (number %)		30 (7.52%)
History of newborn congenital anomalies (number %)		33 (8.27%)
Complicated previous pregnancies (number %)		23 (5.76%)

for HBsAb. No combined HBV/HCV infection was detected (Table 2).

No significant difference was found between HBV or HCV positive cases and those with negative markers as regards demographic or clinical data apart from hypertension that was detected in a significantly higher ratio in HBV positive cases versus those with negative markers or HCV positive cases (16.67% versus 6.78% and 0%) (Table 3).

All positive cases for either HBV or HCV infections did not show any signs of hepatic decompensation. ALT was significantly higher among HBV positive versus negative patients (median (IQR) 13 (10-19) versus 12 (8-15), p = 0.03), while no significant difference was found between HCV positive and negative cases as regards liver enzymes (Tables 4 and 5).

Discussion

Although Egypt is an endemic country to both viral hepatitis C (HCV) and B (HBV) infections, there is limited data on their related burden among pregnant women. In the current study, we aimed to assess the prevalence of chronic HCV and HBV in a cohort of pregnant Egyptian females highlighting the disease burden for better preventive measures.

Table 2 Prevalence of HCV and HBV among the study population (number = 399)

	Number (%)
HCV Ab positivity	28 (7.02%)
HBsAg positive	30 (7.52%)
HBcAb positive	32 (8.02%)
Positive HBcAb and HBsAg	30 (7.52%)
Positive HBcAb and HBsAb	0 (0.0%)
Isolated HBcAb positive	2 (0.50%)

Results of the current study revealed prevalence rates of HCV-Ab and HBsAg positivity of 7.02% and 7.52% respectively. Isolated HBcAb positivity was found in only 2 patients (0.5%). All cases were negative for HBsAb. No combined HBV/HCV infection was detected.

HCV Ab prevalence among pregnant females in the current study (7.02%) matches with the general prevalence of HCV in 2015 Egyptian Health Issues Survey (HIS) for females aged 15-59 years who had HCV antibody and HCV-RNA prevalence rates of 8.1% and 5.5% respectively [3]. On the other side, it is higher than the rate of HCV Ab positivity found in the systematic review and meta-analysis conducted by Binga and collaegues in 2019 to determine the magnitude of HCV and HBV infections among pregnant women living in 30 countries in Africa; they reported a pooled prevalence rate of 3.4% for HCV Ab positivity and 6.8% for HBsAg positivity [11]. High prevalence rate in our study may be explained by the findings that 42.8% of HCV Ab positive females had rural residence, and 46.41% of them had previous pregnancy-related complications including miscarriage and still birth, also 7.14% of them had history of previous operations. In such situations (miscarriage, stillbirth, previous operations), poor implementation of infection control measures in the

Table 3 Demographic, risk factors, and clinical data of females with positive versus negative hepatitis markers

	HCV positive (n = 28)	HBV positive (n = 30)	Negative hepatitis markers (n = 339)	P
Age Median (IQR)	28 (23-29.5)	24.5 (21-29)	28 (22-30)	0.5
Residence Rural/urban	12/16	16/14	190/149	0.4
DM*	4 (14.28%)	4 (13.33%)	31 (9.14%)	0.5
Hypertension*	0	5 (16.67%)	23 (6.78%)	**0.04**
Blood transfusion*	1 (3.57%)	3 (10%)	26 (7.67%)	0.6
Previous operations*	2 (7.14%)	5 (16.67%)	40 (11.80%)	0.6
Family history of liver disease*	2 (7.14%)	1 (3.33%)	33 (9.73%)	0.6
History of abortion*	6 (21.43%)	4 (13.33%)	43 (12.68%)	0.4
History of preterm labor*	2 (7.14%)	0	24 (7.08%)	0.4
History of stillbirth*	2 (7.14%)	3 (10%)	25 (7.37%)	0.8
Complicated previous pregnancies*	3 (10.7%)	0	20 (5.90%)	0.2

*Data are given as number (%)

hospital and especially in the operation rooms and lack of awareness about transmission of these blood born viral infections may contribute to the higher transmission and prevalence rates. This finding necessitates application of strong awareness and screening programs for females in childbearing period prior to marriage or conception to offer treatment with direct acting antiviral therapy with high efficacy and tolerability to avoid risk of vertical transmission and for better maternal outcomes.

In the current study, HBsAg positivity rate (7.52%) is much higher than that detected in 2015 Egyptian Health Issues Survey (HIS) for females aged 15-59 years who had prevalence rate of 1.2% for HBsAg [3]. It is also much higher than the pooled prevalence found in a systematic review and meta-analysis conducted on the frequency of HBsAg in pregnant women from Eastern Mediterranean and Middle Eastern countries by Malekifar and colleagues in 2018, where pooled prevalence in pregnant Egyptian females was 3.2% [12]. This higher rate may reflect lack of awareness and poor compliance of these females to the compulsory HBV vaccination in their childhood especially that 54.89% of them were from rural areas with poor socioeconomic conditions. It also gives insight on the mandatory screening for HBV in pregnant females even with the nationwide application of vaccination programs to save the newborns from getting HBV infected via vertical transmission with application of proper preventive measures including immunoglobulin administration and HBV vaccination of the newborn in the first few hours of his life according to the most recent guidelines [13].

It appears that women in child-bearing period (CBP) have a slower rate of disease progression in viral hepatitis than men and postmenopausal females [7]. This may be attributed to the protective effect of estrogen in females of the CBP. Estrogen in the liver seems to protect the hepatocytes from inflammatory injury, oxidative stress, and cell death [14]. In the current study, no significant difference was found between HCV positive and negative cases as regards liver enzymes. And although ALT was significantly higher among HBV positive versus negative patients, all values were within normal ranges. However, risk of disease progression increases after menopause with loss of hormonal protective effects [8].

Main limitations of our study are being in one center; however, being in a tertiary hospital, it represents a referral center for different destinations, next is the absence of confirmatory PCR results, although all positive patients were referred to specialized clinics for further follow-up for both mothers and neonates.

Table 4 Liver enzymes in HCV positive versus negative cases and HBV positive versus negative cases

	HCV positive	Non-HCV	p value	HBV positive	Non-HBV	p value
ALT (IU/L)	10.5 (7.5-15)	12 (9-15)	0.4	13 (10-19)	12 (8-15)	**0.03**
AST (IU/L)	12 (7-14)	12 (9-17)	0.4	11.5 (9-16)	12 (9-16)	0.8

Table 5 Liver enzymes in HCV positive versus HBV positive versus cases with negative hepatitis cases

	HCV positive (n = 28)	HBV positive (n = 30)	Negative hepatitis markers (n = 339)	P
ALT	10.5 (7.5-15)	13 (10-19)	12 (8-15)	**0.07**
AST	12 (7-14)	11.5 (9-16)	12 (9-17)	0.7

Conclusion

Based on the results of the current study, we can conclude that chronic HCV and HBV infections are prevalent in pregnant Egyptian females, and even more prevalent than general population in HBV infection which highlights the need for national screening programs with clear referral pathways and joint hepatology/obstetrician clinics with applying proper preventive measures and performing further research to prevent vertical transmission and to provide better maternal and fetal outcome.

Abbreviations

HCV: Hepatitis C virus; HBV: Hepatitis B virus; ELISA: Enzyme-linked immunesorbent assay; MTCT: Mother to child transmission

Acknowledgements

No agency to be acknowledged.

Studies involving plants must include a statement specifying the local, national or international guidelines and legislation and the required or appropriate permissions and/or licenses for the study (if applicable)

Not applicable.

Authors' contributions

The authors read and approved the final manuscript. All authors contributed to the work. AF: Idea of the study, revision of the thesis, and manuscript. M abd EL: Supervising the gynecology and obstetrics clinic for the included subjects. RE: Revising the thesis, drafting the manuscript, and the corresponding author. MN: Performing the laboratory studies of ELISA testing for viral markers. M B: Performing the clinical work and data collection for included subjects. NZ: Idea of the study as part of the scientific work of clinic of pregnant females with liver disease activities in Kasr Alainy, revising the manuscript. AY: Idea of the study as part of the scientific work of clinic of pregnant females with liver disease activities in Kasr Alainy. ZA: Doing the statistical tests for the study.

Declarations

Ethics approval and consent to participate

All patients signed informed consent. The study was carried out following the Helsinki Declaration, and was approved by the ethical committee of endemic medicine department, Kasr Alainy Hospital, Cairo University, as a master thesis; hence, it did not have an ethics committee's reference number.

Competing interests

No competing interests

Author details

[1]Endemic Medicine and Hepatogastroentrology Departement, Faculty of Medicine, Cairo University, Cairo, Egypt. [2]Gynecology and Obstetrics Department, Faculty of Medicine, Cairo University, Cairo, Egypt. [3]Clinical and Chemical Pathology Department, Faculty of Medicine, Beni-Suef University, Beni-Suef, Egypt.

References

1. Benova L, Mohamoud Y, Calvert C, Abu-Raddad L (2014) Vertical transmission of hepatitis C virus: systematic review and meta-analysis. CID 59(6):765–773. https://doi.org/10.1093/cid/ciu447
2. Estes C, Abdel-Kareem M, Abdel-Razek W, Abdel-Sameea E, Abuzeid M, Gomaa A, Osman W, Razavi H, Zaghla H, Waked I (2015) Economic burden of hepatitis C in Egypt: the future impact of highly effective therapies. Aliment PharmacolTher. 42(6):696–706. https://doi.org/10.1111/apt.13316
3. Kandeel A, Genedy M, El-Refai S, Funk A, Fontanet A, Talaat M (2017) The prevalence of hepatitis C virus infection in Egypt 2015: implications for future policy on prevention and treatment. Liver Int 37(1):45-53. https://doi.org/10.1111/liv.13186
4. Gomaa A, Allam N, Elsharkway A, El Kassas M, Waked I (2017) Hepatitis C infection in Egypt: prevalence, impact and management strategies. Hepatic Medicine: Evidence and Research. 9:17–25. https://doi.org/10.2147/HMER.S113681
5. Schweitzer A, Horn J, Mikolajczyk RT, Krause G, Ott JJ (2015) Estimations of worldwide prevalence of chronic hepatitis B virus infection: a systematic review of data published between 1965 and 2013. Lancet 386(10003):1546–1555. https://doi.org/10.1016/S0140-6736(15)61412-X
6. Schillie S, Walker T, Veselsky S, Crowley S, Dusek C, Lazaroff J, Morris SA, Onye K, Ko S, Fenlon N, Nelson NP, Murphy TV (2015) Outcomes of infants born to women infected with hepatitis B. Pediatrics 135(5):e1141–e1147. https://doi.org/10.1542/peds.2014-3213
7. Villa E, Vukotic R, Camma C et al (2012) Reproductive status is associated with the severity of fibrosis in women with hepatitis C. PLoS ONE 7(9): e44624
8. Di Martino V, Lebray P, Myers RP et al (2004) Progression of liver fibrosis in women infected with hepatitis C: long-term benefit of estrogen exposure. Hepatology 40(6):1426–1433. https://doi.org/10.1002/hep.20463
9. Jouyandeh Z, Nayebzadeh F, Qorbani M, Asadi M (2013) Metabolic syndrome and menopause. J Diabetes MetabDisord. 12(1):1
10. "Declaration of Helsinki: ethical principles for medical research involving human subjects". JAMA. 2013, 310(20):2191–4. https://doi.org/10.1001/jama.2013.281053
11. Bigna JJ, Kenne AM, Hamroun A, Ndangang MS, Foka AJ, Tounouga DN, Lenain R, Amougou MA, Nansseu JR (2019) SCOPING REVIEW Open Access Gender development and hepatitis B and C infections among pregnant women in Africa: a systematic review and metaanalysis. Infect Dis Poverty journal. 8(1):16. https://doi.org/10.1186/s40249-019-0526-8
12. Malekifar P, Babanejad M, Izadi N, Alavian SM (2018) The frequency of HBsAg in pregnant women from Eastern Mediterranean and Middle Eastern Countries: a systematic review and meta-analysis. Hepat Mon. 18(9):e58830
13. EASL (2017) Clinical Practice Guidelines on the management of hepatitis B virus infection. J Hepatol 67(2):370–398
14. Shimizu I, Mizobuchi Y, Yasuda M, Shiba M, Ma YR, Horie T, Liu F, Ito S (1999) Inhibitory effect of estradiol on activation of rat hepatic stellate cells in vivo and in vitro. Gut 44(1):127–136. https://doi.org/10.1136/gut.44.1.127

21

Detection of liver fibrosis stages in patients with hepatitis C virus infection by non-invasive tool

Waleed Mohamed Serag[1*] and Basem Eysa Elsayed[2]

Abstract

Background: S100A14 is a novel significant individual from S100 proteins family. Its significance is because of its part in tumorigenesis and metastasis process. Elevated level of S100A14 was associated with poor tumor differentiation. A relatively high dose of S100A14 was capable to induce cell injuries. It was discovered that S100A14 is seen at the extracellular medium. S100A14 induces the activation of apoptotic mediators and cell apoptosis. The aim of this study is to assess the clinical response of S100A14 in the detection the stages of liver fibrosis in patients of chronic HCV. ELISA was used to detect the levels of serum S100A14 in both different stages of fibrosis of the liver and control groups, and then, they were noticed together with the results of fibroscan. Other noninvasive markers of fibrosis were calculated such as APRI, AAR, and FIB-4 score.

Results: Protein expression level of S100A14 was positive correlated significantly with stages of fibrosis.

Conclusion: Measurement of serum level of S100A14 is a useful non-invasive marker for detection of the stages of liver fibrosis in patients of chronic HCV. Combinations of measuring S100A14 level to FIB-4 or S100A14 to APRI give a sensitive tool for diagnosing significant fibrosis.

Keywords: Stage of fibrosis, S100A14, FIB-4, APRI, and AAR

Background

Worldwide, morbidity and mortality are caused most likely by hepatic fibrogenesis due to obesity-related disease of the fatty liver and chronic viral hepatitis. The activation of hepatic stellate cell is the inevitable essential event in fibrosis, and they become the primary source of extracellular matrix (ECM) in the liver after injury [1]. Liver diseases with many types lead to liver fibrosis by means of signaling networks integrated that control the sedimentation of extracellular matrix. This cascade of responses drives the activation of hepatic stellate cells (HSCs) into a myofibroblast-like phenotype which is contractile, proliferative, and fibrogenic. Components of ECM including collagen are precipitated as the liver creates an injury-encapsulating a response for wound-healing. Sustained fibrogenesis contributes to cirrhosis, characterized by hepatic parenchyma distortion and vascular architecture. The conception of the complex mechanisms attached to liver fibrogenesis is essential to evolve targeted therapies with anti-fibrotic ability which can enhance the recovery of chronic liver disease patients [2]. The hazard of promote cirrhosis depends on the stages of fibrosis in the liver [3]. Fibroscan is a non-invasive test that replaces liver biopsy [4]. Fibrosis biomarkers can only be direct or indirect markers. Both types of markers can be individually used or in combination which is frequently happening to increase the diagnostic reliability [5, 6]. There are multiple biological processes that the protein family of S100 has been reported to participate, such as cell motility, growth, transcription, signal transduction, apoptosis, and cell survival, which were correlated to

* Correspondence: waleed.ibrahim@suezuniv.edu.eg
[1]Suez University, Faculty of Science, Suez, Egypt
Full list of author information is available at the end of the article

tumorigenesis and normal development [7]. Small calcium binding proteins which are great subgroup of the EF-hand protein family were noticed to be the S100 proteins which have a wide range of extracellular and intracellular functions [8]. The proteins S100 belong to a great subgroup of 25 acidic, small proteins that are described by distinctive homo-or hetero-dimeric architecture and EF hand Ca^{2+}-binding motifs, and which were expressed in a various types of cells [9]. An epic individual from S100 protein is S100A14. In new HCC tissues with and without vascular intrusion, the mRNA and protein levels of S100A4 were found to connect with different tumor hubs and vascular attack. Moreover, S100A14 revelation related with both abbreviated illness free endurance and in general endurance in HCC patients, thus proving its potential as prognostic factor. The part of S100A14 in continuing HCC multiplication, movement, and attack was affirmed in HCC cell culture and in vivo (mice) investigation, hence supporting the function of S100A14 in supporting HCC metastasis [10]. S100A14 is also an objective for p53 and could alter p53 stability and transactivity and by controlling the transcription of matrix metalloproteinase (MMP) 2, and the invasiveness of the cell can be affected by S100A14 in a p53-dependent manner [11]. Higher levels of S100A14 are measured in several types of cancer, including lung, ovarian, cervical, breast, and uterine cancer [8]. We were aiming in this study to discover the clinical efficiency of the level of S100A14 as a marker for detection of the liver fibrosis stages in Egyptian patients.

Methods

This study is a descriptive cross-sectional one had been carried out in the National Hepatology and Tropical Medicine Research Institute (NHTMRI) in the period between April 2019 till December 2019, on ninety person classified into two groups: (I) control group: twenty healthy individuals aged 20–60 years with mean ± SD of 29.85 $\pm$ 8.57 years without any evidence of liver diseases (by normal excretory and synthetic liver function tests, negative HCV PCR, negative HBS Ag, and with ultrasonography that show no hepatic focal lesion , no fatty liver, no ascites, normal liver parenchyma, and normal portal vein diameter); (II) fibrosis group, chronic HCV groups with different stages of fibrosis as inclusion criteria: seventy patients aged 25–60 years with mean ± SD for 49.97 $\pm$ 8.13 years. The subjects in the patients group were selected from in and out patients of NHTMRI, and the healthy relatives of patients were selected as the control group. Fibroscan test detected fibrotic liver patients, and chronic HCV patients were diagnosed by positive HCV antibody by ELISA and positive PCR. Fibrosis stages from (F0–F6) were chosen to be our categories for HCV patients. The non-invasive markers of fibrosis, involving AAR, APRI, and FIB-4 score were measured. Other former studies have announced other noninvasive markers for predicting hepatic fibrosis, including AAR [12], APRI [13], and FIB-4 [14]. The quantitative determination of Human S100A14 concentrations were detected by ELISA Kit of Glory Science Company, Ltd., USA [15]. The exclusion criteria were patients affected by any clinically significant diseases. The sample was taken from both patients and controls with 3 mL of the peripheral blood. For measuring serum S100A14 levels, all the blood samples were centrifuged and stored at 20 °C.

Statistics analysis

The data were statistically analyzed by the IBM SPSS version 20.The chi-squared test was used to compare between two groups with qualitative data. The independent *t* test was used to compare between two groups with quantitative data and parametric distribution. Mann-Whitney test was used to compare between two groups with quantitative data and non-parametric distribution. ANOVA test was used to compare between more than two groups with quantitative data and parametric distribution and Kruskall-Wallis test was used to compare

Table 1 The demographic information of all studied groups

		Fibrosis group (no. = 70)				Control group (no. = 20)		Chi-square test	
		No.		**%**		**No.**	**%**	X^2	*P* value
Sex	Female	34		48.6%		10	50.0%	0.344	0.842
	Male	36		51.4%		10	50.0%		
Age	Mean $\pm$ SD	49.97 $\pm$ 8.13				29.85 $\pm$ 8.57		*T* test 9.37 df = 88	*P* value < 0.001
	Range	25–60				20–60			
Fibroscan (kpa)	**F0–F1**	**F1–F2**	**F2–F3**	**F3–F4**	**F4–F6**				
	5.02 ± 1.03	**7.24 $\pm$ 1.01**	**9.77 ± 0.32**	**24.41 ± 17.68**	**32.23 + 12.2**				

Table 2 S100A14 values in all studied groups

	Fibrosis group (no. = 70)				Control group (no. = 20)				Student's *t* test	
	Mean	SD	Min	Max	Mean	SD	Min	Max	t	*P* value
S100A14 (mg/L)	0.47	0.11	0.27	0.7	0.27	0.06	0.15	0.38	11.19 df = 88	< 0.001

between more than two groups with quantitative data and non-parametric distribution. ROC curve was used to give diagnostic accuracy. The level of probability p value indicated the significant levels where $P < 0.01$: highly significant (HS), $P < 0.05$: significant (S) and $P > 0.05$: non-significant (NS).

Results

In the comparison between the fibrosis group (according to fibroscan) and control group as regards demographic data with age shows a highly statistically significant in the fibrosis group than in the control group, but with sex, there is no statistically significant as regards studied groups. As shown in Table 1.

All basically prepared clinical and biochemical data of patients were collected. Platelets with mean and SD of 111.71 $\pm$ 71.43, AST with 38.14 $\pm$ 20.93, ALT with 38.03 $\pm$ 24.757, and albumin with 2.4 $\pm$ 0.61. Statistically, there is a high significant increase in fibrosis group compared to the control group which can be noticed at Table 2 and Fig. 1 upon the comparison between the fibrosis group and control group as regards S100A14.

Both Table 3 and Fig. 2 present the following: the specificity and sensitivity of S100A14 are 88.57% and 100.0%, respectively, at the cutoff point of > 0.38 ng/ml with AUC of 0.964.

In the relation between S100A14 as regards sex and the stages of fibrosis, in the fibrosis group shows that

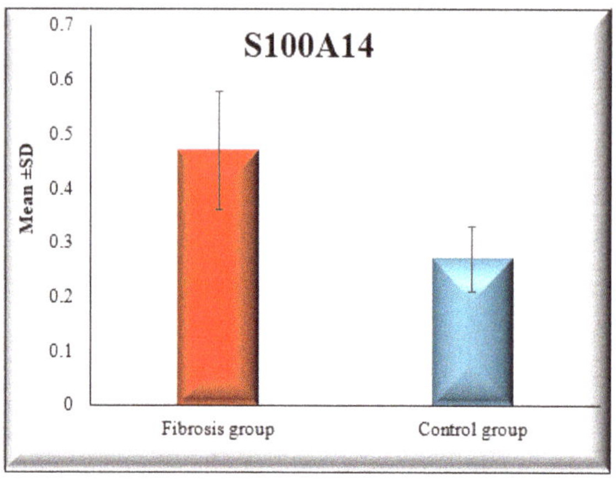

Fig. 1 The error bar graph of S100A14

S100A14 has no significant correlation between males and females and has positive correlation with stages of fibrosis as shown in Table 4.

Table 5 presents the comparison between all non-invasive markers in different fibrosis stages. Overall, there is a positive association between S100A14 and AAR, APRI and FIB-4 in the patient group of fibrosis as shown in Table 5.

APRI is the best performance in our study to differentiate significant fibrosis, with an AUROC of 88%, in comparison to existed models, AAR and FIB-4 with AUROCs of 68% and 81%, respectively, as shown in Fig. 2. Compared to the existing non-invasive assessments, S100A14 is superior to AAR which (AUC = 68%), for predicting significant fibrosis ($F \geq 2$). At the ROC-derived optimum cutoffs, the sensitivity for APRI (> 0.5) is 74% and the specificity is 97% (AUROC, 88%); for AAR (> 0.9), the sensitivity is 72% and the specificity 64% (AUROC, 68%); and for FIB-4 (> 1.6), the sensitivity is 66% and specificity is 94% (AUROC, 81%) as shown in Table 3. S100A14 is performing as the first for detecting the significant fibrosis with AUROC (96.4%), APRI is the second with AUROC (88%), and FIB-4 is the third with AUROC (81%), but after the combination, their diagnostic performance for significant fibrosis enhances with AUROC (98.5%) for S100A14 and APRI and with AUROC (97.5%) for S100A14 and FIB-4 to be higher than AUROC of either one of them alone. AUC of Combination S100A14 and AAR (with AUROC (87.5%)) is lower than combination (S100A14 and APRI) or combination (S100A14 and FIB-4) as shown in Table 6.

Discussion

Amassing proof has indicated that S100 proteins have been ensnared in tumorigenesis and metastasis [16]. Expanding proof demonstrated the significance of S100 family in cell movement, attack, and malignant growth metastasis [17]. In the extracellular medium, many members of S100 family are found with multiple extracellular roles [18, 19]. High dose of S100A14 triggers apoptosis, and the production of ROS was increased. Therefore, exogenous S100A14 induces apoptosis or catalyze cell proliferation at various concentrations via RAGE ligation [20]. A multiligand receptor of the

Table 3 The sensitivity and specificity for S100A14, AAR, APRI, and FIB-4

	Cutoff	Sensitivity (%)	Specificity (%)	PPV (%)	NPV (%)	Accuracy
S100A14	**> 0.38**	100	88.57	100	89.7	96.4% (0.964)
AAR	> 0.9	72	64	74	62	68%
APRI	> 0.5	74	97	97	73	88%
FIB-4	> 1.6	66	94	94	66	81%

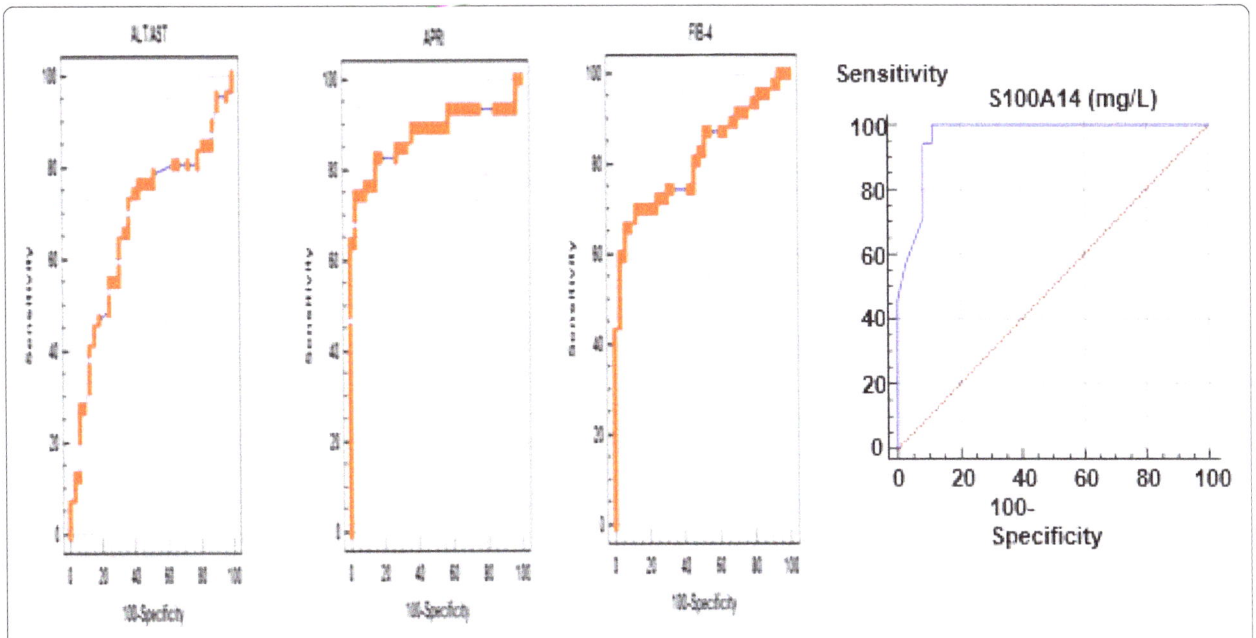

Fig. 2 Receiver operating characteristics analysis for AAR, APRI, FIB-4, and S100A14

Table 4 The relation between S100A14 as regards sex and stages of fibrosis

Variables		S100A14 (mg/L)		Independent *t* test/one-way ANOVA	
		Mean	SD		
Sex	Female	0.46	0.12	*T* test 1.64 df = 68	*P* value >0.1
	Male	0.51	0.16		
Stages of fibrosis	0–1	0.27	0.06	ANOVA *F* 10.849	*P* value 0.001
	1_2	0.38	0.14		
	2_3	0.45	0.17		
	3_4	0.52	0.24		
	4_6	0.70	0.15		

Table 5 Comparison between non-invasive markers at fibrosis stages

Parameters	F0-F1	F1-F2	F2-F3	F3-F4	F4-F6	ANOVA	
						F	*P* value
AAR	0.89 ± 0.28	0.92 ± 0.21	0.93 ± 0.23	1.2 ± 0.33	1.4 ± 0.41	6.092	0.003*
APRI	0.30 ± 0.1	0.71 ± 0.42	1.15 ± 0.81	1.54 ± 1.04	1.97 ± 0.35	11.468	< 0.001*
FIB-4	0.89 ± 0.63	1.7 ± 0.92	2.35 ± 1.80	4.03 ± 4.60	6.23 ± 2.1	8.910	< 0.001*
Fibroscan (kpa)	5.02 ± 1.03	7.24 ± 1.01	9.77 ± 0.32	24.41 ± 17.68	32.23 + 12.2	23.589	< 0.001*
S100A14 (ng/ml)	0.27 ± 0.6	0.38 ± 0.14	0.45 ± 0.17	0.52 ± 0.24	0.7 ± 15	5.416	< 0.002*

* statistically significant at $p < 0.05$

superfamily of immunoglobulin (RAGE) is constitutively secreted during embryonic growth, but its expression in physiological states is downregulated in life of adult [21]. Multiple families of ligands are bond to RAGE, such as amphoterin, S100s, and advanced glycation end products (AGEs), and play a key role in cancer, inflammation, and diabetes [22, 23]. High expression of S100A14 also causes displaying a PARP, cell apoptosis, and caspase-9 cleavage, as well as a decrease in the potential of the mitochondrial membrane. Nac(*N*-acetyl cysteine) is a ROS inhibitor, inhibited high dose of S100A14 induced injuries, point that S100A14-induced apoptosis was likely dependent on accumulation of intracellular ROS [20]. The current work shows that in the patients of liver fibrosis, S100A14 exerts a significant increase than normal people and a significant increase with stages of liver fibrosis. We have explained that S100A14 can react with RAGE, whereas high doses of S100A14 stimulated apoptosis in a RAGE-mediated and oxidant-dependent manner. Liver biopsy is still the gold standard for evaluating liver fibrosis and diagnosing cirrhosis, but being such invasive model with particular unavoidable risks, poor repetitiveness are considered disadvantages, which limit its clinical applications for patients with end-stage liver diseases [24]. Recent years, many methods and models designed for diagnosing liver fibrosis have brought the diagnosis of liver fibrosis into a non-invasive period. Although these diagnosis techniques were not replaced by liver biopsy, they have non-trauma, convenience, and good repetition advantages; moreover, these techniques have high accuracy rate of diagnosis on hepatic fibrosis to prevent some patients from receiving liver biopsy [5, 25]. Between consequent fibrosis stage, we found the mean values of APRI and FIB-4 were significantly higher ($P < 0.05$). For each stage of fibrosis, no differences for AAR were detected ($P > 0.05$, except for S1 VS S2-4, $P = 0.037$). We found a significant correlation between S100A14 and AAR and a positive correlation between S100A14 in different fibrosis stages and APRI, FIB-4[26]. In order to increase the diagnostic effectiveness of non-invasive tests, combined models using two or more tests for liver biopsy have been performed [27].

Conclusion

The study revealed the importance of S100A14 expression protein level as a sensitive tool in detection the stages of liver fibrosis. Combination of S100A14 and APRI or S100A14 and FIB-4 offered a simple potency to diagnose significant fibrosis, and its performance was specific and sensitive tool in comparison to the existing scores AAR, APRI, and FIB-4.

Limitation of study

In our study, there is a limitation relatively small sample sizes of the control group comparing to disease group. Finally, if the number of the control group were at least equal to the diseased group, it would have been more fitting.

Recommendation

To confirm this finding, large sample sizes are recommended.

Table 6 The combination of S100A14 and AAR, APRI, and FIB-4

	P value	Roc				
		Sens.%	Spec.%	PPV%	NPV%	Accuracy
Combination S100A14 and AAR	< 0.001*	96	79	97	78	87.5
Combination S100A14 and APRI	< 0.001*	97	100	100	96	98.5
Combination S100A14 and FIB-4	< 0.001*	96	99	99	95	97.5

* statistically significant at $p < 0.05$

Abbreviations
FIB-4: Fibrosis-4; APRI: AST/platelet ratio index; AAR: Aspartate amino transferase/alanine amino transferase ratio

Acknowledgements
Great confession for all physicians in NHTMRI for their cooperation

Authors' contributions
WS was responsible for the practical part, data analyzing, and wrote the manuscript. BE was responsible for sample collection and classification and revision of the manuscript. The authors read and approved the final manuscript.

Ethics approval and consent to participate
From all study participants, the informed consent was obtained in writing and confirmed under the Ethical Committee of the research of the National Hepatology and Tropical Medicine Research Institute with number 11/2019.

Competing interests
The authors declare that they have no competing interests

Author details
[1]Suez University, Faculty of Science, Suez, Egypt. [2]National Hepatology and Tropical Medicine Research Institute, Cairo, Egypt.

References

1. Virginia H, Scott L (2011) Pathogenesis of liver fibrosis. Annu Rev Pathol Mech Dis 6:425–456. https://doi.org/10.1146/annurev-pathol-011110-130246 PMID: 21073339
2. Ursula E, Scott L (2011) Mechanisms of hepatic fibrogenesis. Best Pract Res Clin Gastroenterol 25(2):195–206. https://doi.org/10.1016/j.bpg.2011.02.005 PMID: 21497738 PMCID: PMC3079877
3. Chengzhao L, Fuchu H, Haijian W, Jie L, Jiyao W et al (2010) Peroxiredoxin 2: a potential biomarker for early diagnosis of hepatitis B virus related liver fibrosis identified by proteomic analysis of the plasma. BMC Gastroenterol 10:115. https://doi.org/10.1186/1471-230X-10-115 PMID: 20939925 PMCID: PMC2959091
4. Nezam H (2012) Fibroscan (transient elastography) for the measurement of liver fibrosis. Gastroenterol Hepatol (N Y) 8(9):605–607 PMCID: PMC3594956; PMID: 23483859
5. Baranova A, Lal P, Birerdinc A, Younossi ZM (2011) Non-invasive markers for hepatic fibrosis. BMC Gastroenterol 11:91. https://doi.org/10.1186/1471-230X-11-91 [PMC free article] [PubMed] [Google Scholar]. PMCID: PMC3176189; PMID: 21849046
6. Ruseva A, Pencheva B, Stoeva D, Mihaylov R (2017) Non-invasive diagnostics of liver fibrosis. Acta Medica Bulgarica 44(1):50–56 https://doi.org/10.1515/amb-2017-0009
7. Min Z, Hongyi W, Jiantao C, Wenmei L, Guo A et al (2017) Calcium-binding protein S100A14 induces differentiation and suppresses metastasis in gastric cancer. Cell Death Dis 8:e2938. https://doi.org/10.1038/cddis.2017.297 PMID: 28726786 PMCID: PMC5550849
8. Wang X, Yang J, Qian J, Liu Z, Chen H, Cui Z (2015) S100A14, a mediator of epithelial-mesenchymal transition, regulates proliferation, migration and invasion of human cervical cancer cells. Am J Cancer Res 5:1484–1495 PMID: 26101712 PMCID: PMC4473325
9. Mizuko T, Naoki I, Namiko S, Keisuke N, Tomiko M et al (2015) Co-expression of S100A14 and S100A16 correlates with a poor prognosis in human breast cancer and promotes cancer cell invasion. BMC Cancer 15:53. https://doi.org/10.1186/s12885-015-1059-6 PMID: 25884418; PMCID: PMC4348405
10. Zhao FT, Jia ZS, Yang Q, Song L, Jiang XJ (2013) S100A14 promotes the growth and metastasis of hepatocellular carcinoma. Asian Pac J Cancer Prev 14:3831–3836. https://doi.org/10.7314/apjcp.2013.14.6.3831 [PubMed] [Google Scholar]
11. Yang Z, Feng Y, Weifeng T, Haiyong G, Heng Z (2017) S100A14 rs11548103 G>A polymorphism is associated with a decreased risk of oesophageal cancer in a Chinese population. Oncotarget 8(49):86917–86923. https://doi.org/10.18632/oncotarget.20868 PMID: 29156846 PMCID: PMC5689736
12. Williams AL, Hoofnagle JH (1988) Ratio of serum aspartate to alanine aminotransferase in chronic hepatitis. Relationship to cirrhosis. Gastroenterology 95:734–739. https://doi.org/10.1016/S0016-5085(88)80022-2 [PubMed] [CrossRef] [Google Scholar]PMID: 3135226
13. Wai CT, Greenson JK, Fontana RJ, Kalbfleisch JD, Marrero JA, Conjeevaram HS (2003) A simple noninvasive index can predict both significant fibrosis and cirrhosis in patients with chronic hepatitis C. Hepatology 38:518–526. https://doi.org/10.1053/jhep.2003.50346
14. Sterling RK, Sulkowski M, Torriani FJ, Dieterich DT, Thomas DL et al (2006) Development of a simple noninvasive index to predict significant fibrosis in patients with HIV/HCV co-infection. Hepatology 43:1317–1325. https://doi.org/10.1002/hep.21178 [PubMed] [CrossRef] [Google Scholar]
15. Pietas A, Schlüns K, Marenholz I, Schäfer BW, Heizmann CW, Petersen I (2002) Molecular cloning and characterization of the human S100A14 gene encoding a novel member of the S100 family. Genomics. 79(4):513–522
16. Lukanidin E, Sleeman JP (2012) Building the niche: the role of the S100 proteins in metastatic growth. Semin Cancer Biol 22:216–225. https://doi.org/10.1016/j.semcancer.2012.006
17. Boye K, Maelandsmo GM (2010) S100A4 and metastasis: a small actor playing many roles. Am J Pathol 176:528–535. https://doi.org/10.2353/ajpath.2010.090526
18. Sparvero SLLJ, Asafu-Adjei D, Kang R, Tang D, Amin N et al (2009) RAGE (Receptor for Advanced Glycation Endproducts), RAGE ligands, and their role in cancer and inflammation. J Transl Med 7:1479–1499. https://doi.org/10.1186/1479-5876-7-17 PMID: 19292913 PMCID: PMC2666642
19. Leclerc E, Fritz G, Vetter S, Heizmann C (2009) Binding of S100 proteins to RAGE: an update. Biochim Biophys Acta 1793:993–1007. https://doi.org/10.1016/j.bbamcr.2008.11.016 PMID: 19121341
20. Jin Q, Chen H, Luo A, Ding F, Liu Z (2011) S100A14 stimulates cell proliferation and induces cell apoptosis at different concentrations via receptor for advanced glycation end products (RAGE). PLoS One 6(4): e19375. https://doi.org/10.1371/journal.pone.0019375 PMCID: PMC3084824; PMID: 21559403
21. Bierhaus A, Humpert P, Morcos M, Wendt T, Chavakis T et al (2005) Understanding RAGE, the receptor for advanced glycation end products. J Mol Med 83:876–886. https://doi.org/10.1007/s00109-005-0688-7 PMID: 16133426
22. Heizmann C, Ackermann G, Galichet A (2007) Pathologies involving the S100 proteins and RAGE. Subcell Biochem 45:93–138. https://doi.org/10.1007/978-1-4020-6191-2_5 PMID: 18193636
23. Logsdon C, Fuentes M, Huang E, Arumugam T (2007) RAGE and RAGE ligands in cancer. Curr Mol Med 7:777–789. https://doi.org/10.2174/156652407783220697 PMID:18331236
24. Jung MK, Cho HJ, Lee HC, Park KS, Seo EH et al (2008) Comparison of transient elastography and hepatic fibrosis assessed by histology in chronic liver disease. Korean J Gastroenterol 51:241–247 [PubMed] [Google Scholar]. PMID: 18516003
25. Anca T, Cojocariu C, Sfarti C, Singeap AM, Stanciu C (2012) Non-invasive evaluation of liver fibrosis in chronic hepatitis C. Rev Med Chir Soc Med Nat Iasi 116:135–138. https://doi.org/10.3748/wjg.v20.i40.14568 PubMed] [Google Scholar]; PMCID: PMC4209524; PMID: 25356021
26. Zhang Z, Wang G, Kang K, Wu G, Wang P (2016) The diagnostic accuracy and clinical utility of three noninvasive models for predicting liver fibrosis in patients with HBV infection. PLoS One 11(4):e0152757. https://doi.org/10.1371/journal.pone.0152757 PMCID: PMC4822783; PMID: 27050531
27. Lederkremer GZ, Webb M, Cytter-Kuint R, Shteingart S, Lurie Y (2015) Non-invasive diagnosis of liver fibrosis and cirrhosis. World J Gastroenterol 21(41): 11567–11583. https://doi.org/10.3748/wjg.v21.i41.11567 PMCID: PMC4631961; PMID: 26556987

22

Microelimination of hepatitis C in patients with chronic hemolytic anemias: a single-center experience

Walaa M. Hashem[1], Manal Hamdy El-Sayed[2], Ossama A. Ahmed[1], Hany M. Dabbous[3], Mohamed Kamal Shaker[3], Ahmed Fouad Sherief[3], Mary Gamal Naguib[4], Shereen Abdel-Monem Ibrahim[5] and Ahmed Mansour[1*]

Abstract

Background: Patients with chronic hemolytic anemias (CHA) are at a high risk for transfusion-transmitted infections. Various studies in Egypt have shown a prevalence of hepatitis C virus (HCV) infection in 24–37% of those patients. Elimination of hepatitis C virus (HCV) in patients with CHA would prevent early progression of liver disease. In this study, we aimed to assess the efficacy, safety, and tolerability of sofosbuvir (SOF) and daclatasvir (DAC) in the special population of HCV-infected patients with CHA. In this prospective study, 21 consenting hepatitis C patients were recruited and treated using ribavirin-free SOF/DAC regimen for either 12 or 24 weeks according to categorization of patients into easy or hard-to-treat in accordance with the national protocols. Sustained virological response was assessed by RT-PCR for HCV-RNA at 12 weeks post-treatment (SVR12). Any treatment-related adverse events were noted.

Results: All patients were adherent to treatment with no discontinuation of therapy. SVR12 was achieved in 19 out of 21 patients (90.5%). There was a significant improvement in levels of ALT ($p<0.009$) after completion of therapy. On the other hand, the hemoglobin, total bilirubin, and ferritin levels showed a non-significant difference ($p<0.501$, $p<0.542$, and $p<0.339$, respectively). Moderate adverse events were observed in 2 out of 21 patients (9.5%), including sickling crisis and hepatic decompensation.

Conclusion: The results of this study substantiate the favorable efficacy, safety, and tolerability of ribavirin-free direct-acting antivirals (DAAs) in the special population of HCV-infected patients with CHA. Micro-elimination of HCV in special patient populations allows for pragmatic delivery of care to patients with co-morbid conditions who are in most need for treatment and allows for achievement of global elimination of HCV worldwide.

Keywords: Microelimination, Hepatitis C, Anemia, Hemolytic, Thalassemia, Antiviral agents, Daclatasvir, Sofosbuvir

Background

CHA is a common blood disorder which occurs either due to hereditary or acquired causes [1]. Survival of most of this group of patients depends mainly upon regular blood transfusion which makes them at risk for iron overload and transfusion-transmitted infections [2].

Hepatitis C is considered to be one of the major transfusion-transmitted infections which represents a serious public health problem worldwide [3]. According to the World Health Organization (WHO), about 71 million people in the world are chronically infected with HCV, with the prevalence of this infection varying throughout the world [4].

Various studies have reported the prevalence of HCV in patients with thalassemia in different countries, e.g., 16.7 % in India, 22.4% in Malaysia, and 63.8% in Iran [5].

* Correspondence: ahmad_magdy@med.asu.edu.eg
[1]Gastroenterology, Hepatology and Internal Medicine Department, Ain Shams University, Cairo, Egypt
Full list of author information is available at the end of the article

In Egypt, studies conducted in different regions showed that the prevalence ranged between 24 and 37% [2].

Pegylated interferon-α (PEG-INF) and ribavirin (RBV) was the only treatment available for HCV infection for several years. It showed a moderate efficacy in patients with chronic hemolytic anemias especially those with thalassemia. Its use was also limited by poor tolerance, and some concerns about RBV-induced hemolysis [6].

The advent of DAAs has brought about a sudden renaissance in the treatment of chronic HCV infection with SVR rates now routinely >90%. The shorter treatment duration and fewer side effects make DAAs the current standard of care for treatment of HCV in adults [7]. According to recent guidelines, patients with chronic hemolytic anemias should be treated with DAAs, preferably by RBV-free regimens [8].

The efficacy of the new DAAs regimens helped WHO to adopt its first Global Health Sector Strategy on Viral Hepatitis in 2016. Its goal was to simply combat hepatitis by calling for the elimination of HCV as a public health threat by 2030. The strategy defined elimination as an 80% reduction in new HCV infections and a 65% reduction in HCV mortality [9].

The most accepted pragmatic approach was to break down the national elimination goals into smaller subgoals uniquely tailored for individual populations, for which treatment and prevention strategies can be delivered more quickly and efficiently. This concept was known as "micro-elimination". Among these individual populations are patients with hemolytic anemias [10].

Micro-elimination strategy was accepted globally, and most high-income countries have already begun its implementation [11]. Other countries including Egypt, Iceland, Portugal, and Spain have also undertaken such strategy as a step to achieve broader elimination goals aimed at the general population [10].

Limited studies addressed the efficacy and safety of the currently available DAAs in this special population. Therefore, this study aimed to assess the efficacy and safety of SOF/DAC regimen in patients with CHA and HCV infection.

Methods

This was a prospective study of patients diagnosed with chronic HCV infection who presented to our institution to receive therapy with DAAs between January 2018 and January 2020. Out of 9500 registered patients, 171 (1.8%) were diagnosed with co-morbid hematological disorders; among those, 21 had chronic hemolytic anemias. Patients with decompensated liver disease, hepatitis B virus (HBV), or human immune-deficiency virus (HIV) co-infection and those with underlying malignancies were excluded. An informed written consent was obtained from all patients before inclusion in this study. The study was approved by the Ethical Review Board of our institution (Reference Number: FMASU M S 67/2019). The study protocol conforms to the ethical guidelines of the 1975 Declaration of Helsinki as reflected in a priori approval by the institution's human research committee.

The demographics of enrolled patients, type of hemolytic anemia, treatment status (naïve or experienced), frequency of blood transfusion, and type of iron chelators before treatment were all recorded both electronically and in a patient report form.

Baseline investigations included complete blood count (CBC), alanine aminotransferase (ALT), aspartate aminotransferase (AST), serum total and indirect bilirubin, serum albumin, international normalization ratio (INR), serum creatinine, alpha-fetoprotein, serum ferritin level, and pelvi-abdominal ultrasound, in addition to non-invasive assessment of liver stiffness by FIB4 and APRI scores. HCV viral load was determined by real-time polymerase chain reaction (RT-PCR) assay.

All patients received SOF 400mg and DAC 60mg daily. None of the patients received RBV in addition to their treatment regimen to avoid the hematological adverse events. The treatment duration ranged between 12 and 24 weeks according to baseline patients' categorization as either easy or hard to treat in accordance with the national protocols.

Patients were categorized as hard to treat if meeting any of the following criteria: PEG-INF treatment-experienced (TE), total bilirubin ≥1.2 mg/dl, serum albumin ≤3.5 g/dl, INR ≥1.2, or platelet count <15,0000/mm^3. The easy to treat group included 8 patients who were treated with SOF/DAC for 12 weeks. The difficult to treat group included 13 patients who were treated with SOF/DAC for 24 weeks.

Patients underwent a 4-weekly follow-up of CBC, serum total and indirect bilirubin, ALT, AST, INR, and serum creatinine. The monthly blood transfusion requirements, as well as any treatment-related adverse events, were recorded every visit. Twelve weeks after the end of SOF/DAC treatment, patients were tested for SVR12 HCV-RNA, serum ferritin level, a pelvi-abdominal ultrasound, and non-invasive assessment of liver fibrosis by FIB-4 and APRI. Change in blood transfusion and iron chelators requirements compared to baseline was also recorded.

The primary aim of our study was to assess the effectiveness of SOF/DAC regimen in this special population of patients by achievement of SVR as defined by undetectable HCV RNA twelve weeks after the end of therapy. The secondary aim was to study the safety and tolerability of DAAs in this special population of patients. All treatment-related adverse events were noted.

All results were collected, tabulated, and statistically analyzed using computer software (IBM SPSS ver. 22).

Descriptive statistical tests of frequency, mean, and standard deviation (SD) were used to describe the obtained data. Moreover, different variables were compared before and after treatment using paired T-test (for parametric data) and related-sample Wilcoxon signed-rank test (for non-parametric data).

Results

Study population

This study included 21 patients with CHA recruited from our institution. These patients included 11 females (52.4%) and 10 males (47.6%), with age ranging between 18 and 62 years (median 33 years). Most of the patients were diagnosed with β-thalassemia (12 patients with thalassemia major [57.1%] and 6 patients with thalassemia intermedia [28.6%]). All patients were treatment-naïve apart from one patient who had been previously treated with PEG-INF (95.2% vs 4.8%, respectively). All patients were either non-cirrhotic or compensated liver cirrhosis (Child A/B). Decompensated cirrhotic patients were excluded from the study. The rest of patients' characteristics and baseline laboratory investigations are summarized in Tables 1 and 2.

Patients received iron chelator therapy as follows: desferoxamine was given intravenously at a dose of 40–50 mg/kg/day over 8–12 h for 5–7 days/week. Deferiperone was given orally at an initial dose of 75mg/kg/day, and a maximum dose of 99 mg/kg/day. The total daily dose was divided twice or thrice daily. No dose adjustment was needed for patients with mild or moderate impairment of hepatic function. Deferasirox was given orally at a dose of 10 mg/kg/day with a maximum dose of 20 mg/kg/day. No dose adjustment was required in patients with Child A, while the dose was decreased by 50% in patients with Child B.

Treatment response

Nineteen out of 21 patients (90.5%) achieved SVR 12 weeks after the end of DAA therapy. The only treatment-experienced (TE) patient in the study achieved SVR (100%), while 18 out of 20 treatment-naïve patients (TN) achieved SVR (90%). According to treatment duration, all 8 patients who received treatment for 12 weeks achieved SVR (100%), while 11 out of 13 patients who received treatment for 24 weeks achieved SVR (84.6%). Both non-responders were β-thalassemia major patients with advanced liver disease treated with SOF 400 mg and DAC 60 mg for 24 weeks. They were ineligible to receive RBV to avoid increased frequency of blood transfusion (mean Hb 7.65 g/dl).

The first non-responder was a 33-year-old female patient who presented with baseline HCV-RNA of 1,458, 963 copies/ml, elevated transaminases (ALT 61 IU/L, AST 116 IU/L), serum ferritin 577 ng/ml, and advanced liver fibrosis (fibroscan liver stiffness 9.6 kPa, F3). She was kept on Deferasirox for iron chelation. The patient was retreated using ritonavir-boosted paritaprevir/ombitasvir and SOF for 24 weeks due to RBV ineligibility and achieved SVR.

The second non-responder was a 32-year-old male patient who presented with baseline HCV-RNA >4 million copies/ml, elevated transaminases (ALT 66 IU/L, AST 99 IU/L), serum ferritin 1670 ng/ml, and advanced liver fibrosis (fibroscan liver stiffness 34.8 kPa, F4). He was kept on deferiprone for iron chelation. The patient was retreated with SOF, DAC, and simeprevir for 24 weeks, and achieved SVR.

Among the studied group, the hemoglobin and ferritin levels did not change after treatment from baseline levels ($p<0.501$ and $p<0.339$, respectively). Similarly, the mean total serum bilirubin did not show a significant difference between baseline and post-treatment levels (2.62± 1.11 vs 2.49±1.48 mg/dl, respectively, $p<0.542$). However, ALT levels dropped significantly at the end of treatment compared to baseline levels (41.41± 24.02 IU/L vs 54.48 ± 22.9, respectively, $p<0.009$).

The non-invasive assessment of liver fibrosis pre- and post-treatment showed significant improvement in APRI (0.44±0.27 vs 0.32±0.22, $p<0.046$) but not in FIB-4 scores (0.78±0.7 vs 0.61±0.5, $p<0.175$) in this population.

The frequency of blood transfusion was assessed by regular monthly follow-up of patient-reported blood transfusion, followed by calculation of mean transfusion amount throughout treatment period and comparing it to baseline mean transfusion requirements. The frequency did not change in the majority of patients. At the end of the DAA treatment period, 12 patients (57.14%) had no change in their blood transfusion requirements and one patient (4.76%) had a decrease in his requirements, while 8 patients (38.1%) had an increase in their requirements, rising from 293.75 ml/month at baseline to 697.89 ml/month at the end of treatment period.

Similarly, the requirements for iron chelation therapy after the end of treatment showed no change among 15 patients (71.4%) and 4 patients (19%) had decreased requirements, while 2 patients (9.5%) had increased requirements.

Safety

Apart from minor adverse events, e.g., dizziness and anorexia (Table 3), one patient with β-thalassemia major who received SOF/DAC for 24 weeks experienced a severe adverse event necessitating immediate withholding of therapy. The patient presented with dyspnea and hepatic decompensation at week 16 and Child-Pugh score deteriorated from A5 to B7. Laboratory investigations revealed hypoalbuminemia (1.9 g/dl vs 3.7 g/dl at

Table 1 Baseline demographic, clinical, and laboratory data for enrolled patients with CHA and HCV infection (n=21)

Characteristics	Frequency (%)/mean±SD
Gender	
Male	10 (47.6%)
Female	11 (52.4%)
Age (years)	18–62 (median 33)
BMI (kg/m^2)	24.4±3.67
Treatment status	
Naïve	20 (95.2%)
Experienced	1 (4.8%)
Treatment duration	
12 weeks	8 (38.1%)
24 weeks	13 (61.9%)
Diagnosis	
β-Thalassemia major	12 (57.1%)
β-Thalassemia intermedia	6 (28.6%)
β-Thalassemia minor	1 (4.8%)
Sickle cell anemia	1 (4.8%)
Hemolytic anemia due to cryoglobulins and cold agglutinins	1 (4.8%)
Child-Pugh score	
A	13 (61.9%)
B	8 (38.1%)
Blood transfusion	
Regular	18 (85.7%)
Sporadic	2 (9.5%)
No	1 (4.8%)
Iron chelators	
No	9 (42.86%)
Deferoxamine	4 (19.05%)
Deferiprone	3 (14.28%)
Deferasirox	5 (23.81%)

Table 2 Comparison between baseline and end-of-treatment laboratory investigations among enrolled patients with CHA and HCV

Lab	Mean ± SD		Significance
	Baseline	End-of-treatment	
Hb (g/dl)	8.51±1.28	8.4±1.2	p<0.501
Ferritin (ng/ml)	1807.63±1480.36	1762.63±1918.7	p<0.339
T.Bil (mg/dl)	2.62±1.11	2.49±1.48	p<0.542
ALT (IU/l)	54.48±22.9	41.41±24.02	p<0.009
Albumin (g/dl)	4.09±0.48	4.3±0.5	p<0.182
INR	1.17±0.09	1.2±0.14	p<0.341
FIB-4	0.78±0.7	0.61±0.5	p<0.175
APRI	0.44±0.27	0.32±0.22	p<0.046

Table 3 Adverse events reported during treatment

Adverse event	Number (%)
No	16 (76.19%)
Dizziness	1 (4.76%)
Anorexia	1 (4.76%)
Sleepiness	1 (4.76%)
Menorrhagia	1 (4.76%)
Sickle cell crisis	1 (4.76%)
Decompensation	1 (4.76%)

baseline) and hyperbilirubinemia (2.6 mg/dl vs 1.9 mg/dl at baseline). A computed tomography of the chest revealed bilateral pleural effusion, and a small rim of pericardial effusion. The patient was admitted to the hospital for management and follow-up. All lab parameters improved thereafter, and the patient achieved SVR.

Another patient experienced a sickle cell crisis at week 12; vaso-occlusive painful crises with generalized severe bone pains and chest pain which resolved by intravenous fluid replacement therapy and packed RBCs. This patient had another episode of sickle cell crisis 3 month following the completion of DAA treatment, which increases the possibility of a non-treatment-related adverse event.

Discussion

HCV infection represents a major clinical health issue in patients with CHA. About 70–80% of infected patients develop chronic hepatitis and up to 20% progress to cirrhosis [12].

The introduction of DAAs has dramatically changed HCV treatment due to its high efficacy (>90%) and superior safety profile compared to INF-based therapy. Although limited data exist on the use of DAAs in hepatitis C patients with chronic hemolytic anemias, current guidelines recommend using DAAs in this group of patients [8].

The current study showed a high SVR of 90.5%, which agrees with other studies done on this special population of patients by Nagral and Alvi and their colleagues showing SVR of 100% using different DAA regimens including fixed dose combination of Ledipasvir (LED/SOF) with and without RBV, and fixed dose combination of Velpatasvir/SOF, in addition to SOF/DAC [7, 13].

Moreover, a large multi-center phase 3 study done on 156 patients with different inherited blood disorders including β-thalassemia and sickle cell anemia reported SVR of 93.5% using fixed dose combination of elbasvir/grazoprevir for 12 weeks [14]. This variability in the treatment regimens used further proves the efficacy of different DAA regimens in management of HCV in patients with CHA.

In contrast, the high SVR in our study differs from a multi-center study done by Di Marco et al. on 230 patients with thalassemia major, which showed very low SVR ranging from 37 to 62% across different HCV genotypes. The main explanation for this contradiction is due to the fact that this study used Peg-interferon (Peg-INF) and RBV not DAAs [15].

Our study achieved complete cure of a single patient with sickle cell anemia, agreeing with a study done by Moon et al. including 10 patients with SVR achieved in 9 patients and failure of only one patient due to drug non-compliance, although in that study, fixed dose combination of LED/SOF was used [16].

Our results therefore confirm that the advent of DAAs has revolutionized the treatment of CHC in subjects with CHA. Not only the rate of premature withdrawal because of adverse events has been reduced to zero while it was as high as 25% with INF-containing regimens, but also the achievement of SVR has dramatically increased from a range of 28 to 66% in patients under INF monotherapy, and from a range of 31 to 93% in patients treated with PEG-INF and RBV to results close to 100% in patients treated with DAAs [15].

This study showed that there was a statistically significant reduction in ALT at end-of-treatment, agreeing with other different studies on patients with thalassemia major ($p<0.009$) [8, 14, 17]. The significant drop in ALT paralleled the drop in the levels of HCV RNA. This could be attributed to the reduction in the liver parenchymal inflammation.

A prospective Indian study assessing the safety and efficacy of SOF-based DAAs including 29 thalassemic patients showed significant decline in serum ferritin levels after treatment despite an increase in transfusion requirements during treatment [18]. Similar results have been presented by Nagral, Alvi, Ponti, and their colleagues [13, 19, 20]. Similarly, the present study showed that there was a decline in serum ferritin at end-of-treatment although it was not statistically significant (1807.63±1480.36 vs 1762.63±1918.7 ng/ml, $p<0.339$). This decline could be due to the use of chelation therapy prior to initiation of DAA therapy to prevent iron overload.

The change in Hb levels was not statistically significant when compared pre- and post-treatment as the study conducted by Nagral and his colleagues [20].

The effect of new antivirals on blood consumption in our cohort was negligible, 38.1% of the patients experienced increase in blood requirements while the majority (57.14%) did not experience any change in transfusion requirements.

In the present study, most patients (71.4%) had no change in their iron chelator requirements, 4 patients (19%) had a decrease, while 2 patients (9.5%) had an increase in their requirements. This comes in accordance with other studies in which there was no significant difference in requirements of iron chelators when compared pre- and 3-month post-treatment [17, 20].

Most patients did not experience any side effects during treatment, and the side effects reported were negligible in comparison with those depicted in previous antiviral regimens including INF. The most relevant side effect was hepatic decompensation in one patient which necessitated treatment discontinuation.

Conclusion

RBV-free DAAs are considered safe, tolerable, and effective modalities in treatment of hepatitis C patients with CHA. Microelimination of HCV in special patients' populations is currently the accepted pragmatic approach to aid in achieving global goals for elimination of HCV worldwide. However, this study was limited by relatively small sample size, and absence of patients with decompensated liver cirrhosis. More studies are needed to address such aspects in the future.

Abbreviations

ALT: Alanine aminotransferase; AST: Aspartate aminotransferase; CBC: Complete blood count; CHA: Chronic hemolytic anemia; DAAs: Direct-acting antivirals; DAC: Daclatasvir; HBV: Hepatitis B virus; HCV: Hepatitis C virus; HIV: Human immune-deficiency virus; INR: International normalization ratio; LED: Ledipasvir; PEG-INF: Pegylated interferon-α; RBV: Ribavirin; RT-PCR: Real-time polymerase chain reaction; SOF: Sofosbuvir; SVR12: Sustained virological response at 12 weeks post-treatment; WHO: World Health Organization

Acknowledgements

None.

Declarations

.

Authors' contributions

WH formulated the research idea and shared in the data collection, analysis, and manuscript revision. ME supervised the data analysis and manuscript drafting. OA shared in the manuscript revision. HD, MS, and AS analyzed the collected data and revised the final manuscript. MN shared in the data collection and manuscript drafting. SI shared in the statistical analysis of collected data, together with manuscript revision. AM shared in formulation of research hypothesis, data processing, statistical analysis, and drafting of final manuscript. All authors have read and approved the final manuscript.

Ethics approval and consent to participate

All subjects involved in the study signed an informed written consent to participate. The study was approved by the Ethical Review Board of our institution (Reference Number: FMASU M S 67/2019). The study protocol conforms to the ethical guidelines of the 1975 Declaration of Helsinki as reflected in a priori approval by the institution's human research committee.

Competing interests

All authors declare that they have no competing interests.

Author details

[1]Gastroenterology, Hepatology and Internal Medicine Department, Ain Shams University, Cairo, Egypt. [2]Department of Paediatrics and Clinical Research Center, Ain Shams University, Cairo, Egypt. [3]Tropical Medicine Department, Ain Shams University, Cairo, Egypt. [4]Clinical Haematology and Internal Medicine Department, Ain Shams University, Cairo, Egypt. [5]Department of Clinical Pathology, Ain Shams University, Cairo, Egypt.

References

1. Haley K (2017) Congenital hemolytic anemia. Med Clin N Am 101:361–374
2. Mahmoud RA, El-Mazary AAM, Khodeary A (2016) Seroprevalence of hepatitis C, hepatitis B, cytomegalovirus, and human immunodeficiency viruses in multitransfused thalassemic children in Upper Egypt. Adv Hematol 2016:1–7. https://doi.org/10.1155/2016/9032627
3. Brown RS, Gaglio PJ (2003) Scope of worldwide hepatitis C problem. Liver Transpl 9(11)
4. WHO. Hepatitis C. 2019 [cited 2019 Nov 1]; Available from: https://www.who.int/news-room/fact-sheets/detail/hepatitis-c
5. Al-Sharifi L, Murtadha J, Shahad A, Mohammed Y, Sura J, Waleed Z, Raheeq M, Sura A, Ehab H, Shahad M, Abbas Q (2019) Prevalence of hepatitis B and C in thalassemic patients and its relation with type of thalassemia, frequency of blood transfusion, and spleen status. Med J Babylon 16(2):108. https://doi.org/10.4103/MJBL.MJBL_6_19
6. Casu S, Balestrieri C, Figorilli F, Onali S, Serra G, Chessa L, Lai ME (2014) P1155 safety and efficacy of PEG-IFNa2a and ribavirin for treatment of hepatitis C in Sardinian adult patients with thalassemia major: a single centre real life experience. J Hepatol 60(1):S468. https://doi.org/10.1016/S0168-8278(14)61315-5
7. Nagral A, Sawant S, Nagral N, Parikh P, Malde P, Merchant R (2017) Generic direct acting antivirals in treatment of chronic hepatitis C infection in patients of thalassemia major. J Clin Exp Hepatol 7(3):172–178 [cited 2019 Aug 8]. Available from: http://www.ncbi.nlm.nih.gov/pubmed/28970702
8. EASL Recommendations: Treatment of hepatitis C (2018) - EASL-The Home of Hepatology. European Association for the Study of the Liver. [cited 2019 Nov 1]. Available from: https://easl.eu/publication/easl-recommendations-treatment-of-hepatitis-c/
9. Hirnschall G, Programme GH. WHO | Global health sector strategy on viral hepatitis 2016-2021. WHO. 2016;(May 2015):1–5. [cited 2020 Aug 31] Available from: http://www.who.int/hepatitis/strategy2016-2021/ghss-hep/en/
10. Lazarus JV, Wiktor S, Colombo M, Thursz M (2017) Micro-elimination – a path to global elimination of hepatitis C. J Hepatol 67:665–666 [cited 2020 Aug 31], Available from: https://pubmed.ncbi.nlm.nih.gov/28760329/
11. Fitzgerald C. Hepatitis C "effectively eradicated" in haemophilia patients who were given contaminated blood. [cited 2020 Aug 31]. Available from: https://www.thejournal.ie/hepatitis-c-3154653-Dec2016/
12. Minola E, Prati D, Suter F, Maggiolo F, Caprioli F, Sonzogni A, Fraquelli M, Paggi S, Conte D (2002) Age at infection affects the long-term outcome of transfusion-associated chronic hepatitis C. Blood 99(12):4588–4591 [cited 2019 Nov 1], Available from: http://www.ncbi.nlm.nih.gov/pubmed/12036892
13. Alvi MA, Arshad Cheema H, Saeed A, Batool S, Pakistan L, Cheema HA, Saeed A, Batool S (2018) Ribavirin free direct-acting antivirals in adolescents with hepatitis C and thalassemia. J Fatima Jinnah Med Univ 12:110–114
14. Hézode C, Colombo M, Bourlière M, Spengler U, Ben-Ari Z, Strasser SI, Lee WM, Morgan L, Qiu J, Hwang P, Robertson M, Nguyen BY, Barr E, Wahl J, Haber B, Chase R, Talwani R, Di Marco V (2017) Elbasvir/grazoprevir for patients with hepatitis C virus infection and inherited blood disorders: a phase III study. Hepatology. 66(3):736–745. https://doi.org/10.1002/hep.29139
15. Di Marco V, D'Ambrosio R, Bronte F, Saracco G, Lanza AG, Fomi G, Poggiali E, Calvaruso V, Borsellino GZ, Cuccia L, Gerardi C, Maggio A, Madonia S, Fiorenza F, Salvo A, Caruso V, Russello MI, Fidone C, Davì A, Squadrito G, Aulenti G, Filosa A, Cianciulli P, Lai ME, Piga A, on behalf ITHACA (Italy for THAalassemia, hepatitis C Advances) Group (2016) Dual therapy with peg-interferon and ribavirin in thalassemia major patients with chronic HCV infection: Is there still an indication? Dig Liver Dis 48(6):650–655
16. Moon J, Hyland RH, Zhang F, Brainard DM, Lanzkron S, McHutchison JG, Sulkowski M (2017) Efficacy and safety of ledipasvir/ sofosbuvir for the treatment of chronic hepatitis c in persons with sickle cell disease. Clin Infect Dis 65(5):864–866. https://doi.org/10.1093/cid/cix441
17. Mehta R, Kabrawala M, Nandwani S, Desai P, Bhayani V, Patel S, Parekh V (2018) Safety and efficacy of sofosbuvir and daclatasvir for hepatitis C virus infection in patients with β-thalassemia major. J Clin Exp Hepatol 8(1):3–6. Available from:. https://doi.org/10.1016/j.jceh.2017.06.002
18. Nagral A, Sawant S, Malde P, Parikh P, Nagral N, Merchant R (2017) Experience with direct acting antivirals (DAA) agents in treatment of chronic hepatitis C virus (HCV) infection in patients of thalassemia major. J Clin Exp Hepatol 7:S14–S15. Available from:. https://doi.org/10.1016/j.jceh.2017.05.035
19. Ponti ML, Comitini F, Murgia D, Ganga R, Canu R, Dessì C, Foschini ML, Leoni GB, Morittu M, Perra M, Pilia MP, Casini MR, Zappu A, Origa R (2019) Impact of the direct-acting antiviral agents (DAAs) on chronic hepatitis C in Sardinian patients with transfusion-dependent Thalassemia major. Dig Liver Dis 51(4):561–567. Available from:. https://doi.org/10.1016/j.dld.2018.12.016

23

Diagnostic and prognostic value of serum soluble CD163 in cirrhotic patients with hepatitis C virus-related hepatocellular carcinoma before and after locoregional therapy

Marwa Ahmed Sakr[1], Khaled Abdel Hamid Mohamed[1], Ahmed Mohamed Hussein[2], Mohamed Hassan Fouad[1], Ahmed Samir Allam[1] and Eslam Safwat[1*]

Abstract

Background: Tumor-associated macrophages (TAMs), inflammatory cells in tumor microenvironment, are crucial for the tumor occurrence and progression which in turn increase the expression of soluble CD163 (sCD163). Nevertheless, not much has been established regarding sCD163 and its connection to HCC diagnosis and prognosis. This study was conducted to evaluate the diagnostic and prognostic role of sCD163 in patients with HCC on top of HCV-related liver cirrhosis. Forty adult patients with HCV-related liver cirrhosis and HCC (HCC group) were randomly selected and subjected to locoregional therapies, either transarterial chemoembolization (TACE) or radiofrequency ablation (RFA). Four patients were excluded because of portal vein invasion. Another group of 20 patients with liver cirrhosis only served as controls (LC group). Routine laboratory studies and abdominal ultrasound were done for all. Alpha-fetoprotein (AFP) and sCD163 were measured twice, at baseline and 1-month post-intervention, using a commercially available enzyme-linked immunosorbent assay kit.

Results: At baseline, sCD163 showed an insignificant higher value in HCC group ($p > 0.05$). The best cutoff value for sCD163 and AFP was 6.2 mg/L and 195 ng/mL, respectively. AFP had a larger area under the curve (0.88 vs. 0.767). An overall significant decline was seen in sCD163 after treatment (6.5±1.5 to 3.1±2.5 mg/L; $p < 0.001$), while AFP showed an insignificant decrease ($p > 0.05$). Also, sCD163 decreased significantly in the eradicated cases (6.1±1.4 mg/L before intervention vs. 2.3±1.4 mg/L after intervention, $p < 0.01$), while there was a significant increase in the recurrent cases (8.4±0.4 mg/L before intervention vs. 10.3±1.6 after intervention; $p < 0.05$). Moreover, sCD163 showed a significant difference in its pre-intervention and post-intervention values between recurrent and eradicated HCC cases ($p < 0.01$).

Conclusions: It is concluded that sCD163 has a minor role as a diagnostic marker for HCC, yet it could be used as a good prognostic marker in predicting the tumor response to locoregional therapies.

Keywords: HCC, Soluble CD163, Transarterial chemoembolization, Radiofrequency ablation

* Correspondence: eslam_safwat@med.asu.edu.eg
[1]Department of Internal Medicine, Faculty of Medicine, Ain Shams University, Cairo, Egypt
Full list of author information is available at the end of the article

Background

Hepatocellular carcinoma (HCC) poses a major global health problem as it is the fifth most common cancer and the second most frequent cause of cancer-related death worldwide, with an estimate of 7% of all cancers and with 5-year survival of 18% [1]. Most of HCC cases arise within chronically inflamed liver tissues, with the majority due to viral hepatitis with HBV (54% of all HCCs) or HCV (31% of all HCCs), cirrhosis (80% of all HCCs), high alcohol consumption, obesity, genetic disorders such as hemochromatosis, and exposure to aflatoxin-contaminated foodstuff [2].

In addition to the underlying liver cirrhosis as a pathogenic precursor of HCC, HCV may unintentionally be a precursor to HCC development through several mechanisms including persistent hepatocyte inflammation and immune-mediated intracellular oxidative stress damage and deregulation of cell signaling pathways induced by viral proteins (HCV core, NS3, and NS5A/B). Moreover, HCV facilitates metabolic re-programming to steatosis, which in turn leads to progressive fibrosis and HCC [3].

As a well-known fact, surgical resection and liver transplantation (LT) are the mainstay curative tools for the long-term survival, yet despite the advances in this field, only 5–15% of HCC lesions are estimated to be readily resectable. This might be attributed to many factors including tumor location and size or severity of the underlying liver disease [4].

Thus, locoregional therapy is considered among the most important and feasible lines of HCC treatment including radiofrequency ablation (RFA) and transarterial chemoembolization (TACE). RFA is the best tool in patients with early stage of HCC who are not eligible for surgical resection or LT [5]. On the other hand, TACE has been shown to be a good therapeutic option in patients with Child-Pugh A-B cirrhosis with no local vascular invasion or extrahepatic cancer-related symptoms, and it could be applied before LT as a neoadjuvant therapy or as a means of downstaging of patient's condition [6].

Hepatocellular carcinoma usually progresses with subclinical events or with minor abnormalities in hepatic functions escaping early diagnosis, which in turn makes screening and surveillance of this fatal disease highly crucial, giving a good chance for early intervention. In standard clinical practice, imaging studies are so long considered the gold standard non-invasive methods, where abdominal ultrasonography is the most widely used screening imaging study, followed by triphasic computed tomography (CT) or dynamic magnetic resonance imaging (MRI) as confirmatory tools [7]. However, the diagnostic performance of imaging technologies is sometimes unsatisfactory, particularly for the diagnosis of small lesions and early-stage HCC [8].

Serological biomarkers can provide a diagnostic support for the imaging results and may provide a crucial breakthrough in detecting biochemical changes prior to the image-based identification of hepatic malignant nodules. Alpha-fetoprotein (AFP) is the most extensively tested biomarker in HCC. However, it has a limited diagnostic performance in HCC surveillance with a sensitivity of only 25% for nodules smaller than 3 cm [9]. Besides, variable levels of AFP might be seen in liver cirrhosis or might reflect flares of underlying viral infection [10]. This raises our need for identification of new more reliable biomarkers for early diagnosis of HCC.

Mounting evidence has shown that macrophages are involved as a key pathogen in many conditions that range from severe sepsis to carcinogenesis [11]. According to their functional status, macrophages are further subclassified into M1 (classically activated) and M2 (alternatively activated), where tumor-associated macrophages (TAM) have an M2 phenotype with pro-tumoral impacts [12]. HCC is a typical example of an inflammation-related tumor, as more than 90% of HCC cases arise in the context of hepatic injury and inflammation, a fact that was shown in some anecdotal studies where an interaction between HCC cells and hepatic macrophages was illustrated by the association between the density of the TAMs and HCC progression. Consequently, macrophages may represent a possible therapeutic target in HCC [13].

Moreover, macrophage-associated markers have raised scientists' interest as possible markers of HCC presence and progression. Among these markers is the hemoglobin-haptoglobin scavenger receptor CD163, which is located exclusively on the cell surface of macrophages and monocytes. Upon macrophage activation, CD163 is shed from the cell surface into the circulation. Thus, the soluble form of CD163 (sCD163) might be considered a promising specific marker of macrophage activation that might have a good capacity as a biomarker of the severity and outcome of various liver diseases, including HCC [14].

In this study, we aimed to evaluate the diagnostic utility of serum sCD163 in HCC and to study its role as a prognostic marker before and after locoregional intervention.

Methods

This study was a prospective single-center study conducted on 40 randomly selected adult patients with HCV-related liver cirrhosis and HCC (HCC group). The diagnosis of HCC was confirmed according to the American Association for the Study of Liver Diseases (AASLD) guidelines in 2011 [15]. Another group of 20 age- and sex-matched subjects with only liver cirrhosis without HCC participated as a control group (LC group). The study was carried out on patients attending the hepatology outpatient clinics or admitted at the internal medicine department, in collaboration with the Radiology Department, Ain Shams University Hospitals, during the interval between September 2018 and May 2019.

During patients' selection, those with any contraindication for locoregional therapies were excluded from the study, including any radiological evidence of major portal or hepatic vein branch invasion, extrahepatic metastases or other non-hepatic malignancies, Child-Pugh class C cirrhosis or impaired coagulation profile (platelet count below 50×10^9/L or prothrombin activity below 50%), active gastrointestinal bleeding, and pregnancy.

The study was performed according to the ethical standards for human experimentation and in accordance with the ethical principles of the 1975 Declaration of Helsinki that was granted by the local Ethics Committee of Ain Shams University. Before enrollment in the study and after explaining the aim of the study and the nature of the investigations and interventions required, an informed written consent was obtained from all participants.

Patients in both groups were subjected to a thorough medical history, clinical assessment, and laboratory investigations including complete blood count, hepatic and renal profiles, and viral markers (HCV Ab and HBsAg). Serum AFP was measured in all subjects using human AFP EIA kit (CanAg Diagnostics; Gothenburg, Sweden) according to the manufacturer's instructions.

Serum sCD163 levels were determined with the Macro163 sandwich ELISA (Trillium Diagnostics, Bangor, Maine, USA) according to the recommendation of the manufacturer. The assay is based on the principle of the sandwich ELISA. A polyclonal antibody recognizing CD163 is immobilized on the surface of a microtiter plate. After incubation with the sample or recombinant CD163 standard, a second biotinylated monoclonal antibody recognizing CD163 is added. Detection of the latter was done by adding streptavidin-horseradish peroxidase (HRP). Using TMB as substrate for the enzyme HRP, the amount of sCD163 protein could be quantified. Before use, all buffers should be allowed to reach room temperature (20–25 °C) except for reagent F (TMB) which is kept at 4 °C. The washing buffer (reagent D) is diluted 10 times with demineralized water before use. The dilution buffer (reagent E) is diluted 10 times with demineralized water before use.

Abdominal ultrasound was done for all patients, and only those in HCC group underwent further confirmatory imaging studies including abdominal triphasic CT or dynamic MRI as a part of HCC diagnosis. Child-Pugh classification was calculated for all studied patients to assess the severity of liver disease, depending on patients' clinical and laboratory data (ascites, hepatic encephalopathy, serum albumin, serum bilirubin, and international normalized ratio INR).

Radiofrequency ablation was applied for patients with very early (BCLC-0) or early (BCLC-A) HCC who are not candidates for liver resection or LT, with tumor size less than 5 cm in diameter or less than three nodules with a maximum diameter of 3 cm. RFA was performed using a specific electrode into the targeted lesion that generates a zone of thermal destruction encompassing the tumor (temperature range 60–100 °C). A heat-sink effect is also generated by the convective cooling by adjacent blood vessels when ablated tissues are heated [16]. TACE was applied in patients with intermediate BCLC stages who had Child-Pugh A-B cirrhosis, large or multifocal HCC, which were not suitable for surgical resection or RFA. It was performed in a super-selective way, depending on the details provided in the imaging studies, by injecting the feeding artery of tumor nodule with the emulsion of lipiodol chemotherapy drug and then use the same vascular embolization to obtain the synergistic effect of cytotoxic activity of drug and ischemia [17]. Both techniques were performed by an expert interventional radiologist.

During follow-up, AFP, sCD163, and imaging studies were performed twice in the HCC cohort (baseline and 1-month post-intervention).

Statistical methods

The collected data were coded, tabulated, and statistically analyzed using the IBM SPSS statistics (Statistical Package for Social Sciences) software version 18.0, IBM Corp., Chicago, USA. Descriptive statistics were done for quantitative data as mean ± SD (standard deviation) for normally distributed data, and median and 1st and 3rd interquartile range for non-normally distributed data, while it was done for qualitative data as number and percentage.

For quantitative variables, independent *t*-test was used in cases of two independent groups with normally distributed data, paired *t*-test in cases of two dependent groups with normally distributed data, Mann-Whitney *U* in cases of two independent groups with non-normally distributed data, and Wilcoxon signed rank test in cases of two dependent groups with non-parametric data.

In qualitative data, analyses for independent variables were done using Chi square test for differences between proportions and Fisher's exact test for variables with small, expected numbers.

ROC curve was constructed to evaluate the performance of different tests and differentiate between certain groups. The level of significance was taken as p-value < 0.05 is significant and < 0.01 is highly significant, otherwise is insignificant.

Results

A total of 60 subjects were recruited in this study, including 40 patients with proved liver cirrhosis and HCC with mean age of 57.1±6.8 years old (28 were males (70%) and 12 females (30%)), and 20 patients with liver cirrhosis only with mean age of 54.8±7.6 years old (12 were males (60%) and 8 females (40%)). Hepatitis C virus (HCV) was the underlying etiology in all included subjects. Child-Pugh A class was found in 32 patients (23 in the HCC group and 9 in the LC group), Child-Pugh B in 27 patients (17 in the HCC group and 10 in the LC group), and Child-Pugh C in 1 patient in the liver cirrhosis group. Demographic and laboratory data of all studied subjects are shown in Table 1.

At baseline, the mean value of sCD163 was higher in the HCC group as compared to the LC group, yet non-significant (6.6±1.6 mg/L vs. 6.1±1 mg/L; $p = 0.079$). On the other hand, AFP showed a significant difference between the 2 groups with a median value much higher in the HCC group (305 ng/ml vs. 25 ng/ml; $p < 0.001$) (Table 2). Among the randomly selected 40 HCC patients, 4 of them were found to have portal vein invasion and were excluded from underlying locoregional therapy. None had PVT in LC group. sCD163 was significantly higher among cases with portal vein thrombosis (8.4±0.2 mg/L vs. 6.0±1.5 mg/L; $p < 0.001$), while AFP showed no significant difference regarding PVT.

For the estimation of diagnostic efficacy, ROC curve was performed for both sCD163 and AFP to get the best cutoff value to discriminate between HCC and LC group. Area under the curve (AUC) for serum sCD163 was 0.767 (95% CI 0.644–0.889) while that of AFP was 0.880 (95% CI 0.79–0.969). Both were statistically significant ($p < 0.01$). According to the curve, the best cutoff value for sCD163 was 6.2 mg/L, above which the sensitivity to discriminate HCC patients was 63.9%, and below which the specificity to discriminate LC patients was 85% with 71.4% diagnostic accuracy (true results for both), while AFP could differentiate HCC from LC cases at a cutoff value of 195 ng/mL, with 75% sensitivity, 85% specificity, and 78.6% diagnostic accuracy (Table 3, Fig. 1).

The approved selection criteria were applied for locoregional therapies, where 26 patients were eligible for TACE and 10 patients for RFA. During follow-up (1 month) after intervention, 6 patients had HCC recurrence (3 in RFA and 3 in TACE). At that time, 1 month after therapeutic intervention, sCD163 showed an overall significant decline from a mean value of 6.5±1.5 to 3.1±2.5 mg/L in all treated case; $p < 0.001$. Also, AFP decreased from a median value of 327 to 280 ng/ml, yet it was an insignificant decline ($p = 0.66$) (Table 4).

For further details, sCD163 and AFP were compared in both recurrent and eradicated HCC cases before and after intervention. sCD163 showed a significant decrease in the eradicated cases (n=30), with a mean value of 6.1±1.4 mg/L before intervention as compared to 2.3±1.4 mg/L after intervention ($p < 0.001$), while it showed a significant increase in the recurrent cases (n=6) (8.4±0.4 mg/L before intervention vs. 10.3±1.6 after intervention; $p = 0.022$). Moreover, sCD163 showed a significant

Table 1 Demographic and laboratory data of studied groups

Parameter		HCC group (n=40)	LC group (n=20)	p
Age (years)		57.1±6.8	54.8±7.6	0.236
BMI (Kg/m^2)		24.7±2.1	25.4±3	0.365
Gender	Male n (%)	28 (70%)	12 (60%)	0.439
	Female n (%)	12 (30%)	8 (40%)	
Child-Pugh class	A n (%)	23 (57.5%)	9 (45%)	0.305
	B n (%)	17 (42.5%)	10 (50%)	
	C n (%)	0 (0.0%)	1 (5%)	
ALT (U/L)		57.0±28.3	40.2±17.3	0.006
AST (U/L)		57.9±31.0	30.9±17.1	< 0.001
ALP (U/L)		79.2±23.6	88.4±30.7	0.25
S. albumin (g/dl)		3.6±0.4	3.4±0.6	0.156
T. bilirubin (mg/dl)		1.5±0.4	1.7±0.6	0.13
D. bilirubin (mg/dl)		0.7±0.2	0.9±0.4	0.117
INR		1.4±0.38	1.31±0.37	0.37
Hemoglobin (g/dL)		11.0±1.5	10.3±0.9	0.022
WBCs (× 10^3/mL)		7±2.3	5.6±1.4	0.28
Platelets (× 10^3/mL)		148.0±36.5	137.4±41	0.313
S. creatinine (mg/dL)		0.85±0.32	0.79±0.32	0.516
S. sodium (mEq/L)		137.6±3.8	136.3±3.1	0.187
S. potassium (mEq/L)		4.0±0.5	4.2±0.4	0.129

Table 2 Comparison between the 2 studied groups as regards baseline sCD163 and AFP

Parameter	sCD163 (mg/L)		*p*	AFP (ng/ml)		*p*
	Mean±SD	Range		Median	IQR	
HCC group (*n*=40)	6.6±1.6	3.7–8.8	0.079	305	145.8–550.5	< 0.001
LC group (*n*=20)	6.1±1	4.9–8.3		25	12.8–110.5	

IQR interquartile range

difference in its pre-intervention mean values between recurrent and eradicated HCC cases ($p < 0.001$), and it had a significant difference between both subgroups post-intervention ($p < 0.001$). On the other hand, AFP showed insignificant changes in both recurrent and eradicated cases ($p > 0.05$) (Table 5).

The diagnostic accuracy of both biomarkers was assessed for the discrimination between patients with recurrent and eradicated HCC. ROC curve was performed showing an AUC of AFP before and after intervention 0.528 (95% CI 0.311–0.744) and 0.642 (95% CI 0.374–0.910), respectively ($p > 0.05$), while that of sCD163 was 0.986 (95% CI 0.000–1.000) and 0.994 (95% CI 0.000–1.000), respectively ($p < 0.001$). A highly significant difference was found between AUROC of AFP and sCD163 ($p < 0.001$). As the AUC of AFP was extremely low, a cutoff value could not be postulated. The best cutoff value of sCD163 at 7.8 mg/L before intervention had a sensitivity of 100% and specificity of 90%, with a positive predictive value of 66.7%, and a negative predictive value of 100%, with a diagnostic accuracy of 91.7%, and at best cutoff value of 5 mg/L after intervention, a sensitivity of 100% and specificity of 86.7% were detected. The positive predictive value of the test was 60%, while the negative predictive value of the test was 100%. The diagnostic accuracy of the test was 88.9% (Fig. 2).

The most relevant demographic, clinical, and biochemical data found in recurrent and eradicated HCC cases were age of patients, Child-Pugh score, s. albumin, and number and size of HCC focal lesions (62.8±3.1 vs. 56.0±6.9 years, $p < 0.001$; 7.2±0.8 vs. 5.9±1.0, $p = 0.008$; 3.3±0.2 vs. 3.7±0.4 g/dl, $p = 0.036$; 3.0±0.0 vs. 1.7±0.7, $p < 0.001$; 6.2±1.6 vs. 3.3±1.2 cm, $p < 0.001$, in recurrent and eradicated HCC cases, respectively) (Table 6).

Discussion

Globally, HCC is reported to be the second most common cause of cancer-related death. Chronic HCV remains on the top of the etiologic factors, considered as a strong promoter of inflammation and hence hepatocarcinogenesis [18]. In recent years, despite the revolution in HCV treatment by the direct-acting antiviral agents (DAAs) with achievement of high rates of sustained virologic response (SVR), the risk of HCV-related HCC could not be fully eradicated, particularly in those with advanced liver disease [19]. Consequently, diagnosis of HCC at early stages seems crucial giving an optimum chance for successful curative treatment, but frequently a challenge due to the scarcity of symptoms until discovered at late stage. Besides, current screening strategies comprising ultrasound for high-risk patients (mainly those with cirrhosis) consume substantial amounts of resources, and sensitivity is often suboptimal [20].

For years, serum AFP has been used as the most useful serum marker for diagnosis of HCC. However, serum AFP is not always elevated to a diagnostic level in all patients, particularly in small HCC, and considerable numbers of patients with more advanced stages would be missed unless another diagnostic tool is used [21]. Thus, it seems implausibly demanding to require a biomarker that helps in diagnosis and follow-up of HCC after locoregional treatment.

Recent studies have raised the significance of the tumor microenvironment in the development, metastasis, and recurrence of HCC. Tumor-associated macrophages (TAMs) are copious in the tumor microenvironment and vital in tumor development and metastasis [22]. Upon activation of the resident liver macrophages (Kupffer cells) by various stimuli including hepatocyte death, it releases a variety of interleukins, cytokines, and reactive oxygen species which modulate hepatocellular growth. Soluble CD163 was shown to reflect macrophage activity in serum and can be regarded as a marker for activated macrophages. Thus, soluble CD163 has shown a promising capacity as a biomarker of the severity and outcome of various liver diseases, including HCC [23].

Table 3 Diagnostic performance of the best cutoff values of sCD163 and AFP in discriminating HCC groups from LC group

Parameter	Cutoff value	AUC (95% CI)	Sensitivity (%)	Specificity (%)	PPV (%)	NPV (%)	Accuracy (%)	*p*
sCD163 (mg/L)	6.2	0.767 (0.644–0.889)	63.9	85	88.5	56.7	71.4	< 0.01
AFP (ng/ml)	195	0.88 (0.790–0.969)	75	85	90	65.4	78.6	< 0.01

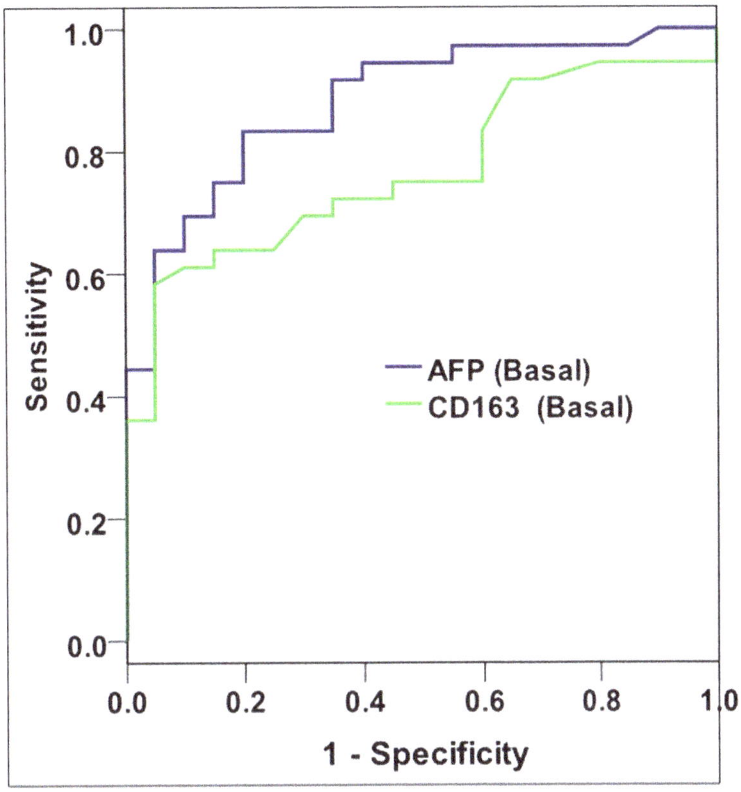

Fig. 1 ROC curve showing comparison of the diagnostic performance of serum sCD163 and AFP for discriminating HCC group from liver cirrhosis group

In this study, we aimed at evaluating the diagnostic value of serum level of sCD163 as a tumor marker for HCC and studying its prognostic performance before and after locoregional therapies.

Sixty subjects were included in the present study, classified into 2 groups: group I (HCC group) including 40 randomly selected patients with HCV-related liver cirrhosis and HCC (excluding BCLC class D) who underwent either RFA or TACE, and group II (LC group) including 20 age- and sex-matched patients with HCV-related liver cirrhosis only. Among the randomly selected HCC patients, 4 were excluded due to portal vein thrombosis; thus, 36 patients were subjected to locoregional treatment according to the selective criteria for intervention.

Among HCC patients, males were predominantly affected (28 males (70%) vs. 12 females (30%)); a result that is in accordance with a recent single-center Egyptian study that aimed at identifying the trend, possible risk factors, and any pattern change of HCC over a decade, [24] showing a significant increase in male proportion from 82.5 to 87.6% (p = 0.009), M/F from 5:1 to 7:1 in periods I (1993–1997) and II (1998–2002), respectively. This finding might be explained in part by exposure to risk factors and sex hormones. It has been speculated that estrogens, androgens, degree of iron deposition, and difference in ethnicity could modulate hepatocarcinogenesis and explain the higher incidence of HCC in men [25].

For HCC diagnosis, the present study did not demonstrate any significant difference in serum sCD163 levels between patients with HCC and LC patients (p =0.079), yet AFP showed a significant difference between the 2 groups with a median value much higher in HCC group

Table 4 Pre- and post-intervention values of AFP and sCD163 in all treated HCC cases (n=36)

Parameter	Pre-intervention value	Post-intervention value	p
AFP (ng/ml) median (IQR)	327 (154.5–687)	280 (202.8–768)	0.66[a]
sCD163 (mg/L) mean ±SD	6.5 ± 1.5 (3.7–8.8)	3.1 ± 2.5 (0.8–9.2)	< 0.001[b]

[a]Wilcoxon signed rank test
[b]Paired t test

Table 5 AFP and sCD163 in recurrent and eradicated HCC cases pre- and post-locoregional intervention

Variable	Recurrent HCC cases (*n*=6)	Eradicated HCC cases (*n*=30)	*p*
AFP (ng/ml)			
Pre-intervention			0.832[a]
Median (IQR)	356 (232.5–502.5)	305 (138.5–742.5)	
Post-intervention			
Median (IQR)	365 (235.8–1999.8)	249 (182–634)	0.279[a]
p	0.832[b]	0.279[b]	
sCD163 (mg/L)			
Pre-intervention			< 0.001[c]
Mean±SD	8.4±0.4	6.1±1.4	
Post-intervention			
Mean±SD	10.3±1.6	2.3±1.4	< 0.001[c]
p	0.022[d]	< 0.001[d]	

[a]Mann-Whitney (*U*) test
[b]Wilcoxon rank sum test
[c]Independent *t* test
[d]Paired *t* test

($p < 0.001$). These results might be explained by the fact that sCD163 expression is significantly increased in liver tissues of chronic HCV patients, correlated well with the degree of hepatic fibrosis and cirrhosis, which is in line with another recent publication confirming sCD163 as a fibrosis predictor [26]. Moreover, an anecdotal study reported elevated levels of plasma sCD163 in patients with acute and chronic viral hepatitis [27]. Taken together, all these findings could explain the poor diagnostic value of sCD163 in differentiating HCC from mere liver cirrhosis.

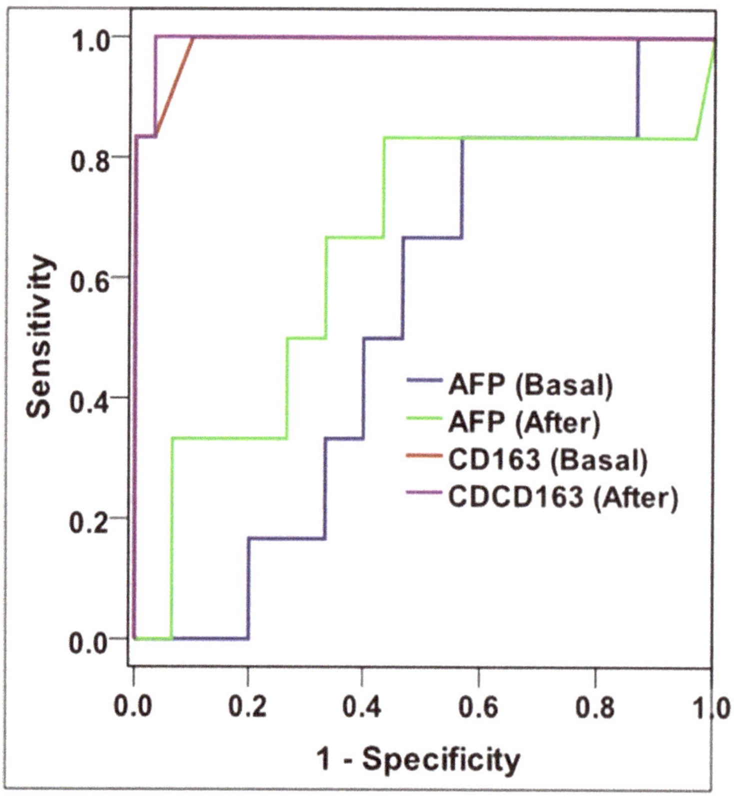

Fig. 2 ROC curve showing comparison of the diagnostic performance of pre- and post-intervention sCD163 and AFP in differentiating recurrent from eradicated HCC cases

Table 6 Demographic, clinical and biochemical parameters among recurrent and eradicated HCC cases

Parameter		Recurrent HCC cases (*n*=6)	Eradicated HCC cases (*n*=30)	*p*
Age (years)		62.8±3.1	56 ±6.9	< 0.001
BMI (Kg/m^2)		24.5±1.6	24.7±2.3	0.869
Gender	Male *n* (%)	5 (83.3)	20 (66.7)	0.643[a]
	Female *n* (%)	1 (16.7)	10 (33.3)	
Child-Pugh score		7.2±0.8	5.9±1.0	0.008
ALT (U/L)		67.8±38.9	54.3±26.2	0.295
AST (U/L)		62.8±41.4	56.8±29.5	0.672
ALP (U/L)		80.0±24.5	79.5±24.7	0.964
S. albumin (g/dl)		3.3±0.2	3.7±0.4	0.036
T. bilirubin (mg/dl)		1.7±0.5	1.5±0.4	0.198
D. bilirubin (mg/dl)		0.8±0.2	0.7±0.2	0.119
INR		1.6±0.4	1.3±0.4	0.118
Hemoglobin (g/dL)		9.6±1.9	10.2±1.4	0.358
WBCs (× 10^3/mL)		4.2±2.4	5.3±2.3	0.301
Platelets (× 10^3/mL)		159.2±21.6	146.2±37.4	0.42
S. creatinine (mg/dL)		0.92±0.33	0.84±0.34	0.598
S. sodium (mEq/L)		137.3±4.1	137.5±3.7	0.907
S. potassium (mEq/L)		4.1±0.7	4.0±0.5	0.841
Number of HCC lesions		3.0±0.0	1.7±0.7	< 0.001
Size of HCC lesions (cm)		6.2±1.6	3.3±1.2	< 0.001

[a]Fisher's exact test

That is why the difference in sCD163 level was insignificant between the 2 groups in our study.

Moreover, sCD163 shows an inferior sensitivity, specificity, and overall accuracy to that of AFP in discriminating HCC from LC groups. The AUC of sCD163 was lower than that of AFP (0.767 vs. 0.880), indicating that AFP had a better diagnosing accuracy.

Interestingly, in the present study, sCD163 was significantly higher among patients with portal vein invasion ($p < 0.001$). That result agreed with those made by Ling-Qun et al. [28] who stated that soluble CD163 was significantly higher among patients with microvascular invasion ($p= 0.037$). Most notably, sCD163 is a specific marker for the M2 macrophage which produces a variety of matrix metalloproteinase and chemokines such as MMP-2, CCL18, and CCL22 that facilitate cancer microvascular invasion [29].

Contradictory to our results, Konstantin et al. [30] stated that there was no association between sCD163 and vascular invasion.

On comparing the values of sCD163 and AFP before and after locoregional intervention, of notice, sCD163 showed a marked decline after intervention (3.1 ± 2.5 post-intervention vs. 6.5 ± 1.5 pre-intervention; $p< 0.001$), while AFP showed insignificant decline after intervention ($p = 0.66$). As observed in previous studies, sCD163 activity in HCC patients had a significant decrease after 1 month of intervention with TACE or RFA. Besides, its activity decreased close to the normal level, showing that serum CD163 activity appeared to be correlated with curative effect, thus might have an important value in post-treatment monitoring of HCC patients [30, 31].

Currently, there is a clinical need for monitoring the outcome of HCC prior to locoregional therapy to assess susceptibility and predict tumor response to locoregional therapies, and thus, an exploration of effective predictive indicators is of great significance and of great value in adopting timely treatment strategies to avoid recurrence and improve outcomes of HCC patients [32, 33]. To our knowledge, there is still limited number of studies that have investigated whether sCD163 could predict the prognosis of HCC patients treated with TACE or RFA. In the present work, sCD163 showed a good predictive value in comparing patients who were successfully eradicated and those who had failed locoregional treatment. At baseline, sCD163 had higher values in patients who had HCC recurrence after intervention as compared to eradicated cases (8.4 ± 0.4 vs. 6.1 ± 1.4 mg/L; $p < 0.001$). Also, during follow-up after intervention, there was a notable decline in sCD163 in eradicated cases from 6.1 ± 1.4 to 2.3 ± 1.4 mg/L ($p < 0.001$), while those who had HCC recurrence showed a significant increase from 8.4 ± 0.4 to 10.3 ± 1.6 mg/L ($p = 0.022$).

The diagnostic accuracy of both AFP and sCD163 was assessed for discriminating between patients with recurrent HCC and those with eradicated HCC. AUC of AFP was low both before and after intervention 0.528 (95% CI 0.311–0.744) and 0.642 (95% CI 0.374–0.910), respectively ($p > 0.05$), while sCD163 showed a significantly higher AUC, 0.986 (95% CI 0.000–1.000) and 0.994 (95% CI 0.000–1.000), respectively ($p < 0.001$). At baseline, the best cutoff of sCD163 to predict HCC recurrence was 7.8 mg/L, and post-intervention, it was 5 mg/L. Thus, this study highlights the importance of sCD163 as a prognostic predictor in ablative therapy for HCC, which has an intrinsic problem of unavailability of histopathological prognostic features. These findings agreed with Konstantin et al. [30] who found that patients with high level of basal soluble CD163 with cutoff ≥8.0 mg/L had shorter progression-free survival. Also, these results were supported by Shabo and Svanvik [34] who reported that soluble CD163 is not only a parameter of macrophage activation but also an indicator of the M2 polarization of tumor-associated macrophage which support tumor progression. Consistently, recent studies introduced by Mark et al. [35] reported that increased plasma concentration of the soluble form of CD163 "a marker of alternatively activated M2" has been associated with poor survival in HCC patients indicating that M2 macrophage may be a potential target for HCC immunotherapy.

Some limitations should be considered in the present work. The number of studied populations was relatively small; CD163 levels were not assessed at different stages of HCC as regards tumor size and number; the follow-up period had to be extended to a more prolonged time.

Conclusions

It is concluded from this study that sCD163 has no reliable role as a diagnostic marker for HCC, yet it has a good prognostic role in predicting the tumor response to locoregional therapies as it showed a significant decline in eradicated cases of HCC after treatment.

Abbreviations

AASLD: American Association for the Study of Liver Disease; AFP: Alpha-fetoprotein; BCLC: Barcelona Clinic Liver Cancer; CT: Computed tomography; EIA: Enzyme immunoassay; ELISA: Enzyme-linked immunosorbent assay; HCC: Hepatocellular carcinoma; HCV: Hepatitis C virus; LT: Liver transplantation; MRI: Magnetic resonance imaging; PVT: Portal vein thrombosis; ROC: Receiver operating characteristic; RFA: Radiofrequency ablation; sCD163: Soluble CD163; TACE: Transarterial chemoembolization; TAM: Tumor-associated macrophage

Acknowledgements

The authors express their gratitude to the members of the clinical Pathology Department, Faculty of Medicine, Ain Shams University, for their valuable participation.

Authors' contributions

MAS had made substantial contribution to the design in this study by collecting and revising the data. She had followed up the patients after treatment and shared in writing the manuscript. KAHM had made substantial contribution to the conception and analysis and revised the work and shared in writing the manuscript. AMH had contributed to the study by doing the interventional radiologic procedures and shared in revising and drafting the work. MHF had revised and tabulated the data and helped in statistical analysis of the collected data. ASA had shared in revising all the manuscript data and participated in its final revisions. ES is the corresponding author. He collected the data, revised the statistical analysis of all data, and shared in writing the manuscript and its publication. All authors have read and approved the submitted version of manuscript. Each author agreed to be personally accountable for his own contributions and ensured that questions related to the accuracy or integrity of any part of the work are appropriately investigated and resolved.

Declarations

Ethics approval and consent to participate

The study was performed according to the ethical standards for human experimentation and in accordance with the ethical principles of the 1975 Declaration of Helsinki that was granted by the local Ethics Committee of Ain Shams University. Before enrollment in the study and after explaining the aim of the study and the nature of the investigations and interventions required, an informed written consent was obtained from all participants. Ethics committee's reference number 000017585.

Competing interests

The authors declare that they have no competing interests.

Author details

[1]Department of Internal Medicine, Faculty of Medicine, Ain Shams University, Cairo, Egypt. [2]Department of Radiology, Faculty of Medicine, Ain Shams University, Cairo, Egypt.

References

1. Akinyemiju T, Abera S, Ahmed M, Alam N, Alemayohu MA et al (2017) The burden of primary liver cancer and underlying etiologies from 1990 to 2015 at the global, regional, and national level. JAMA Oncol 3(12):1683–1691. https://doi.org/10.1001/jamaoncol.2017.3055
2. Yang JD, Hainaut P, Gores GJ, Amadou A, Plymoth A, Roberts LR (2019) A global view of hepatocellular carcinoma: trends, risk, prevention and management. Nat Rev Gastroenterol Hepatol 16(10):589–604. https://doi.org/10.1038/s41575-019-0186-y
3. D'souza S, Lau Ck K, Coffin CS, Patel TR (2020) Molecular mechanisms of viral hepatitis induced hepatocellular carcinoma. World J Gastroenterol 26(38):5759–5783. https://doi.org/10.3748/wjg.v26.i38.5759
4. Zhang ZQ, Meng H, Wang N, Liang LN, Liu LN, Lu SM, Luan Y (2014) Serum microRNA 143 and microRNA 215 as potential biomarkers for the diagnosis of chronic hepatitis and hepatocellular carcinoma. Diagn Patho 9(1):135. https://doi.org/10.1186/1746-1596-9-135
5. Cho YK, Kim JK, Kim MY, Rhim H, Han JK (2009) Systematic review of randomized trials for hepatocellular carcinoma treated with percutaneous ablation therapies. Hepatology 49(2):453–459. https://doi.org/10.1002/hep.22648
6. Xie ZB, Wang XB, Peng YC, Zhu SL, Ma L, Xiang BD, Gong WF, Chen J, You XM, Jiang JH, Li LQ, Zhong JH (2015) Systematic review comparing the safety and efficacy of conventional and drug-eluting bead transarterial chemoembolization for inoperable hepatocellular carcinoma. Hepatol Res 45(2):190–200. https://doi.org/10.1111/hepr.12450
7. Kanwal F, Kramer JR, Mapakshi S, Natarajan Y, Chayanupatkul M et al (2018) Risk of hepatocellular cancer in patients with non-alcoholic fatty liver

disease. Gastroenterology 155(6):1828–1837. https://doi.org/10.1053/j.gastro.2018.08.024
8. Hung YC, Lin CL, Liu CJ, Hung H, Lin SM, Lee SD, Chen PJ, Chuang SC, Yu MW (2015) Development of risk scoring system for stratifying population for hepatocellular carcinoma screening. Hepatology 61(6):1934–1944. https://doi.org/10.1002/hep.27610
9. Hester CA, Rich NE, Singal AG, Yopp AC (2019) Comparative analysis of nonalcoholic steatohepatitis versus viral hepatitis and alcohol-related liver disease-related hepatocellular carcinoma. J Natl Compr Canc Netw 17(4): 322–329. https://doi.org/10.6004/jnccn.2018.7105
10. di Bisceglie AM, Sterling RK, Chung RT, Everhart JE, Dienstag JL, Bonkovsky HL, Wright EC, Everson GT, Lindsay KL, Lok ASF, Lee WM, Morgan TR, Ghany MG, Gretch DR, the HALT-C Trial Group (2005) Serum alpha-fetoprotein levels in patients with advanced hepatitis C: results from the HALT-C Trial. Hepatology 43(3):434–441. https://doi.org/10.1016/j.jhep.2005.03.019
11. Komohara Y, Fujiwara Y, Ohnishi K, Takeya M (2016) Tumor associated macrophages: potential therapeutic targets for anticancer therapy. Adv Drug Deliv Rev 99:180–185. https://doi.org/10.1016/j.addr.2015.11.009
12. Georgoudaki AM, Prokopec KE, Boura VF, Hellqvist E, Sohn S, Östling J, Dahan R, Harris RA, Rantalainen M, Klevebring D, Sund M, Brage SE, Fuxe J, Rolny C, Li F, Ravetch JV, Karlsson MCI (2016) Reprogramming tumor-associated macrophages by antibody targeting inhibits cancer progression and metastasis. Cell Reports 15(9):2000–2011. https://doi.org/10.1016/j.celrep.2016.04.084
13. Shirabe K, Mano Y, Muto J, Matono R, Motomura T, Toshima T, Takeishi K, Uchiyama H, Yoshizumi T, Taketomi A, Morita M, Tsujitani S, Sakaguchi Y, Maehara Y (2012) Role of tumor-associated macrophages in the progression of hepatocellular carcinoma. Surg Today 42(1):1–7. https://doi.org/10.1007/s00595-011-0058-8
14. Gronbaek H, Sandahl TD, Mortensen C, Vilstrup H, Moller HJ et al (2012) Soluble CD163, a marker of Kupffer cell activation, is related to portal hypertension in patients with liver cirrhosis. Aliment Pharmacol Ther 36(2): 173–180. https://doi.org/10.1111/j.1365-2036.2012.05134.x
15. Bruix J, Sherman M (2011) Management of hepatocellular carcinoma: an update. Hepatology 53(3):1020–1022. https://doi.org/10.1002/hep.24199
16. Poulou LS, Botsa E, Thanou I, Ziakas PD, Thanos L (2015) Percutaneous microwave ablation vs radiofrequency ablation in the treatment of hepatocellular carcinoma. World J. Hepatol 7(8):1054–1063. https://doi.org/10.4254/wjh.v7.i8.1054
17. Facciorusso A (2018) Drug-eluting beads transarterial chemoembolization for hepatocellular carcinoma: current state of the art. World J Gastroenterol 24(2):161–169. https://doi.org/10.3748/wjg.v24.i2.161
18. Marengo A, Rosso C, Bugianesi E (2016) Liver cancer: connections with obesity, fatty liver, and cirrhosis. Annu Rev Med 67(1):103–117. https://doi.org/10.1146/annurev-med-090514-013832
19. Ioannou GN, Green PK, Beste LA, Mun EJ, Kerr KF, Berry K (2018) Development of models estimating the risk of hepatocellular carcinoma after antiviral treatment for hepatitis C. J Hepatol 69(5):1088–1098. https://doi.org/10.1016/j.jhep.2018.07.024
20. Tzartzeva K, Obi J, Rich NE, Parikh ND, Marrero JA et al (2018) Surveillance imaging and alpha fetoprotein for early detection of hepatocellular carcinoma in patients with cirrhosis: a meta-analysis. Gastroenterology 154(6):1706–1718 e1
21. Stefaniuk P, Cianciara J, Wiercinska-Drapalo A (2010) Present and future possibilities for early diagnosis of hepatocellular carcinoma. World J Gastroenterology 16(4):418–424. https://doi.org/10.3748/wjg.v16.i4.418
22. Zhou SL, Zhou ZJ, Hu ZQ, Huang XW, Wang Z et al (2016) Tumor-associated neutrophils recruit macrophages and T-regulatory cells to promote progression of hepatocellular carcinoma and resistance to sorafenib. Gastroenterology 150(7):1646–1658 e17
23. Koji M, Kiyokaz H, Shinichi U et al (2018) Prognostic significance of CD68, CD163 and folate receptor-B positive macrophage in hepatocellular carcinoma. Exp and Ther Med 15:4465–4476
24. El-Zayadi AR, Badran HM, Barakat EM et al (2005) Hepatocellular carcinoma in Egypt: a single center study over a decade. World J Gastroenterology 11(33):5193–5198
25. Nishida N, Arizumi T, Hayaishi S, Takita M, Kitai S, Yada N, Hagiwara S, Inoue T, Minami Y, Ueshima K, Sakurai T, Ikai I, Kudo M (2012) Gender differences in the livers of patients with hepatocellular carcinoma and chronic hepatitis C infection. Digestive Diseases 30(6):547–553. https://doi.org/10.1159/000343057
26. Zhao S-X, Li W-C, Na F, Kong L-B, Zhang Q-S, Han F, Ren W-G, Cui P, Jing-Hua D, Wang B-Y, Zhang Y-G, Wang R-Q, Kong L, Nan Y-M (2020) CD14 $^{+}$ monocytes and CD163 $^{+}$ macrophages correlate with the severity of liver fibrosis in patients with chronic hepatitis C. Exp Ther Med 20(6):228. https://doi.org/10.3892/etm.2020.9358
27. Hiraoka A, Horiike N, Akbar SM, Michitaka K, Matsuyama T et al (2005) Soluble CD163 in patients with liver diseases: very high levels of soluble CD163 in patients with fulminant hepatic failure. J Gastroenterol 40(1):52–56. https://doi.org/10.1007/s00535-004-1493-8
28. Ling-Qun K, Xiao-Dong Z, Hua-Xiang X et al (2013) The clinical significance of the CD163 and CD68 macrophages in patients with hepatocellular carcinoma. PLoS ONE 8(3):e59771
29. Fu-Biao K, Ling W, Dong L et al (2015) Hepatocellular carcinomas promote tumor-associated macrophage M2-polarization via increased B7-H3 expression. Oncology Reports 33(1):274–282
30. Konstantin K, Anthony R, Kira S et al (2015) Macrophage activation marker soluble CD163 may predict disease progression in hepatocellular carcinoma. Scand J Clin Lab Invest 76(1):64–73
31. Oliver W, Verena K, Dominik B et al (2013) Diagnostic and prognostic significance of cell death and macrophage activation markers in patients with hepatocellular carcinoma. J Hepatol 59:769–779
32. Schobert IT, Savic LJ, Chapiro J, Bousabarah K, Chen E, Laage-Gaupp F, Tefera J, Nezami N, Lin MD, Pollak J, Schlachter T (2020) Neutrophil-to-lymphocyte and platelet-to-lymphocyte ratios as predictors of tumor response in hepatocellular carcinoma after DEB-TACE. Eur Radiol 30(10): 5663–5673. https://doi.org/10.1007/s00330-020-06931-5
33. Wang Q, Zhao P, He N, Sun JP, Li K, Zang CR, Zhao YN, Zhao Y, Zhang YH (2019) Combination of the gamma-glutamyltransferase-to-prealbumin ratio and other indicators may be a novel marker for predicting the prognosis of patients with hepatocellular carcinoma undergoing locoregional ablative therapies. Infect Agent Cancer 14(1):49. https://doi.org/10.1186/s13027-019-0266-1
34. Shabo I, Svanvik J (2011) Expression of macrophage antigens by tumor cells. Adv Exp Med Biol 714:141–150. https://doi.org/10.1007/978-94-007-0782-5_7
35. Mark Y, Dongmei X, Lan L et al (2017) Characterization of the immune microenvironment in hepatocellular carcinoma. Clin Cancer Res 23(23): 7333–7339

Evaluation of long-term changes of aspartate—platelet ratio index, FIB4 and liver stiffness in chronic hepatitis C patients successfully treated by direct-acting antivirals

Nadia Abdel Ataay Abdelkader[1], Osama Ashraf Ahmed[2], Ahmed Fouad Sherief[1], Doaa Mahmoud Kandil[1], Mohammed Soliman Gado[1] and Amira Mahmoud Al Balakosy[1*]

Abstract

Background: A large number of chronic hepatitis C patients had been successfully treated by directly acting antivirals; therefore, strategies for the long-term follow-up of these patients have to be planned based on the post-treatment fibrosis stage—the main determinant of prognosis. In this study, we aim to evaluate changes in aspartate-platelet ratio index, FIB4, and liver stiffness in chronic hepatitis C patients who achieved SVR and ended treatment more than 1 year by DAAs.

Results: One hundred chronic hepatitis C patients who achieved SVR were enrolled at a median of 16 months after the end of treatment by DAAs. According to the baseline liver stiffness, 63 and 37 patients belonged to early (F0, F1, and F2) and advanced (F3 and F4) fibrosis stages, respectively. Both groups showed a decline of the degree of liver stiffness at follow-up compared to the baseline that was statistically significant in the early fibrosis group (5.9± 1.5 vs 5.4±2.2 Kpcal, p=0.04), while measurements in the advanced group were (18±8.8 vs 15.9 ± 7.8 Kpcal, p=0.07). Also, serum biomarkers of fibrosis improved in both groups, where the recorded APRI and FIB4 before and after treatment were 0.42±0.3 vs 0.24±0.1, p<0.01 and 1±0.6 vs 0.93 ±0.5, p=0.1 in the early group and 0.85 ±0.5 vs 0.4± 0.2, p <0.001 and 2.9±2.3 vs 1.8±1.4, p<0.02) in the advanced group, respectively. Changes in APRI and FIB4 correlated with changes in AST and ALT, but liver stiffness changes were not affected by changes in liver enzymes.

Conclusion: Although long-term improvement of APRI, FIB4, and liver stiffness scores could be achieved in chronic HCV patients after SVR by DAAS. High measurements of liver stiffness before treatment likely persist. We recommend transient elastography as a reliable tool for fibrosis assessment post-treatment.

Keywords: Liver stiffness, APRI, FIB4, Chronic HCV, DAAS, SVR, Long-term

* Correspondence: drbalakosy@gmail.com
[1]Tropical Medicine Department, Faculty of Medicine, Ain Shams University, 38 Abbassia street, Postal code, Cairo 1181, Egypt
Full list of author information is available at the end of the article

Background

Hepatitis C virus (HCV) chronic infection is an important etiology of chronic liver disease that is prevalent worldwide; therefore, discovering an effective antiviral therapy was a major target for research [1]. Additionally, chronic HCV is considered the main risk factor for cirrhosis and development of hepatocellular carcinoma [2].

The introduction of direct-acting antiviral drugs (DAAs) was a revolution in HCV management with great safety and efficacy profile. Also, successful treatment of HCV decreases cirrhosis-related complications [3]. Many studies discussed the possibility of fibrosis regression following sustained virological response (SVR) achievement by DAAs which is debatable [4].

Chronic HCV infection and the resultant hepatocyte injury induce an inflammatory response that produces cytokines leading to stimulation of hepatic stellate cells (HSC) and fibrogenesis initiation, and elimination of the injurious agent would halt this inflammatory process. At later stages, fibrosis regression would depend on apoptosis of activated HSC and degradation of the extracellular matrix which is affected by the duration and components of the scar tissue [5].

CHCV patients with advanced liver fibrosis are at risk of developing hepatocellularcarcinoma (HCC), despite HCV eradication [6]. So the determination of the liver fibrosis stage after treatment is essential to detect the patients' need for continuous surveillance [7].

Liver biopsy is the gold standard for the evaluation of the degree of tissue damage and hepatic fibrosis. Due to its limitations and procedure-related complications, the use of non-invasive methods for fibrosis assessment has become an alternative. Among the most widely used and validated are serum biomarkers and transient elastography. Aspartate to platelet ratio index (APRI) and fibrosis-4-index (FIB4) are serum biomarkers that have high applicability and reproducibility being calculated by using routine laboratory indices. While transient elastography (TE) physically assessed liver fibrosis by measuring liver stiffness with the advantages of being reliable, safe, and easy to perform [8].

In Egypt, the National Committee for Control of Viral Hepatitis (NCCVH) implemented a national strategy aiming to eradicate HCV, and this target became feasible by the availability of DAAs since 2014. Initially, patients with advanced fibrosis stages were only included in the treatment program, but later in 2015, all fibrosis stages (F0–F4) received antiviral therapy without discrimination [9]. By 2018, 40% of the total HCV-infected population (2 million patients) were treated by DAAS with SVR above 90% [10]. So, a strategy for the follow-up of this large number of cured patients has to be planned to put into consideration patients with utmost priority. In the current study, we aim to share our center experience in the follow-up of successfully treated CHCV patients as regards the changes in scores of non-invasive tests of fibrosis APRI, FIB4, and TE.

Methods

This is a single-center retrospective and prospective cohort study, which was conducted at the Viral Hepatitis Treatment Unit, Ain Shams University Hospitals, during the time period from October 2017 to December 2018. Chronic HCV patients who ended treatment with DAAS and attended at our outpatient clinic for follow-up were included if fulfilling the following criteria:

1. Chronic HCV patients who were treated with a complete course of all oral DAAS regimens, achieved SVR and at least 1 year has passed since the end of treatment.
2. Patients who had baseline transient elastography (TE) done before DAAS initiation.
3. Complete data available in files.

Exclusion criteria

Patients who developed ascites and/or HCC at the time of follow-up.

The following workup was done for re-evaluation of included patients:

1. Clinical assessment for symptoms or signs of liver cell failure and laboratory investigations as CBC, AST, ALT, total and direct bilirubin, and albumin and INR.
2. Liver stiffness measurement (LSM) using TE: The device used is FibroScan® (Echosens, Paris, France). The operator placed the transducer in the intercostal space at the mid-axillary line in the right hypochondrium and took at least 10 measurements. An interquartile range of ≤30% and a success rate of >80% were required for a valid interpretation [8].

TE results were correlated to different stages of liver fibrosis according to the histological staging system of METAVIR (Table 1) [11].

Non-invasive serum fibrosis biomarkers

Aspartate aminotransferase-to-platelet ratio index (APRI) and fibrosis-4 index (FIB-4) were calculated at baseline and at follow-up by using the following equations:

1. **APRI score** by Wai's formula [12]: (AST/upper limit of normal)/platelet count (expressed as platelets×109 /L) × 100

Table 1 Histological staging system of METAVIR

Stage	Metavir Scoring System	Fibroscan cut-off values (Kpcal)
F0	No fibrosis	0–5.4
F1	Portal fibrosis without septa	5.5–6.9
F2	Portal fibrosis with few septa	7–9.4
F3	Numerous septa without cirrhosis	9.5–12.4
F4	Cirrhosis	12.5

2. **FIB-4 score** by Sterling's formula [13] : Age (years) × AST (IU/L)/platelet count (×109/L) × √ALT (IU/L)).

Statistical analysis

The collected data was revised, coded, tabulated, and introduced to a computer using Statistical package for Social Science (SPSS 20). Parametric numerical data was presented as mean, standard deviation (± SD), and range while non-parametric numeric data were presented as the median and interquartile range (IQR). Non-numeric data were presented as the frequency and percentage.

We used Student *T* test to compare two paired study group means. Pearson correlation (*r*) was used for measuring a linear dependence between two variables. The McNemar test is used to analyze pretest-posttest fibrosis study groups. Regression analysis was used for estimating the relationships between baseline factors and changes in LSM. Repeated-measures ANOVA was used to compare the changes of LSM across time between the early and advanced fibrosis group.

Results

During the time period from October 2017 to December 2018, 120 chronic HCV patients attended our clinic for follow-up after the end of treatment with DAAs, only 100 patients fulfilled the inclusion criteria and were enrolled in this study while 20 patients were excluded, as 2 were relapsers, 7 developed HCC and/or ascites while 11 patients refused to participate.

Among the included patients, 63 belonged to early fibrosis stages (F0, F1, and F2), while 37 patients belonged to advanced stages (F3 and F4) classified according to baseline TE readings retrieved from patients' files.

The median duration since the end of treatment in included patients was 16 months (minimum and maximum—12 and 33 months, respectively), where most of the patients (75th percentile) were re-examined at 21 months after the end of treatment.

Baseline patient characteristics

The mean age of included patients was 48±15 years: 52 males and 48 females. Diabetes and hypertension were reported in 14 and 12 patients, respectively (Table 2). The mean LSM of patients in the early fibrosis stage was 5.9±1.5 Kpcal while that of the advanced stage was 18± 8.8 Kpcal (Table 3).

Before treatment initiation, the median of HCV RNA quantitative was 2066.45 (IQR=4000), SVR was confirmed by undetectable HCV PCR at week 12 post-treatment in all included patients. Treatment regimens used were Sofosbuvir/Dacltasvir for 12 weeks in 58 patients; most of them (*n*=51) were at early fibrosis stages, while 32 patients including 18 with advanced fibrosis received Sofosbuvir/Dacltasvir/Ribavirin for 12–24 weeks; finally, only 10 patients were treated by PAR/OMB/RBV; and most of them belonged to F0.

Table 2 Baseline patients' characteristics

Age (years)	48 ±15
BMI	26 ±3.7
Female (%)	48
Male (%)	52
Diabetes (%)	14
Hypertension (%)	12
Other co-morbidities*(%)	11
HCV RNA quantitative*	2066.45±4000
ALT (IU/L)	53.5±40
AST (IU/L)	48±29
AFP (IU/L)	4.3±3.4
Albumin (g/dL)	4.1±0.5
Total bilirubin (mg/dL)	0.75±0.4
Indirect bilirubin (mg/dL)	0.48±0.4
WBCx10^3/mm^3	7.1±2.2
Hb (g/dL)	13.5±1.8
Creatinine (mg/dL)	0.9±0.2
INR	1.1±0.1
Platelets×10^3/mm^3	231.7±72
Fibrosis stage (F) by TE (%)	**F0 (23%)**
	F1 (26%)
	F2 (14 %)
	F3 (9%)
	F4 (28%)

*Ischemic heart diseases and bronchial asthma

Table 3 Laboratory and fibrosis score changes in early and advanced groups

	Early stage			Advanced stage		
	Baseline	Follow-up	*P* value	Baseline	Follow-up	*P* value
Stiffness	5.9±1.5	5.4±2.2	0.04	18±8.8	15.9 ±7.8	0.077
APRI score	0.42±0.3	0.24±0.1	<0.01	0.85±0.5	0.4±0.2	<0.001
Fib4	1±0.6	0.93±0.5	0.1	2.9±2.3	1.8±1.4	0.002
ALT (IU/L)	53±42	21±10	<0.01	55±37	26±11	<0.001
AST (IU/L)	42±30	24±10	<0.01	58±26	28±11	<0.001
AFP (IU/L)	3.3±2	3.5±1.8	0.5	6±4.2	5.5±3	0.4
Albumin (g/dL)	4.2±0.35	4.1±0.3	0.35	3.9±0.6	3.9±0.4	0.5
Total bilirubin (mg/dL)	0.6±0.2	0.7±0.2	0.2	0.9±0.5	0.86±0.3	0.4
Indirect bilirubin (mg/dL)	0.4±0.4	0.4±0.2	0.7	0.6±0.3	0.5±0.2	0.5
WBCx10^3/mm^3	7±2.4	6.8±1.7	0.3	7.1±1.8	6.7±2.1	0.2
Hb	13.8± 1.6	12.5±1.2	<0.001	13±1.9	12.4±1.5	0.008
plateletsx10^3/mm^3	251.5 ± 58	265 ± 72	0.05	199±80	215±67	0.08
INR	1±0.09	1 ±0.09	0.3	1.12.	1.16	0.1
Creatinine	0.87±0.2	0.85±0.15	0.6	0.8±0.1	0.9±0.1	0.8

At baseline, AST and ALT of all included patients were elevated 48 ± 30 (IU/L) and 53 ± 40 (IU/L), respectively, while other liver function tests were normal (Table 2).

Changes at the time of follow-up

Laboratory

In both groups, improvement of ALT (53 ± 42 vs 21± 10) and (55 ± 37 vs 26±11 (p<0.01) as well as AST (42± 30 vs 24±10) and (58±26 vs 28±11) (p<0.01) were reported for early and advanced fibrosis stages, respectively. No significant changes of LFTs (total bilirubin, albumin, and INR) were found in both groups. The platelet count improved in both groups, but the increase was statistically significant only in the early fibrosis group (251.5 ± 57 vs 266 ±72, p=0.001) and not the advanced group (199±80 vs 215±67, p=0.08). However, most patients at advanced fibrosis stages (12 out of 16) who had thrombocytopenia at baseline showed an improvement (mean =124 vs 188) (Table 3).

Analysis of changes in FIB4, APRI, and LSM in both groups

Non-invasive biomarkers

Early fibrosis stages APRI score significantly decreased at follow-up compared to baseline (0.42±0.3 vs 0.24±0.1, p<0.01), while non-significant improvement was reported in Fib4 1±0.6 vs 0.93 ±0.5, p=0.1) (Table 3). The change in APRI is correlated with that of FIB4 (p=0.000) but not with the change in LSM (Table 4).

Advanced fibrosis stages APRI and Fib4 score significantly decreased at follow-up compared to baseline (0.85 ±0.5 vs 0.4±0.2, p <0.001) and (2.9±2.3 vs 1.8±1.4, p< 0.02), respectively (Table 3). The change in APRI correlated with that of FIB4 (p=0.000) but not with the change in LSM (Table 4).

In all included patients, the percent of change of APRI is correlated with that of AST and ALT, and the percent of change of Fib4 is correlated with AST (Table 5).

Table 4 Correlation between change in APRI, FIB4, and LSM

	Early stage						Advanced stage					
	APRI diff		Fib4 diff		Stiffness diff		APRI diff		Fib4 diff		Stiffness diff	
	r	*P* value	*r*	*P* value	*r*	*P* value	*r*	*P* value	*r*	*P* value	*r*	*P* value
APRI diff			0.677	0.000	0.105	0.4			0.706	0.000	−0.148	0.4
Fib4 diff	**0.677**	0.000			0.086	0.5	0.7	0.000			0.001	0.1
Stiffness diff	0.105	0.413	0.086	0.505			−0.148	0.381	0.001	0.993		

Table 5 Correlation between the percentage of change of liver enzymes and fibrosis scores

	Percent of change									
	STIFFNESS		ALT (IU/L)		AST (IU/L)		APRI score		Fib4 calculation	
	r	*P* value	*r*	*P* value	*r*	*P* value	*r*	*P* value	*r*	*P* value
STIFFNESS			−0.084	0.408	−0.031	0.758	0.037	0.715	0.095	0.347
ALT (IU/L)	−0.084	0.408			0.394	0.000	0.373	0.000	−0.069	0.494
AST (IU/L)	−0.031	0.758	0.394	0.000			0.820	0.000	0.678	0.000
APRI score	0.037	0.715	0.373	0.000	0.820	0.000			0.743	0.000
Fib4 Calculation	0.095	0.347	−0.069	0.494	0.678	0.000	0.743	0.000		

Transient elastography in early and advanced stages at baseline and follow-up

Early stages LSM markedly improved at the time of follow-up (5.9±1.5 vs 5.4±2.2 Kpcal, *p*=0.04) (Table 3).

Subgroup analysis revealed that LSM significantly decreased in patients classified as F1 at baseline (6±0.4 vs 5±1.2, *p*<0.001) (Table 6).

Advanced stages LSM improved at the time of follow-up, but was statistically insignificant (18±8.8 vs 15.9 ± 7.8 Kpcal, *p=0.07*) (Table 3); however, subgroup analysis demonstrated a significant decrease of LSM in patients classified as F3 at baseline (11.1±0.8 vs 8.5±2 Kpcal, *p*= 0.02) (Table 6).

In all included patients, the percent of change of LSM was not correlated with either AST nor ALT (Table 5).

The distribution of fibrosis stages among the studied patients at baseline and follow-up

The percentage of patients stratified as early fibrosis stages significantly increased at follow-up compared to baseline (*p*<0.001) (Fig. 1).

Comparison between the two groups regarding the degree of change in stiffness score

Although the amount of change was bigger in advanced than early fibrosis stages, the difference was statistically insignificant (*p* value=0.1) (Fig. 2).

Baseline factors affecting fibrosis scores at a long-term follow-up (Table 7)

Baseline FIB4 and liver stiffness measured by fibroscan are the main determinants of fibrosis at the time of follow-up regardless of age, BMI, and existence of diabetes. For patients with high FIB4 and LS before treatment, their scores will remain high in a long term.

Discussion

A long-term follow-up of CHCV patients after being successfully treated with DAAS should be directed to selected patients who still have the risk to develop hepatic complications in spite of achieving SVR. As post-treatment prognosis is mainly determined by the fibrosis stage, many studies have been conducted to evaluate whether regression of fibrosis can be achieved after completion of DAAS therapy; however, most of these studies were done at a short duration after the end of treatment (12 and 24 weeks) [14, 15]. Additionally, the selection of the most reliable method to categorize the fibrosis stage in treated patients would help clinicians to identify those needing regular medical care and HCC surveillance.

In our study, patients were recruited at an average of 16 months after the end of DAAs and classified according to TE done before treatment initiation into 2 groups early and advanced fibrosis. LSM decreased in both early and advanced fibrosis groups (5.9 ±1.5 vs 5.4±2.2 Kpcal and 18.8±8.8 vs 15.9±7.8 Kpcal, respectively).

Our results agree with those of a study that evaluated the long-term changes of liver elasticity in 143 CHCV patients who achieved SVR by DAAs [16], where LSM

Table 6 Subgroup analysis of changes in fibrosis scores

Baseline TE	LSM			APRI			FIB4		
	Baseline	Follow-up	*P* value	Baseline	Follow-up	*P* value	Baseline	Follow-up	*P* value
F0	4.34±0.7	5.05±2.4	0.19	0.46±0.34	0.24±0.13	0.004	1±0.6	0.9±0.6	0.5
F1	6 ± 0.4	5 ± 1.2	<0.001	0.4±0.3	0.26±0.1	0.006	1.1±0.8	0.98±0.5	0.37
F2	8.1±0.8	6.9±3	0.15	0.48±0.2	0.2±0.1	0.001	1.15±0.5	0.95±0.5	0.13
F3	11±0.8	8.5±2	0.02	0.78±0.7	0.3±0.1	0.06	1.47±0.8	0.95±0.4	0.08
F4	21±8.6	18.5±7.5	0.14	0.86±0.5	0.4±0.25	<0.001	3.3±2.5	2±1.5	0.01

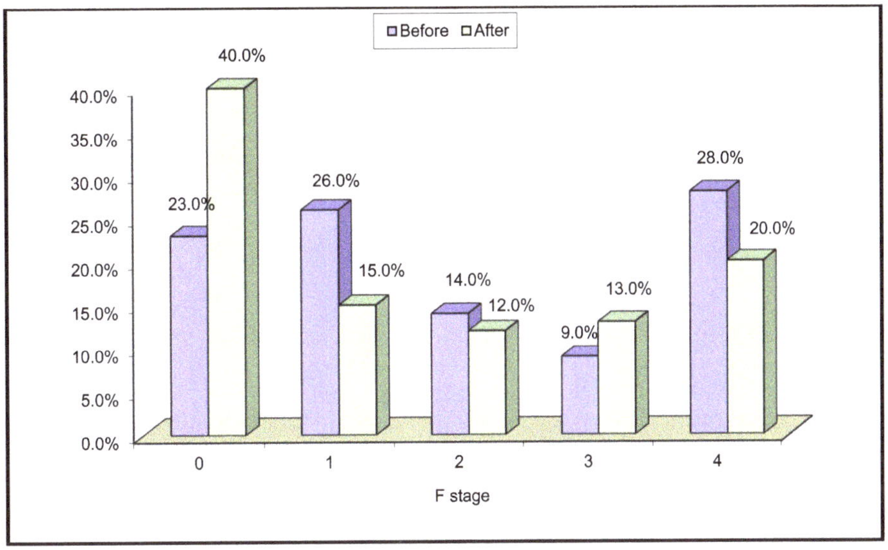

Fig. 1 Comparison of distribution of fibrosis stages among the studied patients at baseline and follow up: difference was statistically significant (<0.001)

improved significantly in cirrhotic and non-cirrhotic patients 25.9 vs 14.5 Kpcal and 7.8 vs 5.4 Kpcal, respectively, at week 96 post-treatment. In the same study, it was reported that patients with early compensated cirrhosis (baseline LSM=20.4pkcal) had significant progressive improvement of LSM at 6 and 24 months ((14.8 Kpcal and 11.2Kpcal), respectively, while patients at more advanced cirrhosis stage denoted by impaired liver function with baseline LSM=32.6pkcal initially achieved a significant decrease in LSM at week 24 post-treatment that was not significantly sustained at week 96 (24 months) after treatment (22.7 vs 19.1 Kpcal). Finally, the change was significantly greater in the cirrhotic group given that they had higher readings at baseline, and

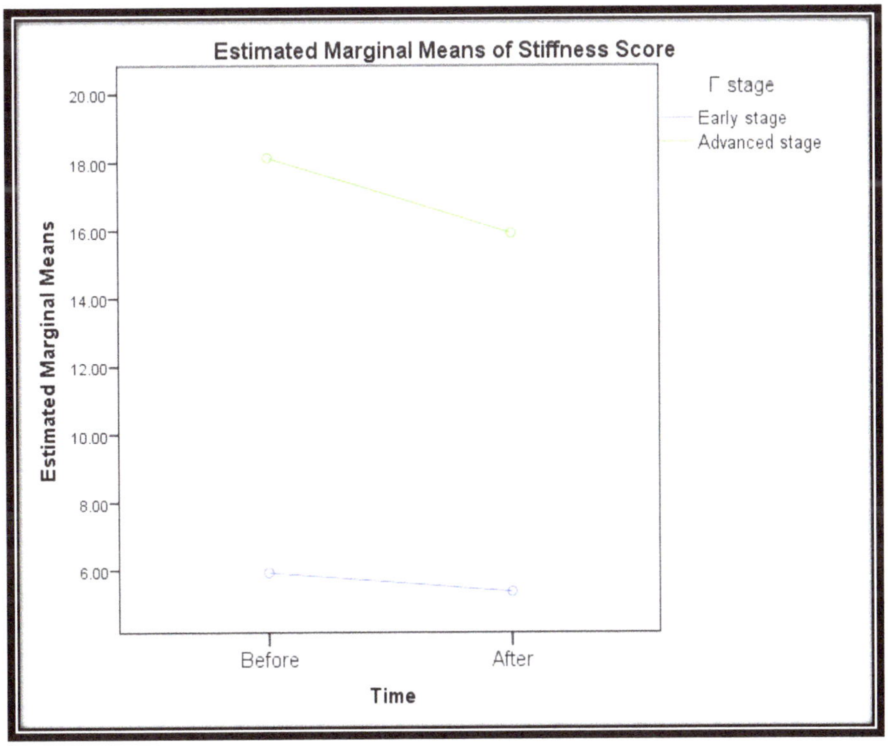

Fig. 2 Estimated marginal means of stiffness score in the early and advanced fibrosis groups

Table 7 Regression analysis for baseline factors affecting stiffness score after treatment

	Unstandardized coefficients		Standardized coefficients	t	Sig.	95% Confidence interval for B	
	B	Std. error	Beta			Lower bound	Upper bound
Age (years)	.044	.036	.092	1.214	.228	−.028	.116
BMI	−.071	.114	−.037	−.624	.534	−.298	.155
Diabetes	−.020	1.265	−.001	−.016	.988	−2.531	2.492
Stiffness score before treatment	.553	.062	.618	8.940	<0.001	.430	.676
APRI Score before treatment	−1.438	1.557	−.088	−.924	.358	−4.531	1.654
Fib4 before treatment	1.304	.489	.313	2.668	.009	.333	2.274

similarly in our study, the amount of change of LSM was bigger in advanced than early fibrosis stages. A meta-analysis attributed the higher decline of liver stiffness in advanced stages after antiviral therapy to a higher inflammatory burden, in which patients with high baseline ALT also showed a higher magnitude of the decline in LSM [17].

In the present study, the subgroup analysis showed that the significant reduction of LSM was reported in patients classified as F1 and F3 (6.1±0.4 vs 5±1.2, $p=$ 0.001 and 11.1±0.8 vs 8.5±2 Kpcal, $p<0.02$). Subsidence of necro-inflammatory reaction is most likely responsible for the improvement reported in early stages [5]. As regards the advanced group, F3 is characterized histologically by numerous immature septae and bridges that precedes nodular formation characteristic of cirrhosis (F4) [18], after withdrawal of the insulting agent (HCV) immature septae might reverse, while mature cross-linked septae rich in elastin and associated with matrix modification are more likely to persist [19].

Clinically elevated liver enzymes are a marker of necro-inflammatory reaction, and in our study, AST and ALT significantly declined and were normalized at follow-up. Also, the non-invasive fibrosis serum biomarker of APRI significantly decreased in both groups and a marked reduction of Fib4 was recorded in advanced stages. The percent of change of APRI is correlated with that of AST and ALT, and the percent of change of Fib4 is correlated with AST; therefore, this improvement of serum biomarkers might be due to normalization of liver enzymes only and not representing fibrosis regression, especially that our results showed that the percent of change of liver stiffness is not correlated with that of liver enzymes, APRI, or Fib4.

Therefore, we could suggest that TE is the reliable method for evaluation of significant fibrosis in the context of follow-up after HCV treatment because as explained above, it is not affected by changes in liver enzymes and also we found that baseline TE scores is the main determinant of liver stiffness at follow-up which means that high scores before treatment are likely to persist after treatment even if a decline was achieved.

Additionally, patients in the advanced fibrosis group at follow-up recorded APRI score of 0.4 ± 0.2 which is lower than the validated cut-off value for significant fibrosis (0.77 and 0.83) [8], and also, the recorded Fib4 for the same group (1.8) is indeterminate [8] for the fibrosis stage.

In a prospective study designed to identify factors influencing fibrosis regression after DAAs, baseline BMI, steatosis, and hepatic stiffness were documented as independent factors [20]; this partially agrees with our study in which baseline LSM but not BMI affected LSM at follow-up; however, in another meta-analysis, BMI was not found to affect change in stiffness [17].

Importantly, LSM of 15.8 Kpcal that was recorded in our advanced group patients alarms us that they are still at an increased risk to develop HCC. As evidenced by a study done by Pons et al. [21] , in which LSM <10 Kpcal at follow-up is correlated with a lower risk of HCC than the higher score of 10–20 Kpcal. He documented that the higher the LSM at follow-up, the greater the risk of HCC.

Conclusion

Although the scores of non-invasive methods of fibrosis assessment (TE, APRI, and FIB4) may improve after successful treatment of CHCV by DAAs, liver stiffness persists high in patients with pre-treatment advanced fibrosis stages. We recommend that TE should be done at least once after treatment to evaluate the further plan of follow-up especially if it is not done before treatment.

The limitations of the current study are the small number of patients specifically those included in the advanced stage group.

Abbreviations

CHCV: Chronic hepatitis C virus; TE: Transient elastography; LS: Liver stiffness; LSM: Liver stiffness measurement; Kpcal: Kilopascal; BMI: Body mass index; LFT: Liver function tests; HCC: Hepatocellular carcinoma

Acknowledgements

Nurse Staff at Ain Shams University Viral hepatitis unit

Authors' contributions

Dr. NA and Dr. OA created the conception and design of the study: Dr. AM, M.S, and D.K were responsible for the acquisition of laboratory and clinical data. Data analysis and/interpretation were done by Dr. A.F. Drafting and revision of the manuscript were done by Dr. A.M, D.K, and A. F. The authors have read and approved the manuscript.

Declarations

Ethics approval and consent to participate

This study was approved by the research ethical committee at Ain Shams University, Faculty of Medicine, MS 124/2020. Verbal and written consent was taken from all participants before inclusion after approval of the research ethical committee at Ain Shams University.

Competing interests

The authors declare that they have no competing interests.

Author details

[1]Tropical Medicine Department, Faculty of Medicine, Ain Shams University, 38 Abbassia street, Postal code, Cairo 1181, Egypt. [2]Internal Medicine Department, Faculty of Medicine, Ain Shams University, Cairo, Egypt.

References

1. Sievert W, Altraif I, Razavi HA, Abdo A, Ahmed EA, Alomair A et al (2011) A systematic review of hepatitis C virus epidemiology in Asia, Australia and Egypt. Liver Int 31(Suppl 2):61–80
2. Dash S, Aydin Y, Widmer KE, Nayak L (2020) Hepatocellular carcinoma mechanisms associated with chronic HCV infection and the impact of direct-acting antiviral treatment. J Hepatocell Carcinoma 15(7):45–76
3. Lombardi A, Mondelli MU (2019) Hepatitis C: is eradication possible? Liver Int 39(3):416–426
4. Rout G, Nayak B, Patel AH, Gunjan D, Singh V, Kedia S, Shalimar (2019) Therapy with oral directly acting agents in hepatitis C infection is associated with reduction in fibrosis and increase in hepatic steatosis on transient elastography. J Clin Exp Hepatol. 9(2):207–214. https://doi.org/10.1016/j.jceh.2018.06.009
5. Sepulveda-Crespo D, Resino S, Martinez I (2021) Strategies targeting the innate immune response for the treatment of hepatitis C virus-associated liver fibrosis. Drugs 81(4):419–443. https://doi.org/10.1007/s40265-020-01458-x
6. Singal AG, Lim JK, Kanwal F (2019) AGA clinical practice update on interaction between oral direct-acting antivirals for chronic hepatitis C infection and hepatocellular carcinoma: expert review. Gastroenterology. 156(8):2149–2157. https://doi.org/10.1053/j.gastro.2019.02.046
7. El-Garem H, Abd-Allah M, Omar H, Cordie A, Abdel Alem S, Mohey Eldin Elzahry MA, Ghaith D, Abou El-Soud NH, Kamal W, Elsharkawy A, Esmat G (2019) DAAs therapy associated with improved hepatic fibrosis in HCV-GT4 patients co-infected with HIV. Expert Rev Gastroenterol Hepatol. 13(7):693–698. https://doi.org/10.1080/17474124.2019.1614441
8. European Association for Study of Liver; Association Latino Americana para el Estudio del Higado. EASL-ALEH Clinical Practice Guidelines (2015) Non-invasive tests for evaluation of liver disease severity and prognosis. J Hepatol. 63(1):237–264
9. El Kassas M, Alboraie M, Omran D, Salaheldin M, Wifi MN, ElBadry M et al (2018) An account of the real-life hepatitis C management in a single specialized viral hepatitis treatment centre in Egypt: results of treating 7042 patients with 7 different direct acting antiviral regimens. Expert Rev Gastroenterol Hepatol. 12(12):1265–1272. https://doi.org/10.1080/17474124.2018.1476137
10. Waked I, Esmat G, Elsharkawy A, El-Serafy M, Abdel-Razek W, Ghalab R et al (2020) Screening and treatment program to eliminate hepatitis C in Egypt. N Engl J Med 382(12):1166–1174
11. Castera L, Forns X, Alberti A (2008) Non-invasive evaluation of liver fibrosis using transient elastography. J Hepatol 48(5):835–847. https://doi.org/10.1016/j.jhep.2008.02.008
12. Wai CT, Greenson JK, Fontana RJ, Kalbfleisch JD, Marrero JA, Conjeevaram HS, Lok AS (2003) A simple noninvasive index can predict both significant fibrosis and cirrhosis in patients with chronic hepatitis C. Hepatology 38(2):518–526. https://doi.org/10.1053/jhep.2003.50346
13. Sterling RK, Lissen E, Clumeck N, Sola R, Correa MC, Montaner J, S. Sulkowski M, Torriani FJ, Dieterich DT, Thomas DL, Messinger D, Nelson M, APRICOT Clinical Investigators (2006) APRICOT Clinical Investigators. Development of a simple noninvasive index to predict significant fibrosis in patients with HIV/HCV coinfection. Hepatology. 43(6):1317–1325. https://doi.org/10.1002/hep.21178
14. Elsharkawy A, Alem SA, Fouad R, El Raziky M, El Akel W, Abdo M et al (2006) Changes in liver stiffness measurements and fibrosis scores following sofosbuvir based treatment regimens without interferon. J Gastroenterol Hepatol 32(9):1624–1630
15. Knop V, Mauss S, Goeser T, Geier A, Zimmermann T, Herzer K, Postel N, Friedrich-Rust M, Hofmann WP, German Hepatitis C-Registry, Ende K, Pathil A, Bauer T, Zeuzem S, Berg T, Cornberg M, Börner N, Ringelhan M, Klinker H, Schlenker T, Lutz T, Heinzow H, Günther R, Busch H, Baumgarten A, Buggisch P, Roessle M, Hüppe D, Manns MP, Niederau C, Sarrazin C, Schirmacher P, Simon KG, Wedemeyer H (2020) Dynamics of liver stiffness by transient elastography in patients with chronic hepatitis C virus infection receiving direct-acting antiviral therapy-results from the German Hepatitis C-Registry. J Viral Hepat. 27(7):690–698. https://doi.org/10.1111/jvh.13280
16. Pietsch V, Deterding K, Attia D, Ringe KI, Heidrich B, Cornberg M, Gebel M, Manns MP, Wedemeyer H, Potthoff A (2018) Long-term changes in liver elasticity in hepatitis C virus-infected patients with sustained virologic response after treatment with direct-acting antivirals. United European Gastroenterol J. 6(8):1188–1198. https://doi.org/10.1177/2050640618786067
17. Singh S, Facciorusso A, Loomba R, Falck-Ytter YT (2018) Magnitude and kinetics of decrease in liver stiffness after anti-viral therapy in patients with chronic hepatitis C: a systematic review and meta-analysis. Clin Gastroenterol Hepatol 16(1):27–38.e4
18. Goodman ZD (2007) Grading and staging systems for inflammation and fibrosis in chronic liver diseases. J Hepatol 47(4):598–607
19. Garcia-Tsao G, Friedman S, Iredale J, Pinzani M (2010) Now there are many (stages) where before there was one: in search of a pathophysiological classification of cirrhosis. Hepatology. 51(4):1445–1449. https://doi.org/10.1002/hep.23478
20. Soliman H, Ziada D, Salama M, Hamisa M, Badawi R, Hawash N, Selim A, Abd-Elsalam S (2020) Predictors for fibrosis regression in chronic HCV patients after the treatment with DAAS: results of a real-world cohort study. Endocr Metab Immune Disord Drug Targets. 20(1):104–111. https://doi.org/10.2174/1871530319666190826150344
21. Pons M, Rodríguez-Tajes S, Esteban JI, Mariño Z, Vargas V, Lens S, Buti M, Augustin S, Forns X, Mínguez B, Genescà J (2020) Non-invasive prediction of liver-related events in patients with HCV-associated compensated advanced chronic liver disease after oral antivirals. J Hepatol. 72(3):472–480. https://doi.org/10.1016/j.jhep.2019.10.005

25

Role of hepatitis C virus core antigen assay in hepatitis C care in developing country

Ouafa Kallala[1,2*], Saoussen Kacem[1,2], Imene Fodha[1,2], Bruno Pozzetto[3,4] and Trabelsi Abdelhalim[1,2]

Abstract

Background: The World Health Organization (WHO) aims to achieve global hepatitis C elimination by 2030, defined as diagnosis of 90% of infected individuals and treating 80% of them. Current guidelines for the screening and diagnosis of hepatitis C infection denote using a relatively cheap screen with anti-hepatitis C virus (HCV) antibody immunoassay, followed by the much costlier molecular test for HCV RNA levels using polymerase chain reaction (PCR) assay to confirm active HCV infection. Simplification of the HCV evaluation algorithm to reduce the number of required tests could considerably expand the provision of HCV treatment especially in a developing country. This study investigates the performance of hepatitis C Core Antigen (HCV Ag) test by comparing HCV Ag results versus the results obtained with HCV ribonucleic acid (RNA) PCR which is considered the gold standard for the diagnosis of HCV infection.

Results: Among the 109 anti-HCV positive sera, 96 were positive for both HCV Ag (> 3 fmol/L) and HCV RNA (> 15 IU/mL); 8 were negative for both tests, while the remaining 5 were positive for HCV RNA only. Considering the HCV RNA as gold standard; the sensitivity, specificity, positive predictive value (PPV) and negative predictive value (NPV) of HCV Ag test were found to be 95.05%, 100%, 100%, and 61.54%, respectively. HCV genotype was performed for 59 patients. The most common HCV genotype was genotype 1 (72.9%). Genotype 2 (15.3%) and genotype 3 (11.9%) were detected in the others samples. A high level of correlation was seen between HCV RNA and HCV Ag (r = 0.958, $p < 0.001$). The correlation for the samples that were genotyped 1 was significant ($r = 0.966$, $p < 0.001$).

Conclusion: In our study, it was found that there was strong correlation between HCV RNA levels and HCV Ag levels. So, it can be used for a one-step HCV antigen test to diagnose active HCV infection.

Keywords: Core Antigen, Hepatitis C, Polymerase chain reaction

Background

Hepatitis C virus (HCV) infection is a global public health problem. Hepatitis C is found worldwide. The most affected regions are Eastern Mediterranean and European Regions, with the prevalence of 2.3% and 1.5%, respectively. Prevalence of HCV infection in other regions varies from 0.5 to 1.0%. Tunisia is a low endemicity country of HCV infection, with an average prevalence of 0.7% and a north-south gradient [1, 2].

HCV causes both acute and chronic infection. Acute HCV infection is usually asymptomatic, and is only very rarely (if ever) associated with life-threatening disease. About 15–45% of infected persons spontaneously clear the virus within 6 months of infection without any treatment. The remaining 55–85% of persons will develop chronic HCV infection. Of those with chronic HCV infection, the risk of cirrhosis of the liver is between 15 and 30% within 20 years [1].

Due to the fact that acute HCV infection is usually asymptomatic, few people are diagnosed during the acute phase. In those people who go on to develop

* Correspondence: ouafa.kallala@gmail.com
[1]Research Laboratory for "Epidemiology and Immunogenetics of Viral Infections" (LR14SP02), Sahloul University Hospital, University of Sousse, Sousse, Tunisia
[2]Faculty of Pharmacy, University of Monastir, Avicenne Street, Monastir, Tunisia
Full list of author information is available at the end of the article

chronic HCV infection, the infection is also often undiagnosed because the infection remains asymptomatic until decades after infection when symptoms develop secondary to serious liver damage [1, 3].

HCV infection is diagnosed in 2 steps. The first one is a screening for anti-HCV antibodies (anti-HCV) with a serological test which identifies people who have been infected with the virus. If the test is positive for anti-HCV, a nucleic acid test for HCV ribonucleic acid (RNA) is needed to determine active/previous infection state. Although no longer infected, they will still test positive for anti-HCV [1, 4, 5]. HCV RNA test should be performed in addition to anti-HCV in acute HCV infections during the window period and also in cases with certain immunodeficiencies [3, 4]. However, due to the expensiveness and high technicality of Polymerase chain reaction (PCR) machinery, it is impractical for low-income countries to routinely administer these tests [5, 6].

Simplification of the HCV evaluation algorithm to reduce the number of required tests could considerably expand the provision of HCV treatment. HCV Core Antigen (Ag) can be detected from 1 to 2 days following HCV RNA detection in serum and 33.2 (range 23–46) days prior to detection of HCV antibodies [7].

The aim of the present study is to evaluate the performance of HCV Ag test by comparing HCV Ag results versus the results obtained with HCV RNA polymerase chain reaction (PCR) which is considered the gold standard for the diagnosis of HCV infection.

Methods

Sample selection and characteristics

A total of 109 patient serum or plasma samples sent from different clinics to the Microbiology Laboratory of Sahloul University Hospital of Sousse, located in the Eastern Centre of Tunisia, for HCV RNA test were included in the study during the 2012–2015 period. Information on patients' diagnoses, treatments, HCV activation markers, and microbiological laboratory data (anti-HCV, HCV RNA) were obtained from the hospital's electronic information system and patient files.

Detection of anti-HCV antibodies

Anti-HCV antibody test was performed by means of a chemiluminescent microparticle enzyme immunoassay (CMIA) (Cobas e411 Elecsys analyser, Roche, USA) in line with manufacturer's recommendations. The "cut-off" value was considered 1.0 as per the kit procedure. It was considered as reactive which value of the test is ≥ 1.0.

HCV RNA assay

Real-time PCR (COBAS AmpliPrep/COBAS Taq Man HCV real-time PCR, Roche Diagnostics, Germany) was used in line with manufacturer's recommendations for HCV RNA quantitation in plasma samples. The assay has a limit of detection of 15 IU/mL with a linear quantitation window of 43–6.9 × 10^7 IU/mL.

HCV Ag assay

HCV Ag quantification were performed using Abbott ARCHITECT HCV Ag Assay (Abbott, Germany) with manufacturer's recommendations. This is a two-step chemiluminescent microparticle immunoassay (CMIA) which is divided into a liquid phase with acridinium labeled murine anti-HCV antibodies, and a solid phase with paramagnetic microparticles. The manufacturer states the "cut-off" value as 3.00 fmol/L (0.06 pg/mL) and the quantitation upper limit as 20,000 fmol/L for this assay.

Genotyping

HCV RNA extraction

The viral nucleic acid from HCV-infected patients' plasmas was extracted using the QIAamp® DSP Virus Kit (QIAGEN) according to manufacturer's instructions.

Reverse Transcription (RT) and Amplification of HCV 5'UTR/Core regions

This step was carried out using the HCV Amplification 2.0 Kit (LiPA) Simens®.

HCV genotyping

A Versant HCV genotype 2.0 assay (INNO-LiPA HCV 2.0) Simens® was performed according to the manufacturer's instructions.

Statistical analysis

Lineal regression analysis was used to assess the linear association between HCV Ag and HCV RNA concentrations as well as anti-HCV and HCV RNA concentrations in logarithmic scales.

Sensitivity, specificity, negative predictive value, positive predictive value, and accuracy values for the HCV Ag test were calculated versus the HCV RNA test (the gold standard). All data were analyzed by using SPSS software (SPSS; version 20.0). Statistical significance level was considered as 0.05.

Results

Sixty-one (56.0%) of the 109 patients included in the study group were females and 48 (44.0 %) were males. Seventy eight (71.6%) were treatment-naive and 31 (28.4%) were under treatment.

HCV genotype was performed for 59 patients. Genotype 1 (43/59, 72.9%), genotype 2 (9/59, 15.3%),

Table 1 Sensitivity and specificity of HCV Ag in predicted HCV RNA in 109 anti-HCV positive patients

		HCV RNA		
		Positive	Negative	Total
HCV Ag	Positive	96	0	96
	Negative	5	8	13
	Total	101	8	109

HCV Ag negative: HCV Ag < 3 fmol/L; HCV RNA negative: HCV RNA < 15 IU/mL
Sensitivity = 96/101 = 95.05%
Specificity = 8/8 = 100%
Positive predictive value (PPV) = 96/96 = 100%
Negative predictive value (NPV) = 8/13 = 61.54%

and genotype 3 (7, 11.9%) were detected in the study samples.

Among the 109 anti-HCV positive sera, 96 were positive for both HCV Ag (> 3 fmol/L) and HCV RNA (> 15 IU/mL); 8 were negative for both tests, while the remaining 5 were positive for HCV RNA only.

Considering the HCV RNA as gold standard, the sensitivity, specificity, positive predictive value (PPV), and negative predictive value (NPV) of HCV Ag test were found to be 95.05%, 100%, 100%, and 61.54% respectively (Table 1).

Figure 1 shows comparison between HCV RNA levels and HCV Ag levels using a logarithmic scale. Pearson's correlation coefficient was 0.958 ($p < 0.001$) indicating good concordance, and the two tests were therefore considered as highly concordant.

The correlation for the samples that were genotyped 1 was significant ($p < 0.001$), given a Pearson coefficient value of 0.966. Figure 2 shows linear regressions for genotypes when plotted on log scales of HCV RNA and HCV Ag levels. Statistical correlation tests could not be performed regarding the genotypes other than genotype 1 due to the small number of non-genotype 1 samples detected in the present study.

Note that the lowest detection level of reactive HCV Ag (4.47 fmol/L) corresponded to 1890 IU/mL HCV RNA.

HCV Ag false negatives occurred at relatively low HCV RNA titers. Five samples (9.26%) positive for HCV RNA (38–813 IU/mL, mean value 406 IU/mL) were found to be negative for the HCV Ag test (0.00–1.08 fmol/L, mean value 0.506 fmol/L). Two of them were under treatment and three were treatment-naïve. HCV genotype could be determined for two samples among

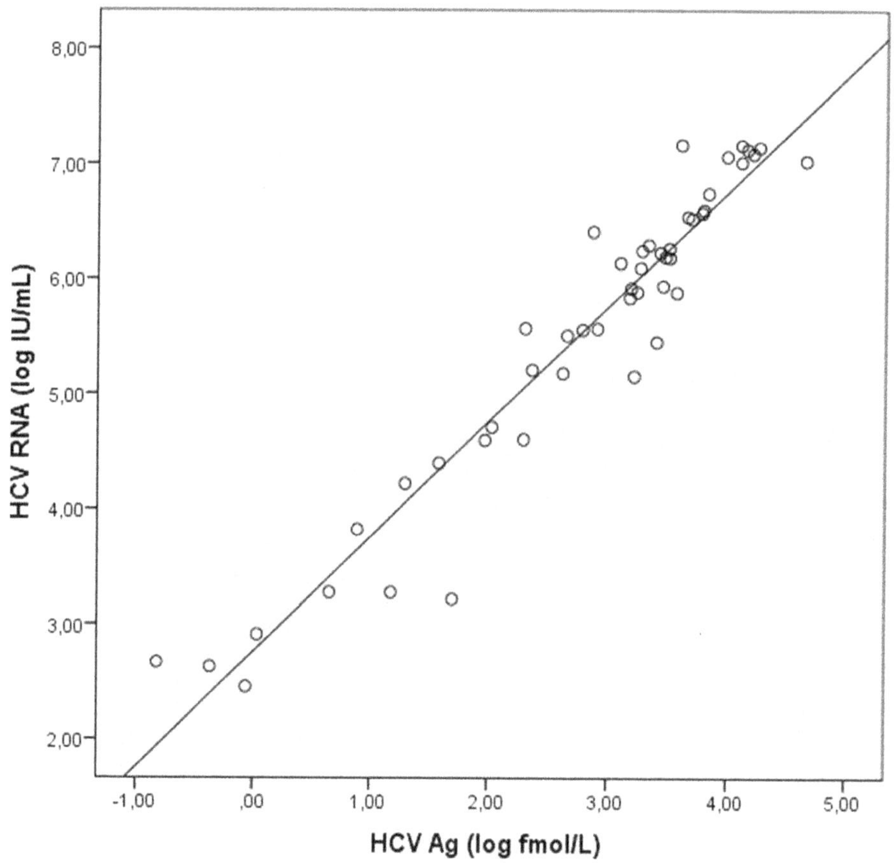

Fig. 1 Correlation diagram of HCV Ag (log10 fmol/L) and HCV RNA (log10 IU/mL), Pearson's correlation ($r = 0.958$, $p < 0.001$)

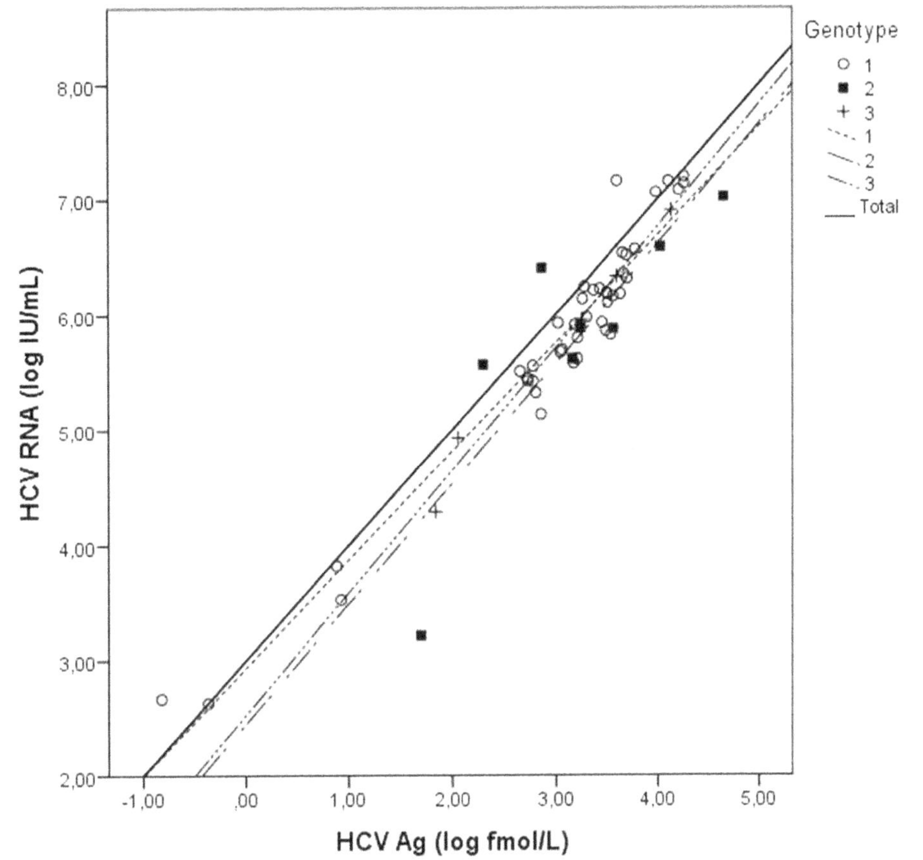

Fig. 2 Correlation diagram of HCV Ag (log10 fmol/L) and HCV RNA (log10 IU/mL) according to genotype for 59 genotyped samples

the five false negative results, and genotype 1 was detected in both cases.

Discussion

Current guidelines for the screening and diagnosis of HCV denote using a relatively cheap screen with anti-HCV anti-body immunoassay, followed by the much costlier molecular test for HCV RNA levels using PCR assay to confirm active HCV infection. HCV Ag assays, which are easier to perform than real time-PCR also save time and are less expensive. Previous cost-effectiveness analysis showed that screening and evaluating HCV viremia using a strategy in which the two-step process is replaced by a one-step process could result in a net cost saving up to $44 per person screened [8, 9].

That is why, there has been a push for a one-step HCV antigen test to diagnose active HCV infection [10].

Detection of HCV Ag was initially described in late 90s. However, first generation antigen tests had soon become unpopular due to their lack of sensitivity [7]. The chemiluminescent immunoassay based new generation HCV Ag test used in this study has a sensitivity of ≤ 3 fmol/L, offering 16- to 25-fold sensitivity compared to preceding tests [11].

In our study, it was found that there was strong correlation between HCV RNA levels and HCV Ag levels. HCV Ag levels were detected, with a corresponding increase in HCV Ag levels to increased titer of viral RNA, with a high correlation coefficient of 0.958 ($p < 0.001$). Similar results were reported by various other studies [10–12]. Due to the excellent correlation between HCV Ag and HCV RNA concentrations, detection of HCV Ag in serum or plasma is useful as an indirect marker of HCV replication [13].

Sensitivity of the HCV Ag test, in the present study, was 95.05% compared to that of the RNA test. Previous studies which utilized the same HCV Ag test have reported a sensitivity of 75.8–99.5% for the HCV Ag test [11, 12, 14–16].

In our study, negative results were obtained with HCV Ag test for five samples with viral load of 38–813 IU/mL. In a study by Çetiner and colleagues [11], seven samples with positive HCV RNA results yielded negative HCV Ag results and viral load were lower than 10,000 IU/mL for these patients (six samples with viral loads of 17–178 IU/mL and one sample with a viral load of 2500 IU/mL). In another study by Ergünay and colleagues [15], the viral load was lower than 10^3 IU/mL in samples which were negative for the HCV Ag test.

In the present study, specificity was found to be 100%. Ross and colleagues [17], Kesli and colleagues [12], Park and colleagues [18], Çetiner and colleagues [11] and Chang and colleagues [10] have also found a specificity level of 100%.

In the present study, PPV was 100% and there is no false positivity with the HCV Ag test. Same result was found by Çetiner and colleagues [11].

However, our negative predictive value (61.54%), similar to result find by Abdelrazik and colleagues [13], was lower than those of the other studies [12, 19]. This result was probably due to the small number of RNA negative samples, that is, 8 out of 109.

Consequently, all positive results found by the HCV Ag assay were also positive with the HCV RNA assay. However, all negative results found by the HCV core Ag assay were not negative with the HCV RNA assay. Thus, it can be concluded that a positive test with the HCV Ag (almost) always represents a true positive since it is highly specific. However, when there is a serum sample showing anti-HCV positivity, the negative results found by the HCV core Ag assay should be also confirmed by a HCV RNA assay [13].

There is increasing, albeit insufficient, evidence that genotype may affect antigen and RNA assay detection results to different extents [20]. In our study, genotype 1 was the predominant detected genotype, corresponding to the genotypic distribution of HCV in Tunisia [21–23]. Specially, there was a strong correlation between HCV RNA levels and HCV Ag levels in genotype 1 (r = 0.966). Similar result was found by Chang and colleagues (r = 0.945) [10]. In contrast, the correlation coefficient was considerably higher than those reported in previous study [24, 25]. This discordance may be explained by the variability of studied population and the use of different assays.

Conclusion

The World Health Organization aims to achieve global hepatitis C elimination by 2030, defined as diagnosis of 90% of infected individuals and treatment initiation of 80% of eligible individuals. In the same directive line, Tunisia launched, in 2016, a national plan for the eradication of hepatitis C by 2023. The development and market approval of novel direct-acting antivirals (DAAs), such as sofosbuvir by itself or in combination with ledipasvir molecules currently available in Tunisia have dramatically changed the hepatitis C virus treatment landscape. Future studies are needed to evaluate the usefulness of HCV Ag quantification for the monitoring and detection of treatment failure, in patients treated with different DAAs.

Abbreviations

Anti-HCV: HCV antibodies; CMIA: Chemiluminescent microparticle enzyme immunoassay; DAAs: Direct-acting antivirals; HCV: Hepatitis C virus; HCV Ag: Hepatitis C core antigen; NPV: Negative predictive value; PCR: Polymerase chain reaction; PPV: Positive predictive value; RNA: Ribonucleic acid; WHO: World Health Organization

Acknowledgements

Not applicable

Authors' contributions

K.S.: study concept and design and Acquisition of data, K.O.: analysis and interpretation of data, statistical analysis and drafting of the manuscript; P.B. and F.I.: critical revision of the manuscript for important intellectual content; T.A.: study supervision. All authors critically revised the manuscript, approved the final version to be published, and agree to be accountable for all aspects of the work.

Declarations

Ethics approval and consent to participate

Not applicable

Competing interests

The authors declare that they have no competing interests.

Author details

[1]Research Laboratory for "Epidemiology and Immunogenetics of Viral Infections" (LR14SP02), Sahloul University Hospital, University of Sousse, Sousse, Tunisia. [2]Faculty of Pharmacy, University of Monastir, Avicenne Street, Monastir, Tunisia. [3]GIMAP EA3064, Faculté de Médecine, Université de Saint-Etienne/Université de Lyon, Lyon, France. [4]Laboratoire des Agents infectieux et d'Hygiène, CHU de Saint-Etienne, Saint-Priest-en-Jarez, France.

References

1. World Health Organization .Hepatitis C. Available at: https://www.who.int/news-room/fact-sheets/detail/hepatitis-c. Accessed 2 May 2019.
2. Debbeche R, Said Y, Ben Temime H, El Jery K, Bouzaidi S, Salem M et al (2013) Epidemiology of hepatitis C in Tunisia. Tunis Med. 91(2):86–90
3. Pawlotsky JM (2002) Use and interpretation of virological tests for hepatitis C. Hepatol Baltim Md. 36(5 Suppl 1):S65–S73. https://doi.org/10.1053/jhep.2002.36815
4. Cloherty G, Talal A, Coller K, Steinhart C, Hackett J, Dawson G et al (2016) Role of serologic and molecular diagnostic assays in identification and management of hepatitis C virus infection. J Clin Microbiol. 54(2):265–273. https://doi.org/10.1128/JCM.02407-15
5. Hu K-Q, Cui W (2016) A highly specific and sensitive hepatitis C virus antigen enzyme immunoassay for One-step diagnosis of viremic hepatitis C virus infection. Hepatol Baltim Md. 64(2):415–424. https://doi.org/10.1002/hep.28663
6. Wang L, Lv H, Zhang G (2017) Hepatitis C virus core antigen assay: an alternative method for hepatitis C diagnosis. Ann Clin Biochem. 54(2):279–285. https://doi.org/10.1177/0004563216661218
7. Hosseini-Moghaddam SM, Iran-Pour E, Rotstein C, Husain S, Lilly L, Renner E, Mazzulli T (2012) Hepatitis C core Ag and its clinical applicability: potential advantages and disadvantages for diagnosis and follow-up? Rev Med Virol. 22(3):156–165. https://doi.org/10.1002/rmv.717
8. van Tilborg M, Al Marzooqi SH, Wong WWL, Maan R, Vermehren J, Maasoumy B et al (2018) HCV core antigen as an alternative to HCV RNA testing in the era of direct-acting antivirals: retrospective screening and

diagnostic cohort studies. Lancet Gastroenterol Hepatol. 3(12):856–864. https://doi.org/10.1016/S2468-1253(18)30271-1
9. Wang JH, Chen CH, Chang CM, Feng WC, Lee CY, Lu SN (2020) Hepatitis C virus core antigen is cost-effective in community-based screening of active hepatitis C infection in Taiwan. J Formos Med Assoc. 119(1 Pt 3):504–508. https://doi.org/10.1016/j.jfma.2019.07.011
10. Chang C, Hung C-H, Wang J-H, Lu S-N (2018) Hepatitis C core antigen highly correlated to HCV RNA. Kaohsiung J Med Sci. 34(12):684–688. https://doi.org/10.1016/j.kjms.2018.08.002
11. Çetiner S, Çetin Duran A, Kibar F, Yaman A (2017) Performance comparison of new generation HCV core antigen test versus HCV RNA test in management of hepatitis C virus infection. Transfus Apher Sci. 56(3):362–366. https://doi.org/10.1016/j.transci.2017.02.005
12. Kesli R, Polat H, Terzi Y, Kurtoglu MG, Uyar Y (2011) Comparison of a newly developed automated and quantitative hepatitis C virus (HCV) core antigen test with the HCV RNA assay for clinical usefulness in confirming anti-HCV results. J Clin Microbiol. 49(12):4089–4093. https://doi.org/10.1128/JCM.05292-11
13. Abdelrazik AM, Abozaid HE, Montasser KA (2018) Role of hepatitis C virus (HCV) core antigen in improving blood transfusion safety in high prevalence, resource limited countries, a step forward. Transfus Apher Sci. 57(4):566–568. https://doi.org/10.1016/j.transci.2018.06.006
14. Morota K, Fujinami R, Kinukawa H, Machida T, Ohno K, Saegusa H, Takeda K (2009) A new sensitive and automated chemiluminescent microparticle immunoassay for quantitative determination of hepatitis C virus core antigen. J Virol Methods. 157(1):8–14. https://doi.org/10.1016/j.jviromet.2008.12.009
15. Ergünay K, Sener B, Alp A, Karakaya J, Hasçelik G (2011) Utility of a commercial quantitative hepatitis C virus core antigen assay in a diagnostic laboratory setting. Diagn Microbiol Infect Dis. 70(4):486–491. https://doi.org/10.1016/j.diagmicrobio.2011.04.011
16. Miedouge M, Saune K, Kamar N, Rieu M, Rostaing L, Izopet J (2010) Analytical evaluation of HCV core antigen and interest for HCV screening in haemodialysis patients. J Clin Virol Off Publ Pan Am Soc Clin Virol. 48(1):18–21. https://doi.org/10.1016/j.jcv.2010.02.012
17. Ross RS, Viazov S, Salloum S, Hilgard P, Gerken G, Roggendorf M (2010) Analytical performance characteristics and clinical utility of a novel assay for total hepatitis C virus core antigen quantification. J Clin Microbiol. 48(4):1161–1168. https://doi.org/10.1128/JCM.01640-09
18. Park Y, Lee J-H, Kim BS, Kim DY, Han K-H, Kim H-S (2010) New automated hepatitis C virus (HCV) core antigen assay as an alternative to real-time PCR for HCV RNA quantification. J Clin Microbiol. 48(6):2253–2256. https://doi.org/10.1128/JCM.01856-09
19. Koroglu M, Sibel Ak, Muharrem Ak, Yakupoğulları Y, Özer A (2012) Evaluation of diagnostic performance of new antigen based enzyme immune assay for diagnosis of Hepatitis C virus (HCV) infections. Afr J Microbiol Res. 6(4):809–812. https://doi.org/10.5897/AJMR11.1130.
20. Khan H, Hill A, Main J, Brown A, Cooke G (2017) Can hepatitis C virus antigen testing replace ribonucleic acid polymearse chain reaction analysis for detecting hepatitis C virus? A systematic review. Open Forum Infect Dis 4(2):ofw252
21. Ben Moussa M, Barguellil F, Bouziani A, Amor A (2003) Comparison of two hepatitis C virus typing assays in a Tunisian population. Ann Biol Clin. 61(2):234–238
22. Djebbi A, Triki H, Bahri O, Cheikh I, Sadraoui A, Ben Ammar A et al (2003) Genotypes of hepatitis C virus circulating in Tunisia. Epidemiol Infect. 130(3):501–505. https://doi.org/10.1017/S095026880300846X
23. Souii A, Elargoubi A, Fallecker C, Mastouri M, Drouet E (2016) Hepatitis C genotype prevalence in Monastir Region, Tunisia: correlation between 5′ untranslated region (5′UTR), non-structural 5B (NS5B), and core sequences in HCV subtyping. Curr Microbiol. 73(3):324–334. https://doi.org/10.1007/s00284-016-1064-2
24. Bouzgarrou N, Fodha I, Othman SB, Achour A, Grattard F, Trabelsi A, Pozzetto B (2005) Evaluation of a total core antigen assay for the diagnosis of hepatitis C virus infection in hemodialysis patients. J Med Virol. 77(4):502–508. https://doi.org/10.1002/jmv.20485
25. Durante-Mangoni E, Vallefuoco L, Sorrentino R, Iossa D, Perna E, Molaro R, Braschi U, Zampino R, Sodano G, Adinolfi LE, Utili R, Portella G (2013) Clinico-pathological significance of hepatitis C virus core antigen levels in chronic infection. J Med Virol. 85(11):1913–1918. https://doi.org/10.1002/jmv.23672

26

Vascular endothelial growth factor in relation to the development of hepatocellular carcinoma in hepatitis C virus patients treated by direct-acting antivirals

Ahmed Mohamed ElGhandour[1], Essam Mohamed Bayoumy[1], Wesam Ahmed Ibrahim[1], Moataz Mohamed Sayed[1], Ashraf Bekheet Salama[1,2], Nahla Mohamed Teama[3*] and Mohamed Magdy Salama[1]

Abstract

Background: Hepatocellular carcinoma (HCC) comprises 5.6% of all cancers worldwide representing the sixth most common cancer. It is also the fourth most common cause of cancer-related mortality. Angiogenesis is a main factor in the development of HCC. Vascular endothelial growth factor (VEGF) is considered as the force for physiological and pathological angiogenesis, and overexpression of VEGF is prominent in HCC. We aimed to study the effect of direct-acting antivirals (DAAs) on VEGF considered as the key regulator of angiogenesis in HCC. This cross-sectional study involved fifty patients who were divided into two groups: group I—twenty-five chronic hepatitis C virus (HCV) patients as (cases) subjected to treatment with direct-acting antiviral drugs for 3 months; group II—twenty-five chronic HCV patients developed HCC as (controls). Serum VEGF level was measured in of group I at baseline, at end of treatment, and 3 months after the end of treatment by sofosbuvir 400 mg plus daclatasvir 60 mg for 3 months in the HCV patient group, also VEGF was assessed in group II with HCC.

Results: Serum VEGF was high in both groups, but it was higher in the HCC group with a statistically significant difference ($p < 0.001$), also serum VEGF in the HCV group decreased after 3 months at the end of DAA treatment from 209.5 ± 137.6 to 44.1 (31.8–55.3) mg/ml, and all patients who received DAAs achieved sustained virologic response (SVR).

Conclusion: We found that change in serum VEGF in HCV patients treated with DAAs in this study cannot explain the risk of HCC after treatment by DAAs.

Keywords: Vascular endothelial growth factor A, HCV, DAAs, HCC

* Correspondence: nahlateama@med.asu.edu.eg
[3]Division of Nephrology, Department of Internal Medicine, Faculty of Medicine, Ain Shams University, Ramsis Street 38, Abbasia, Cairo 11566, Egypt
Full list of author information is available at the end of the article

Background

Liver cancer occupies the sixth rank among common cancers and the fourth among the leading causes of cancer-associated mortalities [1]. Hepatocellular carcinoma (HCC) is considered the commonest liver cancer worldwide [2]. Chronic infection with HCV is considered the most common etiology for HCC [3]. The direct-acting antiviral agents (DAAs) recently improve the standards of therapy that achieve complete cure of hepatitis C virus infection, which in turn leads to a decreased risk of developing HCC and its associated high mortality [4].

Although the novel therapies are effective in treatment, they did not manage to reduce the risk of HCC in those with higher degrees of liver cirrhosis to zero percent [5]. Cirrhosis plays an important role in the occurrence of HCC since the majority of HCV patients who develop HCC are cirrhotic, and patients with advanced cirrhosis are highly prone to develop HCC even after achieving sustained virologic response (SVR) [6]. Many studies have shown the effect of DAA regimens on HCC recurrence and development; however, neither of them could confirm this relation [1, 7–9].

AFP has limited sensitivity (41–65%) for the detection hepatocellular carcinoma especially in its early phases. It is not secreted in all cases of HCC, and its serum levels may be within normal ranges in about 40% of patients with HCC. So, detection of serum AFP only is not a reliable indicator in the early phases of HCC [10]. Therefore, the presence of an alternative marker for HCC is important. It was reported that vascular endothelial growth factor (VEGF) is only detected in HCC cells but not in benign liver tissues, and can thus be used as an excellent marker for the diagnosis of early HCC [11].

VEGF signaling is the main regulator of angiogenesis, which is impaired in most solid types of cancer as liver tumors' growth needs high vascularity through new blood vessel formation to suffice its increased metabolic demands [12]. HCV can affect the process of angiogenesis through triggering of hypoxia-inducible factor 1 alpha (HIF-1α) that turns into increased VEGF expression [13]. Also, HCV activates the signal transducer and activator of transcription 3 (STAT3) which stimulates both the transcriptional activity of androgen receptors and VEGF expression [14].

We aimed to study the impact of DAAs on VEGF expression which is the key regulator of angiogenesis in HCC.

Methods

We included fifty adult patients from Ain Shams University Hospitals; they were divided into two groups:

- Group I (case group): twenty-five chronic HCV patients as evidenced by positive HCV Ab (at least 6 months duration) and detectable quantitative HCV-RNA were subjected to the treatment of hepatitis C virus by sofosbuvir 400 mg plus daclatasvir 60 mg for 3 months (HCV HCC-free group) and all patients achieved SVR.
- Group II (control group): twenty-five HCV patients who developed HCC. HCC was confirmed by triphasic abdominal CT with contrast verifying criteria of HCC (HCV related HCC patients).

Any causes of chronic liver disease other than HCV such as hepatitis B virus (HBV) were excluded. We also excluded patients with morbid obesity, dyslipidemia, diabetes mellitus, and patients with any malignancy other than HCC. Also, patients with rheumatoid arthritis, pregnant females, and patients with decompensated liver disease (Child-Pugh C) were excluded from the study.

All patients were subjected to the following:

Full history and clinical examination and the following laboratory tests:

- Complete blood count (CBC).
- Serum creatinine.
- Aspartate aminotransferase (AST), alanine aminotransferase (ALT), and serum albumin.
- PCR quantitative for HCV.
- Serum alpha-fetoprotein level (AFP).
- Serum vascular endothelial growth factor normal range (27–30 ng/ml) was assessed for all patients included in both groups.
  - For group I, VEGF was assessed before starting antiviral treatment (baseline) then at the end of treatment, 1 month after the end of treatment, and 3 months after the end of treatment (SVR).
  - For group II, VEGF was assessed at the beginning of the study.
- Radiological examination: pelviabdominal ultrasound.

Sample size calculation

After reviewing the literatures [15, 16], we used G*POWER statistical programming version 3.1.9.4 (Franz Faul, University at Kiel, Germany) to calculate the sample size per group. Using a = 0.05, a power of 90%, an effect size of 0.628, and an allocation ration of 1:1 showed that the minimum required sample size to avoid type II error is 58 patients (29 patients in each group) was needed. Four patients were lost to follow-up from each group. So, there were 25 patients in each group.

Statistical analysis

We used SPSS (Statistical Package for Social Sciences) for Windows version 24 (SPSS Inc., Chicago, IL, USA).

Numerical data were expressed in terms of mean and standard deviation (mean ± SD) if normally distributed or median and inter-quartile range if not normally distributed. Normality was tested using the Shapiro-Wilk test. Pearson and Spearman correlations were used to test the association between the numerical dependent and independent variables. The Friedman test was used to test the difference between paired numerical data. We conducted a linear regression analysis to test the absolute relations between dependent and independent variables. *P* value less than 0.05 was sufficient enough to show the statistical significance.

Results

This study was conducted on fifty patients. Both groups were age- and sex-matched. They were subdivided into two groups.

- Group I (HCV HCC-free group): twenty-five HCV patients were subjected to the treatment of chronic hepatitis C virus by DAAs.
- Group II (HCV-related HCC group): twenty-five HCV patients who developed HCC.

As regards the demographic data, there were no statistically significant differences in age and sex, although all patients had normal body weight but significantly higher median BMI in the HCC group compared with the other ($p < 0.001$). Concerning laboratory findings, patients in the HCC group had statistically significantly lower levels of hemoglobin and platelets than others in the HCV group ($p < 0.001$, $p < 0.001$, respectively), but serum creatinine levels were significantly higher in the HCC group than in the HCV group ($p < 0.001$).

Also, AFP was dramatically higher in the HCC group ($p < 0.001$) than in the HCV group. Concerning liver functions, bilirubin levels were significantly higher in HCC group ($p < 0.001$), both groups had similar ALT and AST levels ($p = 0.15$, $p = 0.39$, respectively). However, albumin levels were significantly higher in the HCV group ($p < 0.001$) as shown in Table 1.

HCC patients had significantly higher levels of VEGF compared to HCV patients (488.01 ± 194.5 versus 209.5 ± 137.6, respectively).

For HCV patients, there was a positive correlation between baseline VEGF levels and BMI, bilirubin, AST, PCR, and AFP levels. VEGF was negatively correlated with age, Hb levels, platelet count, albumin level, ALT level, and creatinine levels. However, none of those correlations was statistically significant as shown in Table 2.

For HCC patients, there was a positive correlation with age, bilirubin levels, ALT levels, AST levels, and AFP levels. There was a negative correlation between baseline VEGF levels and BMI of patients, Hb levels, platelets count, Alp levels, and creatinine levels. Only AST levels showed a significant correlation with baseline VEGF in HCC patients ($p < 0.001$) as shown in Table 2.

On follow-up of HCV patients, treatment with DAAs could significantly decrease VEGF values at the end of the treatment period, 1 month after treatment ($p < 0.001$), and even 3 months post-treatment (Table 3).

There was a positive correlation between VEGF values and age of patients, platelets count, bilirubin levels Alp levels, and PCR values. Age of patients and PCR values

Table 1 Comparison between the 2 groups regarding demographic and laboratory findings

	HCV group (n = 25)	HCC group (n = 25)	*P* value
Gender[#]			
Male	17 (50)	17 (50)	1.00
Female	8 (50)	8 (50)	
Age (years)	58.6 ± 4.4*	59 ± 4.2*	0.74
BMI	20 (19–22)**	24 (22–25)**	< 0.001
Hemoglobin (gm/dl)	13 (11.75–15)**	9.54 ± 1.33*	< 0.001
Platelets (10^3/Ul)	220 (153.5–240)**	89.8 ± 17.76*	< 0.001
Bilirubin (mg/dl)	0.8 (0.7–0.95)**	2.4 (1.9–3.9)**	< 0.001
Albumin (g/dl)	3.82 ± 0.34*	2.99 ± 0.45*	< 0.001
ALT (U/L)	46 (27.5–65) **	41.72 ± 9.66*	0.15
AST (U/L)	45.28 ± 22.4*	40.88 ± 12.09*	0.39
Creatinine (mg/dl)	1 (0.8–1.03) **	1.3 (1–1.75) **	0.001
AFP (ng/ml)	4.5 (3.2–6.65) **	311.4 ± 209.43*	< 0.001
VEGF (ng/ml)	209.5 ± 137.6*	488.01 ± 194.5*	< 0.001

*Data represented in terms of mean ± SD
**Data represented in terms of median (Q1–Q3)
[#]Data represented in terms of frequency (percentage), *n* (%)

Table 2 Correlation between baseline VEGF and laboratory findings in both groups

Variable	HCV group (*n* = 25)		HCC group (*n* = 25)	
	Correlation coefficient	*P* value	Correlation coefficient	*P* value
Age (years)	− 0.238[P]	0.251	0.281[P]	0.174
BMI	0.06[S]	0.77	− 0.142[P]	0.5
Hb (gm/dl)	− 0.12[S]	0.56	− 0.344[P]	0.09
Platelets (10^3/Ul)	− 0.14[S]	0.5	− 0.07[P]	0.72
Bilirubin (mg/dl)	0.05[S]	0.83	0.07[P]	0.74
Albumin (g/dl)	− 0.161[P]	0.441	− 0.37[P]	0.07
ALT (U/L)	− 0.02[S]	0.93	0.07[P]	0.713
AST (U/L)	0.086[P]	0.68	0.67[P]	< 0.001
Creatinine (mg/dl)	− 0.215[S]	0.3	− 0.03[P]	0.89
HCV-PCR	0.11[S]	0.6		
AFP (ng/ml)	0.325[S]	0.113	0.02[P]	0.93

[P]Pearson correlation
[S]Spearman correlation

were significant determinants of SVR VEGF values (p = 0.04, p = 0.03, respectively) as shown in Table 4.

After adjustment of the co-founding factors through linear regression analysis, we found that neither age of patients nor PCR values were significant predictors of the VEGF value 3 months post-treatment by DAAs (p = 0.064, p = 0.219, respectively) as shown in Table 5.

Discussion

The modern use of direct-acting antiviral drugs (DAAs) in the treatment of HCV has a major advantage in achieving more than 90% SVR despite the degree of liver cirrhosis. This allowed the treatment of many more patients, some of them with more advanced liver function impairment and more susceptibility for HCC [17]. However, the impact of DAA-based treatment on HCC occurrence in patients with cirrhosis is still controversial.

In this study, we found high statistically significant higher VEGF serum level in HCC patients than in HCV patients reflecting the pro-inflammatory and pro-angiogenic state that continued from benign to malignant liver disease and the impact of VEGF in addition to other angiogenic and growth factors on the growth, propagation, and spread of HCC as previously reported by Villani et al. [16], Debes et al. [18], and Faillaci et al. [19].

In spite of the great advancement in the HCV treatment after DAA introduction and achievement of more than 90% SVR in respective of fibrosis stage, which will improve the HCV natural history of infection, however, several recent reports have raised concerns about DAA treatment because of higher rates of HCC recurrence observed after DAA therapy [16, 20] and even early occurrence of HCC after treatment by DAAs [21].

We addressed in this study the possibility that serum VEGF after successful viral eradication by DAAs may be one of the molecular mechanisms responsible for early occurrence and recurrence of HCC as reported by Villani et al. [16]; however, we found that serum VEGF in our studied patients dropped after 1 month and 3 months after DAA treatment in controversy to the finding of Villani et al. who reported that although DAAs reduce the inflammation, they increase serum VEGF level and they considered this as a rationale for HCC occurrence risk during anti-HCV treatment; however, due to different finding in the present study in our patients, this reflects the different population number and characteristics

Table 3 VEGF through the study period

HCV group	VEGF1	VEGF2	VEGF3
Values (median (Q1–Q3))	173.4 (146.6–199.3)	42.2 (31.3–78.3)	44.1 (31.8–55.3)
P value	< 0.001		
Post hoc			
VEGF1–VEGF2	< 0.001		
VEGF1–VEGF3	< 0.001		
VEGF2–VEGF3	0.09		

VEGF1 measured at the end of treatment, VEGF2 measured one month after the end of treatment, and VEGF3 measured 3 months after the end of treatment

Table 4 Correlation between 3 months VEGF values and laboratory findings in HCV HCC-free patients

Variables	Correlation coefficient	*P* value
Age (years)	0.414^{P}	0.04*
BMI	-0.34^{S}	0.09
Hemoglobin (g/dl)	-0.16^{S}	0.44
Platelets(10^3/Ul)	0.11^{S}	0.59
Bilirubin (mg/dl)	0.003^{S}	0.99
Albumin (g/dl)	0.13^{P}	0.54
ALT (U/L)	-0.037^{S}	0.86
AST (U/L)	-0.025^{P}	0.9
Creatinine (mg/dl)	-0.067^{S}	0.75
HCV-PCR	0.44^{P}	0.03*

^{P}Pearson correlation
^{S}Spearman correlation
*Statistically significant

included in different studies and reflect the multi-factorial explanation for HCC occurrence after DAA therapy.

It is known that platelets can produce many growth factors for HCC including VEGF [22]. We found statistically significant thrombocytopenia ($p < 0.001$) in the HCC group in contrast to the HCV group; this comes in agreement with the study by Carr et al. who demonstrated that non-cirrhotic HCC patients have lower levels of thrombocytopenia than cirrhotic HCC patients specially in those patients who had larger tumors [23]. In the current study, there was statistically significant anemia ($p < 0.001$) in the HCC group, and this reflect the impact of developing HCC on the deterioration of liver function reserve and deterioration of portal hypertension with increased anemia whether related to malignancy or portal hypertension related to blood loss and reduced platelet count expected in cirrhotic patients with or without malignancy.

In this study, we found highly statistically significantly higher serum AFP in the HCC group in comparison with the HCV infection group; this comes in agreement with Zhang et al. who estimated the performance of AFP in diagnosing HCC and they found that AFP serum level is a good sensitive biomarker to diagnose HCC whether used alone or combined with ultrasound, they found that 400 ng/mL was better than 200 ng/mL as a cutoff value for diagnosis of HCC [24].

Table 5 Linear regression analysis to predict SVR VEGF values in HCV patients

Variables	*B*	*P* value	Confidence interval	
			Lower bound	Upper bound
Age	1.94	0.064	− 0.123	4.006
PCR	− 0.000017	0.219	− 0.000045	0.000011

Also, we found that BMI was significantly higher in HCC patients than in HCV group ($p < 0.001$); this comes in agreement with study by Divella et al. who explores the risk of obesity in the development of HCC whether due to the post-viral cirrhosis or in NAFLD [25].

As regards the serum creatinine level, it was significantly higher in the HCC group ($p < 0.001$). Shariff et al. suggested that this increase may be due to the increased metabolic activity that resulted in the increased rate of cellular turnover causing overproduction of carnitine to be sufficient for beta-oxidation and excessive needs of energy [26]. However, reduced serum creatinine in case of chronic liver disease can be due to a 50% decline in hepatic production of creatine; it can be also attributed not only to accumulation of extracellular fluid in the form of edema and ascites which increases the volume of distribution but also to malnutrition and decrease in muscular mass related to recurrent attacks of sepsis affecting satiety of patients [20].

Regarding serum albumin, it was significantly lower in the HCC group also ($p < 0.001$); this result agrees fully with Carr and Guerra who studied the association between serum albumin levels and HCC severity [27]. Albumin production is a marker for hepatocyte function differentiation; low serum albumin level may denote poorly differentiated and more aggressive HCC; on the other hand, normal serum albumin level can be a good indicator for well-differentiated, slowly growing HCCs [28]. However, low albumin level reflects also poor nutrition and could be an indicator of bad prognosis [29]

In this study, we found significantly higher bilirubin in HCC patients compared to the HCV patients' group, and this comes in contact with the study by Carr et al. who also stated that abnormal levels of bilirubin in HCC patients reflect a poor prognosis in contrast to those with normal levels [30].

In our Egyptian cohort of cirrhotic HCV-related and HCC patients, the number is relatively small and genotype 4 is different from other genotypes in other studies, and in addition, other molecular mechanisms may be more involved in our Egyptian patients as alteration of immune system function and inflammatory cytokines.

Conclusion

After successful viral eradication by DAAs, VEGF, the one responsible for both physiological and pathological angiogenesis in HCC, significantly decrease at end of treatment, after 1 month and 3 months of treatment. So, we can conclude that VEGF is not incriminated in the debate of increased incidence of HCC after treatment by DAAs.

Abbreviations

HCC: Hepatocellular carcinoma; VEGF: Vascular endothelial growth factor; DAAs: Direct-acting antivirals; HCV: Hepatitis C virus; SVR: Sustained virologic response; AFP: Alpha-fetoprotein; HIF-1α: Hypoxia-inducible factor 1 alpha; STAT3: Signal transducer and activator of transcription 3; HBV: Hepatitis B virus; CBC: Complete blood count; AST: Aspartate aminotransferase; ALT: Alanine aminotransferase; PCR: Polymerase chain reaction

Acknowledgements

Not applicable

Authors' contributions

MMS, AME, and ABS analyzed and interpreted the patient data. EMB, WAI, and MMS put the study design. NMT and AME were the major contributors in writing the manuscript. All authors read and approved the final manuscript.

Ethics approval and consent to participate

This study was approved according to the ethical standards of Ain Shams University Research Committee (committees reference number 387/2017) and the 1964 Helsinki declaration and its later amendments or comparable ethical standards.

A written informed consent was obtained from all patients in the study.

Competing interests

The authors declare that they have no competing interests.

Author details

[1]Division of Gastroenterology and Hepatology, Department of Internal Medicine, Faculty of Medicine, Ain Shams University, Cairo, Egypt. [2]Tanta University, Tanta, Egypt. [3]Division of Nephrology, Department of Internal Medicine, Faculty of Medicine, Ain Shams University, Ramsis Street 38, Abbasia, Cairo 11566, Egypt.

References

1. Yang JD, Hainaut P, Gores GJ, Amadou A, Plymoth A, Roberts LR (2019) A global view of hepatocellular carcinoma: trends, risk, prevention and management. Nat. Rev. Gastroenterol. Hepatol. 16:589–604
2. Bray F, Ferlay J, Soerjomataram I, Siegel RL, Torre LA, Jemal A (2018) Global cancer statistics 2018: GLOBOCAN estimates of incidence and mortality worldwide for 36 cancers in 185 countries. CA Cancer J. Clin. 68:394–424
3. Axley P, Ahmed Z, Ravi S, Singal AK (2018) Hepatitis C virus and hepatocellular carcinoma: a narrative review. J. Clin. Transl. Hepatol. 6:79–84
4. Hsu SJ, Yang SS, Kao JH (2020) Risk of hepatocellular carcinoma development after hepatitis C virus eradicated by direct-acting antivirals: fact or fiction? J. Formos. Med. Assoc 119(Pt 1):3–11.
5. Ioannou GN, Green PK, Beste LA, Mun EJ, Kerr KF, Berry K (2018) Development of models estimating the risk of hepatocellular carcinoma after antiviral treatment for hepatitis C. J. Hepatol. 69:1088–1098
6. Ioannou GN, Beste LA, Green PK, Singal AG, Tapper EB, Waljee AK et al (2019) Increased risk for hepatocellular carcinoma persists up to 10 years after HCV eradication in patients with baseline cirrhosis or high FIB-4 scores. Gastroenterology 157:1264–1278 e4
7. Carrat F, Fontaine H, Dorival C, Simony M, Diallo A, Hezode C et al (2019) Clinical outcomes in patients with chronic hepatitis C after direct-acting antiviral treatment: a prospective cohort study. Lancet 393:1453–1464
8. Baumert TF, Juhling F, Ono A, Hoshida Y (2017) Hepatitis C-related hepatocellular carcinoma in the era of new generation antivirals. BMC Med. 15:52
9. Waziry R, Hajarizadeh B, Grebely J, Amin J, Law M, Danta M et al (2017) Hepatocellularcarcinoma risk following direct-acting antiviral HCV therapy: a systematic review, meta-analyses, andmeta-regression. J. Hepatol. 67:1204–1212
10. Capurro M, Filmus J (2005) Glypican-3 as a serum marker for hepatocellular carcinoma. Cancer Res 65(1):372–373
11. Hamdy MN, Shaheen KY, Awad MA, Barakat EMF, Shalaby SI, Gupta N et al (2020) Vascular endothelial growth factor (VEGF) as a biochemical marker for the diagnosis of hepatocellular carcinoma (HCC). Clinical Practice. 17(1): 1441–1453
12. Zhu AX, Duda DG, Sahani DV, Jain RK (2011) HCC and angiogenesis: possible targets and future directions. Nat. Rev. Clin. Oncol. 8:292–301
13. Hassan M, Selimovic D, Ghozlan H, Abdel-kader O (2009) Hepatitis C virus core protein triggers hepatic angiogenesis by a mechanism including multiple pathways. Hepatology 49:1469–1482
14. Kanda T, Steele R, Ray R, Ray RB (2008) Hepatitis C virus core protein augments androgen receptor-mediated signaling. J. Virol. 82:11066–11072
15. Mukozu T, Nagal H, Matsui D, Kanekawa T, Sumino Y (2013) Serum VEGF as a tumor marker in patients with HCV-related liver cirrhosis and hepatocellular carcinoma. ANTICANCER RESEARCH. 33:1013–1022
16. Villani R, Facciorusso A, Bellanti F, Tamborra R, Piscazzi A, Landriscina M et al (2016) DAAs rapidly reduce inflammation but increase serum VEGF level: a rationale for tumor risk during anti-HCV treatment. PLoS ONE. 11(12): e0167934
17. Roche B, Coilly A, Duclos-Vallee JC, Samuel D (2018) The impact of treatment of hepatitis C with DAAs on the occurrence of HCC. Liver Int. 38(1):130–145
18. Debes JD, Tilborg MV, Groothuismink ZMA, Hansen BE, Wiesch JSZ, Felden JV et al (2018) Levels of cytokines in serum associate with development of hepatocellular carcinoma in patients with HCV infection treated with direct-acting antivirals. Gastroenterology. 154(3):515–517
19. Faillaci F, Marzi L, Critelli R, Milosa F, Schepis F, Turola E et al (**2018**) Liver angiopoietin-2 is a key predictor of *de novo* or recurrent hepatocellular cancer after hepatitis C virus direct-acting antivirals. Hepatology. 68(3):1010–1024
20. Takabatake T, Ohta H, Ishida Y, Hara H, Ushiogi Y, Hattori N (1988) Low serum creatinine levels in severe hepatic disease. Arch Intern Med. 148: 1313–1315
21. Cheung MCM, Walker AJ, Hudson BE, Verma S, McLauchlan J, David J, Mutimer DJ et al (2016) Outcomes after successful direct-acting antiviral therapy for patients with chronic hepatitis C and decompensated cirrhosis. J Hepatol. 65(4):741–747
22. Nalesnik MA, Michalopoulos GK (2012) Growth factor pathways in development and progression of hepatocellular carcinoma. Front Biosci (School Educ) 4:1487–1515
23. Carr BI, Guerra V (2013) Thrombocytosis and hepatocellular carcinoma. Dig Dis Sci. 58(6):1790–1796
24. Zhang J, Chen G, Zhang P, Zhang J, Li X, Gan D et al (2020) The threshold of alphafetoprotein (AFP) for the diagnosis of hepatocellular carcinoma: a systematic review and meta-analysis. PLoS ONE 15(2):e0228857
25. Divella R, Mazzocca A, Daniele A, Sabbà C, Paradiso A (2019) Obesity, non-alcoholic fatty liver disease and adipocytokines network in promotion of cancer. Int J Biol Sci. 15(3):610–616
26. Shariff MI, Gomaa AI, Cox IJ, Patel M, Williams HR, Crossey MM et al (2011) Urinary metabolic biomarkers of hepatocellular carcinoma in an Egyptian population: a validation study. J Proteome Res. 10:1828–1836
27. Carr BI, Guerra V (2017) Serum albumin levels in relation to tumor parameters in hepatocellular carcinoma patients. Int J Biol Markers 32(4):e391–e396
28. Hernandez-Gea V, Toffanin S, Friedman SL, Llovet JM (2013) Role of the microenvironment in the pathogenesis and treatment of hepatocellular carcinoma. Gastroenterology. 144(3):512–527
29. Schütte K, Tippelt B, Schulz C (2015) Malnutrition is a prognostic factor in patients with hepatocellular carcinoma (HCC). Clin Nutr. 34:1122–1127
30. Carr BI, Guerra V, Giannini EG, Farinati F, Ciccarese F, Rapaccini GL et al (2014) Association of abnormal plasma bilirubin with aggressive HCC phenotype. Semin Oncol. 41(2):252–258

27

Serum level of cytokeratin 19 as a diagnostic and prognostic marker in patients with HCV-related hepatocellular carcinoma

Maissa El Raziky[1*], Hanan Abdel Hafez[1], Aisha Elsharkawy[1], Tarek Ahmed Moneer[2], Suzan M. EL-Sheikh[3], Rabab M. Maher[4] and Sahar A. Sharaf[3]

Abstract

Background: The heterogeneous nature of human hepatocellular carcinoma (HCC) impedes both treatment strategies and prognostic predictions. Several markers have been proposed for the diagnosis of HCC. Cytoskeleton-associated proteins have been known as cellular integrators in neoplasm formation. Hepatic progenitor cells are thought to express alpha-fetoprotein (AFP) and hematopoietic as well as biliary markers such as cytokeratin 19 (CK 19) and cytokeratin 7. The aim of this study was to verify the role of serum CK 19 alone or in combination with AFP as a diagnostic marker of HCC and to assess the changes in its levels after ablation of HCV-related HCC to evaluate its role as a predictor marker for recurrence of HCC after ablation. The study was conducted on 102 HCV-related cirrhotic patients categorized into three different groups according to the clinical, laboratory, and radiological evaluation: group I—62 patients with early or intermediate HCC who underwent locoregional intervention, group II—20 patients with advanced HCC not fit for any intervention apart from best supportive treatment, and group III—20 cirrhotic patients with no evidence of HCC as proved by two imaging techniques.

Results: The mean serum levels of CK 19 were 6.5 ± 5.7, 10.5 ± 12.5, and 6.8 ± 2.8 ng/ml in groups I, II, and III, respectively, with no significant difference between groups. Sensitivity, specificity, positive, and negative predictive values of combined AFP and human CK 19 at cutoff levels of 25.5 ng/ml and 6.25 ng/ml were 93.9%, 45%, 87.5%, and 64.3%, respectively. In group I patients, CK 19 levels were comparable in patients with ablated focal lesion and those who did not at baseline; then, it was significantly higher in ablated patients than in patients with residual tumor 1 and 6 months after the intervention.

Conclusions: Combination of both AFP and CK 19 levels could increase the diagnostic accuracy of suspected HCCs. CK 19 levels are good predictors of ablation/recurrence in patients who underwent interventional procedures minimizing the need for follow-up imaging modalities.

Keywords: Cytokeratin 19, Hepatocellular carcinoma, Ablation, Prognostic

* Correspondence: maelraziky@yahoo.com
[1]Department of Endemic Medicine, Faculty of Medicine, Cairo University, Cairo 11562, Egypt
Full list of author information is available at the end of the article

Background

The heterogeneous nature of human hepatocellular carcinoma (HCC), which represents a serious health problem being the fifth most common malignancy worldwide, and a common cause of death in patients with chronic liver disease [1], impedes both treatment strategies and prognostic predictions [2].

HCC emerges through a process of multistep carcinogenesis [3], and its formation is a subject of discussion and controversy. In fact, other than the different etiological factors, an important cause of its heterogeneity may be the cell type of origin. Formerly, it was suggested that preneoplastic lesions arise from mature hepatocytes subjected to neoplastic transformation [4]. Lately, it has also been proposed that a subset of HCC originates from hepatic progenitor cells (HPCs) [5]. This subset of HCC results enriched for genes expressed earlier in fetal hepatoblasts, including some progenitor cell markers. A continuous upregulation of HPCs was also shown in hepatocellular adenoma [6] and dysplastic nodules [7]. HPC activation was demonstrated to be the most relevant liver carcinogenic condition in chronic viral hepatitis, alcoholic, and non-alcoholic fatty liver disease [8].

Several biliary markers have been proposed for HPCs in HCC including cytokeratin 19 (CK 19) and cytokeratin 7 (CK 7). These cells also express alpha-fetoprotein (AFP) and hematopoietic markers (c-kit, CD34) [9–11].

Cytokeratins are the major filament proteins in the liver where any hepatocyte membrane integrity damage causes their release into the circulation [12]. Moreover, CKs have been known as cellular integrators in several neoplastic changes. Characteristic combinations of CKs are expressed by different epithelia according to the organ of origin and differentiation [13]. An experimental model showed that in vitro primary human CK19-positive tumor cells showed increased invasiveness and that CK-19 knockdown significantly reduced HCC invasive ability [14].

The aim of this study was to verify the role of serum CK 19 alone or in combination with AFP as a diagnostic marker of HCC, to assess the changes in its levels after ablation of HCV-related HCC, and to evaluate the role of CK 19 as a predictor marker for recurrence of HCC after ablation.

Methods

This prospective study was conducted on HCV-induced liver cirrhosis patients with and without HCC according to their clinical, laboratory, and radiological evaluation. They were recruited from the HCC unit at National Hepatology and Tropical Medicine Research Institute (NHTMRI) and the Endemic Medicine Department, Faculty of Medicine, Cairo University.

Study participants

The included groups were as follows: *group I*: 62 cirrhotic patients, 41 males and 21 females, with a mean age (±SD) of 56.6 (±5.6) years with early HCC defined as single or three nodules each less than 3-cm diameter with Child-Pugh score A or B. These patients underwent one of the locoregional interventions. *Group II*: 20 cirrhotic patients, 17 males and 3 females, with a mean age (±SD) of 55.9 (±5.9) years, with advanced HCC more than 5 cm, they were not fit for any intervention apart from best supportive treatment according to BCLC classification. *Group III*: 20 cirrhotic patients, 9 males and 11 females, with a mean age (±SD) of 48.1 (±4.2) years with no evidence of HCC as proved by two imaging techniques (abdominal ultrasound and triphasic CT with contrast) serving as a control group.

Inclusion criteria were (1) males and females above the age of 18 years; (2) post-HCV chronic liver disease, with positive anti-HCV by third-generation enzyme-linked immunosorbent assay (ELISA), detectable serum HCV-RNA by RT PCR and abdominal ultrasonography; and (3) patients in groups I and II with HCC as proved by triphasic CT ± AFP. Patients with focal lesions other than HCC, history, or evidence of other malignancies; those suffering from any organ failure other than the liver, spontaneous bacterial peritonitis, and hepato-renal syndrome; and previously treated HCC patients were excluded from the study. The protocol was approved by the ethical committee of NHTMRI. After giving an informed consent, the selected patients were subjected to clinical biochemical and imaging assessments; AFP levels were tested by ELISA.

Interventions for patients in group I

Interventional procedure aiming for HCC cure based on BCLC staging system and treatment strategy was performed, for patients with stage A HCC: 45 patients underwent radiofrequency ablation (RFA), and 17 patients underwent microwave ablation (MWA) as the tumor had a close relation to a vessel. Follow-up for tumor recurrence and levels of AFP and CK 19 was carried 1 and 6 months after interventions.

Clinical chemistry analysis

Blood samples were collected and investigated for serum total and direct bilirubin, alanine transaminase (ALT), aspartate transaminase (AST), and albumin on the automated BECKMAN COULTER AU680 autoanalyzer (Beckman Coulter, Inc., 250 S. Kraemer Blvd., Brea, CA 92821, USA).

Quantitative detection of CK 19

Serum CK 19 levels were assayed in all patients using the double antibody sandwich ELISA technique supplied by Sun Red Biotechnology (Shanghai, China). Patients who did not undergo any therapeutic modality were tested only one time at the beginning of this study. Patients who underwent therapeutic interventions were tested for CK 19 at baseline, after 1 month, and 6 months in the follow-up.

Statistical analysis

Data was analyzed using IBM SPSS advanced statistics version 25 (SPSS Inc., Chicago, IL). Numerical data were expressed as mean and standard deviation or median and range as appropriate. Qualitative data were expressed as frequency and percentage. The chi-square test or Fisher's exact test was used to examine the relation between qualitative variables. For not normally distributed quantitative data, comparison between two groups was done using the Mann-Whitney test. Comparison between 3 groups was done using the Kruskal-Wallis test; then, post hoc "Schefe test" was used for pair-wise comparison based on Kruskal-Wallis distribution. Freidman's test was used to compare 3 consecutive measures of numeric variables followed by the Wilcoxon-signed ranks test used to compare two consecutive measures of numerical variables. The receiver operating characteristic (ROC) curve was used for the prediction of cutoff values of markers. All tests were two-tailed. A p value < 0.05 was considered significant.

Results

The comparison of demographic data showed that there was a statistically significant difference between HCC groups and control group in regard to age; the control group was significantly younger than the other 2 HCC groups (p-value < 0.001). Also, the percent of male in group II was significantly higher than controls (p-value 0.024).

Clinical and abdominal ultrasonography data showed that jaundice, pallor, ascites, and lower limb edema were present in 25%, 30%, 50%, and 30%, respectively, of the HCC group not fit for intervention but not present in other groups.

The liver biochemical profile of the studied groups showed that there was a significant difference between group II and the other two groups regarding the mean value of albumin and total bilirubin. Albumin in this group was significantly lower than the other two groups (p < 0.001) while total bilirubin was significantly higher. On the other hand, there was no significant difference between all groups regarding the mean value of ALT, AST, and platelet count.

Mean AFP levels were 190.6 ± 852, 951.9 ± 2323.9, and 29.3 ± 44.3 ng/ml in groups I, II, and III, respectively, with a significant difference between groups (p value < 0.001). Regarding the CK 19 levels, there was no significant difference between all groups before any intervention (Table 1).

Using the receiver operating characteristic (ROC) curve, to determine the specificity and sensitivity of human CK 19/AFP alone or combined, the cutoff value of 6.25 ng/ml and 25.5 ng/ml, respectively, were found to be the most suitable (best cutoff) (Table 2).

Studying the characteristics of the focal lesions (FLs), group I showed solitary FL in 90.3% of patients, and size was less than 5 cm in 100% of this group and mainly seated in the right lobe in 82.3%. On the other hand, the FLs were mainly multiple in 70% of group II, and the size of lesions in this group was less than 5 cm in 70% and bi-lobar in 70% of cases.

To assess the prognostic value of CK 19 in HCC patients, the outcome of interventions in group I is displayed in Fig. 1 and the relation of these outcomes to changes in CK 19 levels is shown in Table 3. The CK 19 level was comparable in ablated and residual FL patients at baseline and then was significantly higher in ablated patients than in residual tumor 1 and 6 months after the intervention. Follow-up at 1 month of the intervention, CK 19 median level was 2.9 ng/ml in patients who had no ablation for their FLs compared to it was 15 ng/ml in patients who had ablation. In the follow-up after 6 months, the CK 19 median level was 5.5 ng/ml in patients who had recurrence compared to 17 ng/ml in patients who showed ablation for their focal lesions (p value < 0.001).

Discussion

Early diagnosis of HCC heavily affects the clinical outcome of patients. The widely accepted serological marker for HCC diagnosis is AFP. However, its diagnostic accuracy is controversial and unsatisfactory because of its low sensitivity. Therefore, there is an increasing demand for the discovery of new HCC-specific biomarkers [15]. Moreover, HCCs expressing the biliary/HPC marker CK 19 have been linked with a poor prognosis. Therefore, in this study, we addressed the question of the possibility of using CK 19 as a diagnostic and prognostic marker in HCC [16].

It is established that the incidence of HCC increases progressively with advancing age and it is more

Table 1 Levels of CK 19 in the studied patients

CK 19 levels (ng/ml)	Group I N = 62	Group II N = 20	Group III N = 20	P value
Mean ± SD	6.5 ± 5.7	10.5 ± 12.5	6.8 ± 2.8	0.054
Median	3.2	5.4	7.2	
Minimum	1.6	2	3	
Maximum	20	45	11.4	

CK 19 cytokeratin 19

Table 2 Sensitivity, specificity, positive, and negative predictive values of AFP and CK 19 in studied patients

	Best cutoff	SN	SP	PPV	NPV
AFP	25.5 ng/ml	80.5%	75%	93%	48.4%
CK 19	6.25 ng/ml	63.4%	55%	85.2%	26.8%
Combined AFP and CK 19	25.5 ng/ml and 6.25 ng/ml	93.9%	45%	87.5%	64.3%

AFP alpha-fetoprotein, *CK 19* cytokeratin 19, *SN* sensitivity, *SP* specificity, *PPV* positive predictive value, *NPV* negative predictive value

predominant in males [17]. This comes in agreement with the demographic data of the studied patients. In this study, we found a statistically significant difference between the HCC group not fit for intervention (group II) and the other two groups regarding the mean value of albumin and total bilirubin, this could be explained by the fact that lower albumin and higher bilirubin levels are indicators of a higher Child-Pugh score hindering the possibility of interventional therapy.

In the current study, the AFP levels were significantly elevated in the HCC groups compared to the cirrhosis group. This is in agreement with several previous studies [18, 19]. However, this was not universally agreed [20]. The cutoff value for diagnosis, sensitivity, and specificity showed wide variability among different studies. Our results showed the sensitivity and specificity of serum AFP were 80.5% and 75%, respectively, with a cutoff value of 25.5 ng/ml for HCC diagnosis. A study demonstrated that the sensitivity and specificity of AFP at a cutoff value of 10.86 ng/ml were 75% and 92%, respectively [21]. Spangenberg et al. reported that at a cutoff value of 20 ng/ml, serum AFP showed 60–80% sensitivity, although this sensitivity decreases to about 40% for the detection of small tumors [22]. The use of a higher cutoff value such as 200 ng/ml drops the sensitivity to 22% while increases the specificity [23]. Therefore, the use of AFP in clinical practice is limited by the low sensitivity at cutoff values maintaining sufficiently high specificity. These discrepant results warranted exploring the usage of additional biomarkers to improve the diagnostic accuracy.

CK 19 is an HCC-cancer stem cell marker that plays an integral role in carcinogenesis, metastases, and recurrence [24]. In our study, although there was no significant difference in baseline serum CK 19 levels among the three groups, its combination with AFP improved their sensitivity to 93.9%.

To verify the prognostic role of CK 19, we demonstrated that baseline CK 19 levels in group I were significantly lower than 1- and 6-month levels post-intervention in those who showed ablation of FLs.

A large meta-analysis was done by *Da-wei Sun and his colleagues in 2015* to investigate the association between CK 19 expression in tissue and the prognosis of HCC patients. It included 17 studies with a total of 2943 patients. The results showed that tissue CK 19

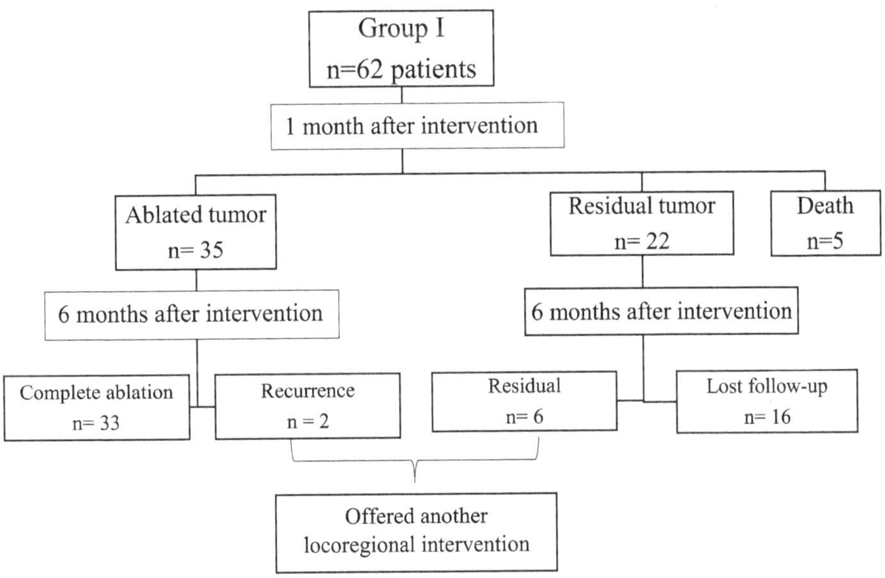

Fig. 1 Flowchart of the outcome of patients 1 and 6 months after intervention in group I

Table 3 Relationship between CK 19 levels and the status of the focal lesions according to the final outcome after 6 months

	Focal lesions by CT						
	Residual tumor (*n* = 8)			**Ablated (*n* = 33)**			
	Median	**Minimum**	**Maximum**	**Median**	**Minimum**	**Maximum**	***p* value**
CK 19 before intervention	3.4	1.6	16.0	3.0	1.7	20.0	0.706
CK 19 1 month after intervention	2.9	2.0	10.0	15.0	7.8	46.0	< 0.001*
CK 19 6 months after intervention	5.5	3.0	9.0	17.0	4.0	40.0	< 0.001*
p value	0.223			< 0.001*			

*p value is significant. *CK 19* cytokeratin 19

overexpression was significantly associated with poor overall survival rate and early tumor recurrence rate in HCC patients [25].

This difference in results may be attributed to many factors: one of them is the number of candidates that was smaller in our study, and another factor is the method of detection of CK 19 which was by measuring its serum level by ELISA in our study but in other studies was immunohistochemistry of surgically excised tumors or using microarrays. Another factor is a longer period of follow-up in other studies, and this may reveal cases of recurrence or new lesions on long follow-up period.

In our study, we found elevation of serum level of CK 19 after ablation of tumor by single or combined locoregional intervention modalities. These interventions led to damage of tumor cells by necrosis and apoptosis which in turn may have led to the release of CK 19 in serum and this may explain partially our results especially that patients with residual tumors did not show a significant increase of CK 19 levels. This explanation is supported by a study performed by *Vanagas* and his colleagues who detected apoptosis in the transition zone at a distance of 9–10 mm from the rim of the necrotic zone 1 h after local ablation procedure [26]. Another theory for the increased levels of CK 19 as a stemness marker is the occurrence of hypoxia post-intervention [27]. However, more studies are needed to see the effect of liver resection on the level of CK 19 before and after resection.

Limitations of this study include the short duration of and loss of some patients during the follow-up period. The strength of this study is the use of serum CK 19 levels measured by simple ELISA technique instead of the repeatedly reported tissue expression method.

Conclusions

Measurement of both CK 19 and AFP combined could be a simple, noninvasive way to increase the diagnostic accuracy of suspected HCCs and evaluate treatment response and prognosis in patients with HCC amenable for intervention. Post-ablation elevation of serum CK 19 levels can predict complete HCC ablation before doing imaging modalities.

Abbreviations

AFP: Alpha-fetoprotein; CK 19: Cytokeratin 19; FL: Focal lesion; HCC: Hepatocellular carcinoma; HPC: Hepatic progenitor cell; MWA: Microwave ablation; RFA: Radiofrequency ablation; ROC: Receiver operating characteristic

Acknowledgements

Not applicable.

Authors' contributions

MER, HA, and AE were responsible for the concept, plan of the work, interpretation of results, and final revision. TAM was responsible for patients' inclusion, intervention performance, and follow-up. RMM was responsible for writing the manuscript. SME and SAS were responsible for laboratory work. All authors have read and approved the final manuscript.

Declarations

Ethics approval and consent to participate

This study was conducted after approval of the ethical committee of the National Hepatology and Tropical Medicine Research Institute. No available reference number. All procedures followed were in accordance with the ethical standards of the responsible committee on human experimentation (institutional and national) and with the Helsinki Declaration of 1975, as revised in 2008. Written informed consent was obtained from all participants included in the study.

Competing interests

The authors declare that they have no competing interests.

Author details

[1]Department of Endemic Medicine, Faculty of Medicine, Cairo University, Cairo 11562, Egypt. [2]National Tropical Medicine & Hepatology Institute, Cairo, Egypt. [3]Department of Clinical and Chemical Pathology, Faculty of Medicine, Cairo University, Cairo, Egypt. [4]Fellow of Tropical Medicine, Cairo University Student Hospital, Cairo, Egypt.

References

1. Forner A, Reig M, Bruix J (2018) Hepatocellular carcinoma. Lancet 391(10127):1301–1314. https://doi.org/10.1016/S0140-6736(18)30010-2
2. Thorgeirsson SS, Grisham JW (2002) Molecular pathogenesis of human hepatocellular carcinoma. Nat Genet 31(4):339–346. https://doi.org/10.1038/ng0802-339
3. Ho DWH, Lo RCL, Chan LK, Ng IOL (2016) Molecular pathogenesis of hepatocellular carcinoma. Liver Cancer 5(4):290–302. https://doi.org/10.1159/000449340

4. Bralet MP, Pichard V, Ferry N (2002) Demonstration of direct lineage between hepatocytes and hepatocellular carcinoma in diethylnitrosamine-treated rats. Hepatology 36(3):623–630. https://doi.org/10.1053/jhep.2002.35540
5. Tummala KS, Brandt M, Teijeiro A, Graña O, Schwabe RF, Perna C, Djouder N (2017) Hepatocellular carcinomas originate predominantly from hepatocytes and benign lesions from hepatic progenitor cells. Cell Rep 19(3):584–600. https://doi.org/10.1016/j.celrep.2017.03.059
6. Williams MJ, Clouston AD, Forbes SJ (2014) Links between hepatic fibrosis, ductular reaction, and progenitor cell expansion. Gastroenterology 146(2): 349–356. https://doi.org/10.1053/j.gastro.2013.11.034
7. Libbrecht L, Desmet V, Van Damme B, Roskams T (2000) The immunohistochemical phenotype of dysplastic foci in human liver: correlation with putative progenitor cells. J Hepatol 33(1):76–84. https://doi.org/10.1016/S0168-8278(00)80162-2
8. Rogler CE, Bebawee R, Matarlo J, Locker J, Pattamanuch N, Gupta S, Rogler LE (2017) Triple staining including FOXA2 identifies stem cell lineages undergoing hepatic and biliary differentiation in cirrhotic human liver. J Histochem Cytochem 65(1):33–46. https://doi.org/10.1369/0022155416675153
9. Lee JS, Heo J, Libbrecht L, Chu IS, Kaposi-Novak P, Calvisi DF, Mikaelyan A, Roberts LR, Demetris AJ, Sun Z, Nevens F, Roskams T, Thorgeirsson SS (2006) A novel prognostic subtype of human hepatocellular carcinoma derived from hepatic progenitor cells. Nat Med 12(4):410–416. https://doi.org/10.1038/nm1377
10. Rhee H, Kim H, Park YN (2020) Clinico-radio-pathological and molecular features of hepatocellular carcinomas with keratin 19 expression. Liver Cancer 9(6):663–681. https://doi.org/10.1159/000510522
11. Roskams T (2003) Progenitor cell involvement in cirrhotic human liver diseases: from controversy to consensus. J Hepatol 39(3):431–434. https://doi.org/10.1016/S0168-8278(03)00333-7
12. Bateman AC, Hübscher SG (2010) Cytokeratin expression as an aid to diagnosis in medical liver biopsies. Histopathology 56(4):415–425. https://doi.org/10.1111/j.1365-2559.2009.03391.x
13. Turley EA, Veiseh M, Radisky DC, Bissell MJ (2008) Mechanisms of disease: epithelial-mesenchymal transition - does cellular plasticity fuel neoplastic progression? Nat Clin Pract Oncol 5(5):280–290. https://doi.org/10.1038/ncponc1089
14. Govaere O, Komuta M, Berkers J, Spee B, Janssen C, De Luca F, Katoonizadeh A, Wouters J, Van Kempen LC, Durnez A, Verslype C, De Kock J, Rogiers V, Van Grunsven LA, Topal B, Pirenne J, Vankelecom H, Nevens F, Van Den Oord J, Pinzani M, Roskams T (2014) Keratin 19: a key role player in the invasion of human hepatocellular carcinomas. Gut 63(4):674–685. https://doi.org/10.1136/gutjnl-2012-304351
15. Stefaniuk P, Cianciara J, Wiercinska-Drapalo A (2010) Present and future possibilities for early diagnosis of hepatocellular carcinoma. World J Gastroenterol 16(4):418–424. https://doi.org/10.3748/wjg.v16.i4.418
16. Govaere O, Petz M, Wouters J, Vandewynckel YP, Scott EJ, Topal B, Nevens F, Verslype C, Anstee QM, Van Vlierberghe H, Mikulits W, Roskams T (2017) The PDGFRα-laminin B1-keratin 19 cascade drives tumor progression at the invasive front of human hepatocellular carcinoma. Oncogene 36(47):6605–6616. https://doi.org/10.1038/onc.2017.260
17. Kew M (2014) Hepatocellular carcinoma: epidemiology and risk factors. J Hepatocell Carcinoma 1:115
18. Worland T, Harrison B, Delmenico L, Dowling D (2018) Hepatocellular carcinoma screening utilising serum alpha-fetoprotein measurement and abdominal ultrasound is more effective than ultrasound alone in patients with non-viral cirrhosis. J Gastrointest Cancer 49(4):476–480. https://doi.org/10.1007/s12029-017-0006-y
19. Lersritwimanmaen P, Nimanong S (2018) Hepatocellular carcinoma surveillance: benefit of serum alfa-fetoprotein in real-world practice. Euroasian J Hepato-Gastroenterology 8(1):83–87. https://doi.org/10.5005/jp-journals-10018-1268
20. Han LL, Lv Y, Guo H, Ruan ZP, Nan KJ (2014) Implications of biomarkers in human hepatocellular carcinoma pathogenesis and therapy. World J Gastroenterol 20(30):10249–10261. https://doi.org/10.3748/wjg.v20.i30.10249
21. Zhang SY, Lin BD, Li BR (2015) Evaluation of the diagnostic value of alpha-l-fucosidase, alpha-fetoprotein and thymidine kinase 1 with ROC and logistic regression for hepatocellular carcinoma. FEBS Open Bio 5(1):240–244. https://doi.org/10.1016/j.fob.2015.03.010
22. Spangenberg HC, Thimme R, Blum HE (2006) Serum markers of hepatocellular carcinoma. Semin Liver Dis 26(4):385–390. https://doi.org/10.1055/s-2006-951606
23. Schütte K, Schulz C, Link A, Malfertheiner P (2015) Current biomarkers for hepatocellular carcinoma: surveillance, diagnosis and prediction of prognosis. World J Hepatol 7(2):139–149. https://doi.org/10.4254/wjh.v7.i2.139
24. Kawai T, Yasuchika K, Ishii T, Katayama H, Yoshitoshi EY, Ogiso S, Kita S, Yasuda K, Fukumitsu K, Mizumoto M, Hatano E, Uemoto S (2015) Keratin 19, a cancer stem cell marker in human hepatocellular carcinoma. Clin Cancer Res 21(13):3081–3091. https://doi.org/10.1158/1078-0432.CCR-14-1936
25. Wei SD, Yi ZY, Dong SX, Guo CY, Qiu W, Ji M, Yue LG (2015) Prognostic value of cytokeratin 19 in hepatocellular carcinoma: a meta-analysis. Clin Chim Acta 448:161–169. https://doi.org/10.1016/j.cca.2015.06.027
26. Vanagas T, Gulbinas A, Sadauskiene I, Dambrauskas Z, Pundzius J, Barauskas G (2009) Apoptosis is activated in an early period after radiofrequency ablation of liver tissue. Hepatogastroenterology 56(93):1095–1099
27. Nahm JH, Rhee H, Kim H, Yoo JE, Lee JS, Jeon Y, Choi GH, Park YN (2017) Increased expression of stemness markers and altered tumor stroma in hepatocellular carcinoma under TACE-induced hypoxia: a biopsy and resection matched study. Oncotarget 8(59):99359–99371. https://doi.org/10.18632/oncotarget.22078

28

Gut microbiome in cirrhotic hepatitis C virus patients with and without hepatocellular carcinoma

Khaled Mohieldeen[1], Soraya Abdel Fatah Hamoda[1], Shwikar Mahmoud Ahmed[2], Abdurrahman Najeeb[1*] and Walid Ismail Ellakany[1]

Abstract

Background: Chronic hepatitis C is the most common cause of chronic liver disease and hepatocellular carcinoma in Egypt. A pathogenic link with gut microbial dysbiosis has been described in different diseases. The aim of the study is to elucidate changes in gut microbiome in cirrhotic HCV Egyptian patients with and without HCC.

Results: The study included 50 cirrhotic HCV patients; 25 with and 25 without HCC and 25 healthy controls with matched age and sex. Stool specimens were taken from all participants. Quantitative SYBR Green real-time PCR technique targeting 16S rRNA was done for the identification and quantitation of selected bacterial phylum, genera, and/or species. Both HCC and cirrhosis groups showed decrease in *Firmicutes*, F/B ratio, *A. mucinophilia*, and *F. prausnitzii* compared to the control group. However, the HCC group only showed statistically significant increase in *Bacteroides* and *Lactobacilli*, and decrease of *Prevotella* relative abundance and P/B ratio compared to both cirrhosis and control groups. As regard the relation between the gut microbiome and stages of HCC, BCLC stage D showed significantly the lowest relative abundance of *Ruminococcus*.

Conclusion: Patients with HCV-related cirrhosis and HCC exhibit microbial dysbiosis; altered microbial relative abundance and diversity with HCC patients showing higher proinflammatory bacteria compared to cirrhotics.

Keywords: Cirrhosis, Hepatitis C virus, Hepatocellular carcinoma, Gut dysbiosis

Background

Hepatitis C virus (HCV) prevalence is estimated to be 71 million cases globally [1]. Infection is often asymptomatic, but chronic infection can lead to cirrhosis, liver failure, and hepatocellular carcinoma (HCC) and the need for liver transplantation.

Egypt has high prevalence of HCV genotype 4 [2]. However, after the state-wide test-and-treat program, the prevalence was found to be lower than previously thought [3]. HCV treatment with the new direct-acting antivirals (DAAs) offered high SVR rates (> 95%) and short treatment course with minimal side effects.

The past few years witnessed an increased interest in the gut microbiota, its composition and its role in health and diseases [4]. Gut dysbiosis was associated with local and distal carcinogenesis either directly or indirectly [5–8]. Microbiota carcinogenic and toxic metabolites potentiate inflammation or immunosuppression [9, 10]. They also enhance our anti-tumor immunity against various cancers [11–13].

The gut microbiota comprises mainly the phylotypes, *Bacteroidetes*, and *Firmicutes*. *Actinobacteria* (like *Bifidobacterium* spp.), *Proteobacteria* (like *Escherichia coli*), and *Verrucomicrobia* (like *Akkermansia muciniphila*) are less abundant but are associated with some diseases. The microbiota synthesize vitamins, help digestion, and

* Correspondence: a_najeeb13@alexmed.edu.eg
[1]Tropical Medicine Department, Faculty of Medicine, Alexandria University, Alexandria, Egypt
Full list of author information is available at the end of the article

boost immunity [14, 15]. They strengthen gut barrier epithelial integrity [16], harvest energy [17], and protect against external pathogens [18].

Association of the gut microbiota with development of hepatic diseases has drawn interest [19]. Most gastrointestinal tract drains into portal vein that enters the liver carrying about two thirds of its blood supply. Besides absorbed nutrients, it can contain gut microbial metabolites, lipopolysaccharides, bacterial endotoxins, or other substances, especially when the intestinal barrier is deranged by dysbiosis. Translocation of products can lead to hepatic inflammation, with release of key inflammatory mediators such as NF-kB and TLR4. This chronic inflammation can foster the initiation and progression of malignancies [20–23].

Aim of the work

The aim of this study was to elucidate changes in gut microbiome in cirrhotic HCV Egyptian patients. This may help in the development of new approaches for treatment and prevention of HCC by modulating the gut microbiome.

Subjects

The study was carried out in Alexandria Main University Hospital. The study included 50 cirrhotic HCV Egyptian patients; 25 with and 25 without HCC who were recruited from the Tropical Medicine Department at Alexandria Main University Hospital and 25 Egyptian healthy subjects with matched age and sex as control group.

Exclusion criteria

Malignancy other than HCC, HBV, and other hepatic diseases; recent surgical intervention of the intestines either small or large within the last 6 months; infectious diarrhea including bacterial, viral, and parasitic diarrhea; history of prolonged use of antibiotics, rifaximin, nonsteroidal anti-inflammatory drugs abuse, corticosteroids for the last 3 months; other autoimmune diseases, pregnancy, chronic renal diseases, diabetes mellitus, alcohol or substance addiction; patients unable to give consent as mentally challenged.

Methods

Clinical data and investigations

Detailed history was taken from patients and controls with special emphasis on dietary and drug history. All patients and controls were subjected to full clinical examination. Body weight and height were measured, and body mass index was calculated. Cirrhotics were classified by Child-Pugh class (CPC) [24] into class A, B, and C and the updated Barcelona Clinic Liver Cancer (BCLC) classification [25] was used to stratify HCC patients (Table 1). Laboratory investigations including serum Albumin, ALT, AST, bilirubin, AFP, INR, and CBC was obtained. Ultrasound was done for all patients. HCC cases were defined by AFP and triphasic CT.

Table 1 Demographic, clinical, and laboratory characteristics of participants

	HCC (n = 25)	Cirrhosis (n = 25)	Controls (n = 25)
Age	57.20 ± 6.26	61.80 ± 9.34	61.0 ± 7.07
Males	15 (60%)	19 (76%)	11 (44%)
BMI	26.68 ± 3.44	28.04 ± 2.68	28.28 ± 4.26
Child-Pugh			
A	3 (12%)	6 (24%)	
B	12 (48%)	13 (52%)	
C	10 (40%)	6 (24%)	
BCLC			
A	2 (8%)		
B	10 (40%)		
C	8 (32%)		
D	5 (20%)		
Hb	12.82 ± 14.02	10.38 ± 2.24	
Platelets	79.0 (55.0-101.0)	104.0 (62.0-136.0)	
WBC	4.56 (2.83-5.20)	5.70 (3.51-8.43)	
AST	75.0 (42.0-91.0)	44.0 (30.0-59.0)	
Albumin	2.50 ± 0.89	2.51 ± 0.52	
Bilirubin	2.40 (1.30-4.30)	1.70 (1.0-3.10)	
INR	1.46 ± 0.44	1.41 ± 0.22	
ALT	37.0 (33.0-42.0)	26.0 (19.0-42.0)	
AFP	777.5 ± 451.1		

Mean ± SD is expressed as $n \pm n$ while median (IQR) is expressed as n (n-n)

Gut microbiome analysis

Specimen collection, preservation, and transport

Stool samples collected from cases and controls were delivered immediately to Alexandria University Main Microbiology Laboratory and stored at −80 °C for further processing. Whenever a delay in transfer is anticipated, the subject was asked to keep it in the freezer at −18 °C to be delivered frozen within the same day to the laboratory.

DNA extraction

DNA was extracted from 180-220 mg stool sample using QIAamp® Fast DNA Stool Mini Kit (Qiagen, Germany) according to the manufacturers' instructions. DNA extracts were stored at −80 °C until PCR testing.

SYBR Green real-time PCR

Specific oligonucleotide primers were used to target the 16S rRNA gene (rDNA) sequences of selected phyla, genera, or species constituting the gut microbiota (*A.*

mucinophilia, Bacteroides, Prevotella, Ruminococcus, Bacteroidetes, Firmicutes, F. prausnitzii, Bifidobacterium, and *Lactobacillus*). In addition to a broad-range primer targeting conserved 16S rRNA sequence of total bacteria, the amplification of which served as the denominator against which the amplification of other bacteria was estimated. All of the primer sequences used are listed in Suppl. Table 1 [26–30]. Primers were commercially obtained (Invitrogen, USA).

Amplification was performed in a light cycler (Rotor Gene Q, Qiagen, Germany) using a SensiFAST ^{TM} SYBR No-ROX PCR kit (Bioline Co., UK). In short, forward and reverse primers (4 pmol each) were used in 20 µl reactions containing 2 µl of the DNA extract.

PCR amplification was performed with initial denaturation at 95 °C for 10 min, followed by 40 cycles of denaturation at 95 °C for 30 s, annealing at 60 °C for 30 s, and extension at 72 °C for 30 s. Melting curve analysis was performed from 40 to 95 °C with a plate-reading step after every 1 °C and held at a temperature for 10 s to check the specificity of the product formed. Quantitation of specific bacterial DNA was expressed as relative quantitation (the cycle threshold (C_t) at which DNA for a specific target was detected relative to the cycle threshold (C_t) at which universal bacterial DNA was detected). This relative quantification is calculated automatically by the Rotor Gene software and expressed as relative fold difference [31].

The enterotype of all participants was determined according to the dominant type present of the three bacteria: *Bacteroides* (Enterotype 1), *Prevotella* (Enterotype 2), or *Ruminococcus* (Enterotype 3).

Statistical analysis of the data

Data entry and analysis were carried out using the Statistical Package for Social Sciences version 20 (SPPS PASW Statistics, Chicago). Quantitative variables were presented in the form of range, mean, median, and standard deviation. On the other hand, studied qualitative variables were presented as frequency and percentage from total. Comparisons between the different study groups were carried out using Chi-square, Fisher's exact, and Monte Carlo tests for qualitative variable and Mann-Whitney, Kruskal-Wallis tests for quantitative ones. For assessing correlations between different quantitative variables, Spearman correlation coefficient was calculated. All results were interpreted at 5% level of significance where the difference between the study groups is considered significant if P is ≤ 0.05. To evaluate the degree of variation of the microbial community structure within a sample, we measured the alpha diversity by employing the Shannon diversity index [32], and to evaluate the degree of similarity between patients and control group, we employed the Bray-Curtis similarity index [33].

Results

Characteristics of the participants

Out of the 25 HCC patients, 15 (60%) were males and 10 (40%) were females, with male to female ratio of 1.5: 1. Their mean age ± SD was 57.20 ± 6.26 years, and their age ranged from 40-65 years. The BMI ranged between 20.0-32.0 kg/m^2 with mean 26.68 ± 3.44 SD. Out of the 25 cirrhotic patients, 19 (76%) were males and 6 (24%) females, with male to female ratio of 3.1:1. Their mean age ± SD was 61.80 ± 9.34 years, and their age ranged from 33-77 years. The BMI ranged between 22 and 32 kg/m^2 with mean ± SD of 28.04 ± 2.68. Out of the 25 control subjects, 11 (44%) were males and 14 (56%) were females, with male to female ratio of 1:1.2. The mean age ± SD of the cases was 61.0 ± 7.07, and their age ranged from 49-80 years. The BMI ranged between 19.28 and 37.11 kg/m^2 with mean ± SD of 28.28 ± 4.26. There was no statistically significant difference between the 3 groups. In HCC, 3 (12%) were CPS A, 12 (48%) were CPS B, and 10 (40%) were CPS C. In cirrhosis group, 6 (24%) were CPS A, 13 (52%) were CPS B, and 6 (24%) were CPS C. There was no statistically significant difference between the 3 groups regarding these clinical parameters (Table 1). For BCLC staging of HCC, 2 (8%) were in stage A, 10 (40%) were in stage B, 8 (32%) were in stage C, and 5 (20%) were in stage D. Serum level of alanine aspartate aminotransferase (AST) was significantly higher in HCC cases compared to cirrhosis group ($p = 0.035$). Although the serum levels of alanine aminotransferase (ALT) and bilirubin were higher in HCC cases, the difference was not statistically significant ($p > 0.05$). Also, the albumin and platelets levels were lower in HCC cases and the difference was not statistically significant (Table 1).

Gut microbiome analysis

Quantitation of specific bacteria DNA was not expressed as an absolute number but was expressed relative to the total bacteria DNA present in the stool sample. The relative abundance values of the various bacteria were shown in the following manner (4.75×10^{-5} was shown as 4.75E−05).

Phylum level analysis

Bacterial phylum analysis showed that both patients with HCC and cirrhosis showed a statistically significant decrease in *Firmicutes* ($p < 0.001$), and although the *Bacteroidetes* was increased, the difference was not statistically significant in comparison to the control group. As regard the *Firmicutes* to *Bacteroidetes* ratio (F/B ratio), it was significantly lower in HCC (0.465) and cirrhosis patients (0.260) versus 1.310 in the control subjects (Table 2, Fig. 1).

Table 2 Comparison between the three studied groups according to *Firmicutes* to *Bacteroidetes* (F/B) ratio, *Prevotella* to *Bacteroides* (P/B) ratio, diversity index, and dissimilarity index (%)

	HCC (n = 25)	Cirrhosis (n = 25)	Control (n = 25)	Test	p
F/B ratio					
Min.-max.	0.018-3.715	0.020-10.550	0.350-2.470	H = 15.699*	< 0.001*
Mean ± SD	0.799 ± 0.970	1.229 ± 2.562	1.312 ± 0.669		
Median (IQR)	0.465 (0.207-0.769)	0.260 (0.100-0.600)	1.310 (0.710-1.870)		
Significance between groups	p_1 = 0.337, p_2 = 0.004*, p_3 < 0.001*				
P/B ratio					
Min.-max.	0.000-2.205	0.000-8.300	0.010-4.490	H = 14.111*	0.001*
Mean ± SD	0.303 ± 0.643	1.519 ± 2.270	0.992 ± 1.236		
Median (IQR)	0.012 (0.001-0.195)	0.710 (0.090-1.590)	0.510 (0.170-1.400)		
Significance between. groups	p_1 = 0.001*, p_2 = 0.001*, p_3 = 0.953				
Diversity index					
Min.-max.	0.75-1.68	0.22-1.70	1.14-1.70	F = 12.789*	< 0.001*
Mean ± SD	1.25 ± 0.27	1.18 ± 0.33	1.53 ± 0.12		
Median (IQR)	1.31 (1.06-1.45)	1.23 (0.98-1.36)	1.56 (1.48-1.60)		
Significance between. groups	p_1 = 0.611, p_2 = 0.001*, p_3 < 0.001*				
Dissimilarity index (%)					
Min.-max.	24.0-85.0	17.0-93.0	0.0-0.0	F = 101.434*	< 0.001*
Mean ± SD	41.44 ± 13.37	43.64 ± 16.38	0.0 ± 0.0		
Median (IQR)	39.0 (32.0-47.0)	40.0 (35.0-48.0)	0.0 (–)		
Significance between groups	p_1 = 0.800, p_2 < 0.001*, p_3 < 0.001*				

IQR, inter quartile range; *SD*, standard deviation; *H*, H for Kruskal-Wallis test, pairwise comparison between each 2 groups was done using post hoc test (Dunn's for multiple comparisons test); *F*, F for ANOVA test, pairwise comparison bet. each 2 groups was done using post hoc test (Tukey); *p*, *p* value for comparing between the studied groups; p_1, *p* value for comparing between HCC and cirrhosis; p_2, *p* value for comparing between HCC and control; p_3, *p* value for comparing between cirrhosis and control

*Statistically significant at $p \leq 0.05$

On the other hand, there was no statistically significant difference between HCC and cirrhosis group as regard *Firmicutes, Bacteroidetes,* and F/B ratio (Table 2, Fig. 1).

Genus level analysis

There was a statistically significant increase in *Bacteroides* and decrease of *Prevotella* relative abundance in HCC group compared to both cirrhosis and control groups. However, both cirrhosis and HCC groups showed a statistically significant decrease in *Ruminococcus,* in comparison to the control group. Also, there was no statistically significant difference between cirrhosis and control groups as regard *Bacteroides* and *Prevotella,* and between HCC and cirrhosis groups as regard *Ruminococcus* (Table 2, Fig. 1).

For the *Prevotella*-to-*Bacteroides* (P/B) ratio, there was no statistically significant difference between cirrhosis and the control groups. However, it was significantly lower in HCC (0.012) versus cirrhosis patients (0.71) and control subjects (0.51) (Table 2).

Species level analysis

As regard the beneficial bacteria, there was a statistically significant decrease in *A. mucinophilia* and *F. prausnitzii* in HCC and cirrhosis groups compared to the control group. Meanwhile, there was no statistical difference between HCC, cirrhosis, and control groups as regard *Bifidobacteria.* Also, there was no statistical difference between cirrhosis and control groups as regard *Lactobacilli.* On the other hand, there was a statistically significant increase in *Lactobacilli* relative abundance in HCC group compared to both the cirrhosis and control groups (Fig. 1).

Alpha diversity

Shannon diversity index, that considers both species richness and evenness, demonstrated a statistically significant low microbial diversity in both the HCC (1.25) and cirrhosis (1.18) groups compared to the control group (1.53). However, there was no statistically significant difference between the diversity index of HCC and cirrhosis patients (Table 2).

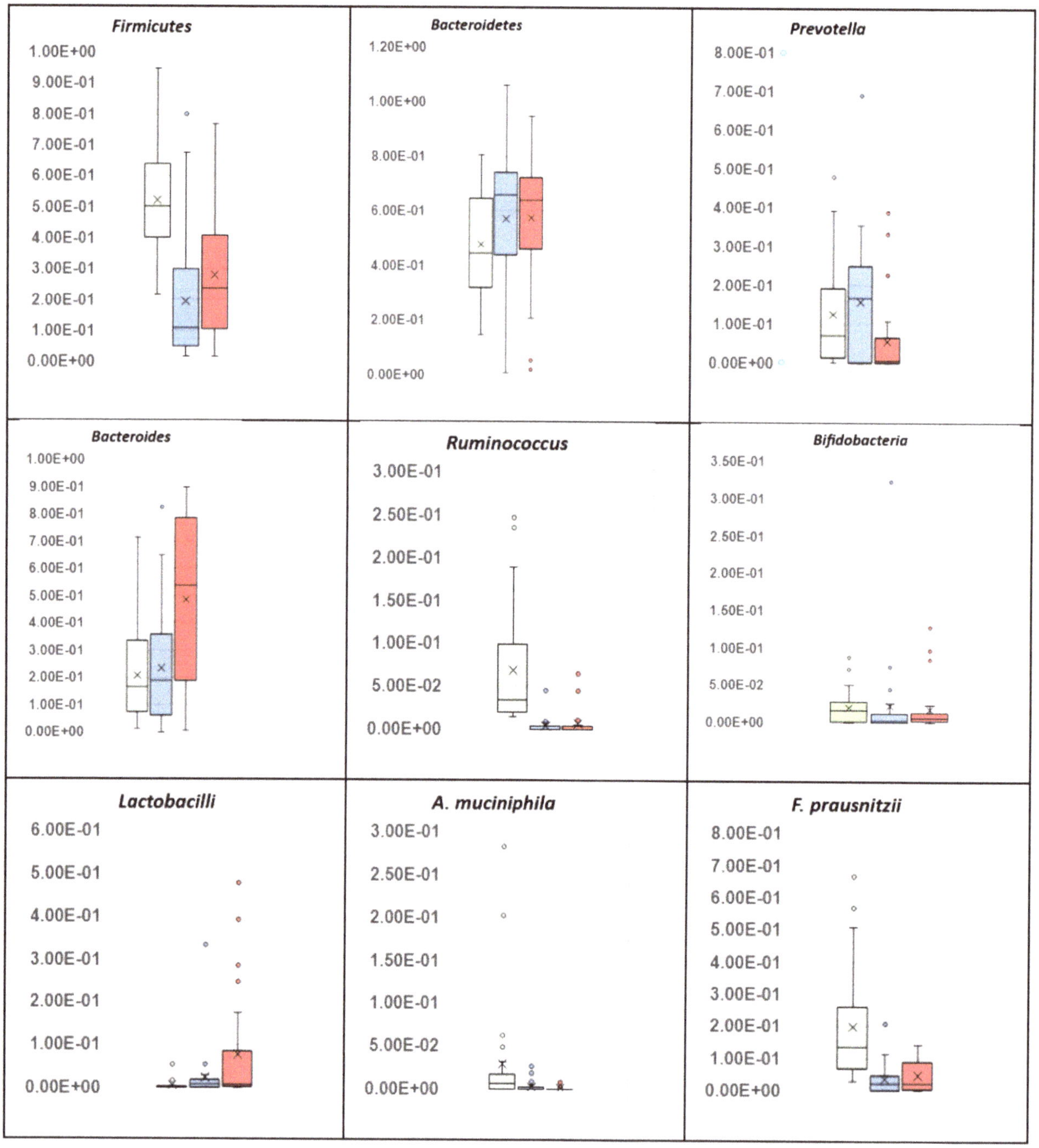

Fig. 1 Box and whisker graph of gut microbiome in the studied groups. The thick line in the middle of the box represents the median, the box represents the inter-quartile range (from 25th to 75th percentiles) and the whiskers represent the minimum and maximum. Control ☐ Cirrhosis ☐ HCC ☐

Bray-Curtis dissimilarity index

Bray-Curtis dissimilarity index was performed to study the degree of dissimilarity between microbiota in the HCC and cirrhosis groups compared to the control group. The dissimilarity index between HCC cases and healthy controls was 41.44%. The dissimilarity index between cirrhosis group and healthy controls was 43.64%. Comparing dissimilarity index between HCC and cirrhosis groups demonstrated no statistically significant difference (p = 0.8). On the other hand, the dissimilarity index between HCC and cirrhosis groups was only 26%. This means that they are 74% like each other (Table 2).

Gut microbiome and the clinical stage

In HCC group, there was no statistically significant difference between Child-Pugh class and the relative abundance of the studied microbiota, F/B ratio, P/B ratio, diversity index, or dissimilarity index (Suppl. Table 2).

There was statistically significant difference between the BCLC stages of HCC and *Ruminococcus* relative abundance (p = 0.023). There was no statically significant difference between the BCLC stage of HCC and other bacteria, F/B ratio, P/B ratio, diversity index, and dissimilarity index (%) (Suppl. Table 3).

In cirrhosis group, there was no statistically significant correlation between the Child-Pugh class and the relative abundance of each of the studied microbiota. Also, there was no statistically significant correlation between the Child-Pugh class and F/B ratio, P/B ratio, diversity index, and dissimilarity index (%) (Suppl. Table 4).

The enterotypes of the study participants

Enterotype 1 was the most common enterotype detected in all study participants. Twenty-two (88%) of the 25 HCC patients were assigned to Enterotype 1, 3 (12%) were assigned to Enterotype 2, and none to Enterotype 3. For the 25 cirrhosis group cases, 15 (60%) were assigned to Enterotype 1, 8 (32%) were assigned to Enterotype 2, and 2 (8%) were Enterotype 3. On the other hand, 13 (52%) of the 25 control subjects were assigned to Enterotype 1, 9 (36%) were assigned to Enterotype 2, and 3 (12%) were Enterotype 3. There was no statistically significant difference between the 3 groups regarding the enterotype distribution. (P value = 0.053). However, Enterotype 1 was higher in HCC group than the control group (P value = 0.016*). Also, Enterotype 1 is the predominant enterotype in HCC group (P value = 0.022*), while the control group showed insignificant higher Enterotype 1 followed Enterotype 2 (P value < 0.05).

Discussion

Hepatocellular carcinoma (HCC) is the second leading cause of cancer-related mortality worldwide. Cirrhosis is the most important risk factor for HCC. However, the exact factors that impact cirrhosis progression to HCC need to be determined [34].

Recent studies have noticed that Hepatitis C virus (HCV) infection and the progression of hepatic cirrhosis are associated with gut dysbiosis. Progressive changes in the gut microbiome have been observed accompanying the progression of liver disease [35, 36].

The present study agrees with the previous studies as regard decreased diversity and gut dysbiosis [35, 37, 38]. All HCV infected cases whether cirrhotic or with HCC showed gut dysbiosis and decreased diversity compared to healthy controls. The pattern of dysbiosis in both HCC and cirrhosis groups showed a significantly lower relative abundance of butyrate-producing bacteria *Firmicutes*, F/B ratio, and the bacteria maintaining the gut barrier function by enhancing mucus production, *A. mucinophilia* and *F. prausnitzii*, compared to the control group. However, the HCC group differed from the cirrhotic in that they showed statistically significant more increase in the proinflammatory genus *Bacteroides* and *Lactobacilli* and marked decrease of butyrate producer and anti-inflammatory genus *Prevotella* relative abundance and P/B ratio compared to both cirrhosis and control groups. The decrease of *Prevotella* and P/B ratio is a potential biomarker for liver disease progression. *Bacteroides and Lactobacilli* were associated with deconjugating bile acids by their bile salt hydrolase enzyme and causing liver damage [39].

Other studies showed a similar pattern of dysbiosis that is linked to inflammation. Pinero et al. (2019) in their study of 25 cirrhotic and 25 HCC cases noticed decreased *Prevotella* and P/B ratio in HCC compared to cirrhotic. However, in their study, there was no significant change in *Bacteroides* which may be due to different dietary pattern of their population [40].

Ponziani et al. (2019) found that NAFLD-related HCC patients had increased inflammatory cytokines related with a higher abundance of *Bacteroides* and *Ruminococcaceae* and a fall in beneficial bacteria such as *Akkermansia*. They also noticed decrease in the P/B ratio in these HCC patients compared to liver cirrhosis and healthy subjects [41]. Also, Chen et al. (2011), in their study of 36 cirrhotic and 24 controls, also noticed decreased *F. prausnitzii* in cirrhotic but no decreased *Firmicutes* [35].

In an Egyptian study (2016) on six HCV patients and eight healthy individuals, Aly et al. found that HCV patients showed a significantly lower relative abundance of *Firmicutes*. However, in contrast to our study, *Prevotella*, *Faecalibacterium*, and *Bacteroidetes* were more abundant in HCV patients compared to healthy individuals which may be related to the sample size [42].

As regard *Lactobacilli*, our results coincide with that of Inoue et al. (2018) who found that chronic hepatitis C patients had an increase in *Lactobacillus* [22]. Also, Sydor S et al. (2020) found that *Lactobacilli* was more abundant in NASH-related HCC than in cirrhotics [43].

As regard the relation between the gut microbiome and stages of HCC, BCLC stage D showed significantly the lowest relative abundance of *Ruminococcus*. This supports the suggestion that the progression of disease is associated with the decrease of anti-inflammatory butyrate producing bacteria and increase of proinflammatory bacteria.

Understanding the composition of gut microbiota in HCV patients may help in the development of new approaches for treatment and prevention of HCC by modulating the gut microbiome. GM-CSF can protect against HCC by its effect on immunity and microbiota composition and metabolism as demonstrated in mice [44].

Our diet influence the enterotype in our gut; high-fat and protein diet enhances the growth of Enterotypes 1, while a diet rich in carbohydrates supports the raise of Enterotype 2 and high fiber diet vegetables with Enterotype 3 [45]. Many studies showed the abundance of Enterotype 1 in countries depending on the Western diet which is associated with increased inflammation and increased gut inflammatory cells [46].

In the present study, Enterotype 1 is the dominant in all our study groups and significantly higher in HCC cases than control group (88% versus 52%). On the other hand, Enterotype 2 was the least enterotype encountered in HCC group; only 3 cases are Enterotype 2.

The gut microbiota may reduce cancer progression by regulating the ICD (immunogenic cell death) pathway, and increase the anticancer effects of drugs. Strategies making use of the gut microbiota such as probiotics and fecal microbiota transplantation (FMT) may act as potential adjuvants for tumor immunotherapy [47]. Yamamoto et al. found that gut microbiota in HCC patients before sorafenib may aid to prevent or delay its side effects [48].

Our results contribute to the knowledge of the possible association between the gut microbiota and the progression of hepatic diseases. Understanding the composition of gut microbiota in HCV patients may help in the development of new approaches for treatment and prevention of HCC by modulating the gut microbiome.

Our study is a single-center study and was performed on 75 subjects. Multi-center studies on heterogeneous larger population can be done in the future.

Conclusions

The overall results of the present study confirmed that patients with HCV-related cirrhosis and HCC exhibit microbial dysbiosis. Altered microbial relative abundance and diversity was noted vs controls. At the genus level, the HCC patients showed higher proinflammatory bacteria pattern compared to cirrhotic patients. These data imply that the changed gut microbiota may represent a potential target to monitor and prevent HCC development by the gut-microbiota-liver axis. The decrease of *Prevotella* and P/B ratio could be used as potential biomarker for liver disease progression.

Abbreviations

HCC: Hepatocellular carcinoma; HCV: Hepatitis C virus; DAAs: Direct-acting antivirals; SVR: Sustained virological response; CPC: Child-Pugh class; BCLC: Barcelona Clinic Liver Cancer; F/B ratio: *Firmicutes* to *Bacteroidetes* ratio; P/B ratio: *Prevotella* to *Bacteroides* ratio

Acknowledgements

The authors would like to thank all patients for their participation in this research.

Authors' contributions

KM: Research design, draft writing, data analysis, and critically reviewed the manuscript. SH: Research design, draft writing, and critically reviewed the manuscript. AN: Research design, recruitment of patients, data collection, and draft writing. SA: Research design, performed the lab work, analysis and interpretation of the gut microbiome PCR results, participated in draft writing, and critically reviewed the manuscript. WE: Concept, draft writing, data analysis, and critically reviewed the manuscript. All authors have read and approved the manuscript.

Declarations

Ethics approval and consent to participate

The study follows the principles of the Declaration of Helsinki (6th revision, 2008). After approval of the Ethical Committee, Faculty of Medicine, Alexandria University (serial no. 0201306), informed consents were obtained from all patients expressing their acceptance to participate in the study and have the results published.

Competing interests

The authors declare that they have no competing interests.

Author details

[1]Tropical Medicine Department, Faculty of Medicine, Alexandria University, Alexandria, Egypt. [2]Medical Microbiology and Immunology Department, Faculty of Medicine, Alexandria University, Alexandria, Egypt.

References

1. Organization WH (2017) Global hepatitis report 2017. Geneva: World Health Organization
2. Centers for Disease Control and Prevention (CDC) (2012) Progress toward prevention and control of hepatitis C virus infection--Egypt, 2001-2012. MMWR Morb Mortal Wkly Rep 61(29):545–9.
3. Waked I, Esmat G, Elsharkawy A, El-Serafy M, Abdel-Razek W, Ghalab R et al (2020) Screening and treatment program to eliminate hepatitis C in Egypt. N Engl J Med 382(12):1166–1174. https://doi.org/10.1056/NEJMsr1912628
4. Cresci GA, Bawden E (2015) Gut microbiome: what we do and don't know. Nutr Clin Pract 30(6):734–746. https://doi.org/10.1177/0884533615609899
5. Dzutsev A, Badger JH, Perez-Chanona E, Roy S, Salcedo R, Smith CK, Trinchieri G (2017) Microbes and cancer. Annu Rev Immunol 35(1):199–228. https://doi.org/10.1146/annurev-immunol-051116-052133
6. Shahanavaj K, Gil-Bazo I, Castiglia M, Bronte G, Passiglia F, Carreca AP, del Pozo JL, Russo A, Peeters M, Rolfo C (2015) Cancer and the microbiome: potential applications as new tumor biomarker. Expert Rev Anticancer Ther 15(3):317–330. https://doi.org/10.1586/14737140.2015.992785
7. Arthur JC, Perez-Chanona E, Mühlbauer M, Tomkovich S, Uronis JM, Fan T-J, Campbell BJ, Abujamel T, Dogan B, Rogers AB, Rhodes JM, Stintzi A, Simpson KW, Hansen JJ, Keku TO, Fodor AA, Jobin C (2012) Intestinal inflammation targets cancer-inducing activity of the microbiota. Science 338(6103):120–123. https://doi.org/10.1126/science.1224820
8. Zitvogel L, Galluzzi L, Viaud S, Vétizou M, Daillère R, Merad M et al (2015) Cancer and the gut microbiota: an unexpected link. Sci Transl Med 7(271): 271ps1-ps1

9. Yu L-X, Schwabe RF (2017) The gut microbiome and liver cancer: mechanisms and clinical translation. Nat Rev Gastroenterol Hepatol 14(9): 527–539. https://doi.org/10.1038/nrgastro.2017.72
10. Helmink BA, Khan MAW, Hermann A, Gopalakrishnan V, Wargo JA (2019) The microbiome, cancer, and cancer therapy. Nat Med 25(3):377–388. https://doi.org/10.1038/s41591-019-0377-7
11. Morkūnas E, Skiecevičienė J, Kupčinskas J (2020) The impact of modulating the gastrointestinal microbiota in cancer patients. Best Pract Res Clin Gastroenterol 101700:101700. https://doi.org/10.1016/j.bpg.2020.101700
12. Zitvogel L, Daillère R, Roberti MP, Routy B, Kroemer G (2017) Anticancer effects of the microbiome and its products. Nat Rev Microbiol 15(8):465–478. https://doi.org/10.1038/nrmicro.2017.44
13. Daillère R, Vétizou M, Waldschmitt N, Yamazaki T, Isnard C, Poirier-Colame V, Duong CPM, Flament C, Lepage P, Roberti MP, Routy B, Jacquelot N, Apetoh L, Becharef S, Rusakiewicz S, Langella P, Sokol H, Kroemer G, Enot D, Roux A, Eggermont A, Tartour E, Johannes L, Woerther PL, Chachaty E, Soria JC, Golden E, Formenti S, Plebanski M, Madondo M, Rosenstiel P, Raoult D, Cattoir V, Boneca IG, Chamaillard M, Zitvogel L (2016) Enterococcus hirae and Barnesiella intestinihominis facilitate cyclophosphamide-induced therapeutic immunomodulatory effects. Immunity. 45(4):931–943. https://doi.org/10.1016/j.immuni.2016.09.009
14. Gensollen T, Iyer SS, Kasper DL, Blumberg RS (2016) How colonization by microbiota in early life shapes the immune system. Science. 352(6285):539–544. https://doi.org/10.1126/science.aad9378
15. Guarner F, Malagelada J-R (2003) Gut flora in health and disease. Lancet 361(9356):512–519. https://doi.org/10.1016/S0140-6736(03)12489-0
16. Natividad JMM, Verdu EF (2013) Modulation of intestinal barrier by intestinal microbiota: pathological and therapeutic implications. Pharmacol Res 69(1): 42–51. https://doi.org/10.1016/j.phrs.2012.10.007
17. den Besten G, van Eunen K, Groen AK, Venema K, Reijngoud D-J, Bakker BM (2013) The role of short-chain fatty acids in the interplay between diet, gut microbiota, and host energy metabolism. J Lipid Res 54(9):2325–2340. https://doi.org/10.1194/jlr.R036012
18. Bäumler AJ, Sperandio V (2016) Interactions between the microbiota and pathogenic bacteria in the gut. Nature. 535(7610):85–93. https://doi.org/10.1038/nature18849
19. Acharya C, Sahingur SE, Bajaj JS (2017) Microbiota, cirrhosis, and the emerging oral-gut-liver axis. JCI Insight 2(19):e94416. https://doi.org/10.1172/jci.insight.94416
20. Bhat M, Arendt BM, Bhat V, Renner EL, Humar A, Allard JP (2016) Implication of the intestinal microbiome in complications of cirrhosis. World J Hepatol 8(27):1128–1136. https://doi.org/10.4254/wjh.v8.i27.1128
21. Tsochatzis EA, Bosch J, Burroughs AK (2014) Liver cirrhosis. Lancet 383(9930): 1749–1761
22. Inoue T, Nakayama J, Moriya K, Kawaratani H, Momoda R, Ito K, Iio E, Nojiri S, Fujiwara K, Yoneda M, Yoshiji H, Tanaka Y (2018) Gut dysbiosis associated with hepatitis C virus infection. Clin Infect Dis 67(6):869–877. https://doi.org/10.1093/cid/ciy205
23. Darnaud M, Faivre J, Moniaux N (2013) Targeting gut flora to prevent progression of hepatocellular carcinoma. J Hepatol 58(2):385–387. https://doi.org/10.1016/j.jhep.2012.08.019
24. Pugh RN, Murray-Lyon IM, Dawson JL, Pietroni MC, Williams R (1973) Transection of the oesophagus for bleeding oesophageal varices. Br J Surg 60(8):646–649. https://doi.org/10.1002/bjs.1800600817
25. Forner A, Reig M, Bruix J (2018) Hepatocellular carcinoma. Lancet 391(10127):1301–1314. https://doi.org/10.1016/S0140-6736(18)30010-2
26. Nadkarni MA, Martin FE, Jacques NA, Hunter N (2002) Determination of bacterial load by real-time PCR using a broad-range (universal) probe and primers set. Microbiology 148(Pt 1):257–266
27. Collado MC, Derrien M, Isolauri E, de Vos WM, Salminen S (2007) Intestinal integrity and Akkermansia muciniphila, a mucin-degrading member of the intestinal microbiota present in infants, adults, and the elderly. Appl Environ Microbiol 73(23):7767–7770. https://doi.org/10.1128/AEM.01477-07
28. Bergström A, Licht TR, Wilcks A, Andersen JB, Schmidt LR, Grønlund HA, Vigsnaes LK, Michaelsen KF, Bahl MI (2012) Introducing GUt low-density array (GULDA): a validated approach for qPCR-based intestinal microbial community analysis. FEMS Microbiol Lett 337(1):38–47. https://doi.org/10.1111/1574-6968.12004
29. Rinttilä T, Kassinen A, Malinen E, Krogius L, Palva A (2004) Development of an extensive set of 16S rDNA-targeted primers for quantification of pathogenic and indigenous bacteria in faecal samples by real-time PCR. J Appl Microbiol 97(6):1166–1177. https://doi.org/10.1111/j.1365-2672.2004.02409.x
30. Ramirez-Farias C, Slezak K, Fuller Z, Duncan A, Holtrop G, Louis P (2009) Effect of inulin on the human gut microbiota: stimulation of Bifidobacterium adolescentis and Faecalibacterium prausnitzii. Br J Nutr 101(4):541–550. https://doi.org/10.1017/S0007114508019880
31. Tomova A, Husarova V, Lakatosova S, Bakos J, Vlkova B, Babinska K, Ostatnikova D (2015) Gastrointestinal microbiota in children with autism in Slovakia. Physiol Behav 138:179–187. https://doi.org/10.1016/j.physbeh.2014.10.033
32. Shannon CE (1948) A mathematical theory of communication. Bell Sys Techn J 27(3):379–423. https://doi.org/10.1002/j.1538-7305.1948.tb01338.x
33. Bray JR, Curtis JT (1957) An ordination of the upland forest communities of Southern Wisconsin. Ecol Monogr 27(4):325–349. https://doi.org/10.2307/1942268
34. Balogh J, Victor D 3rd, Asham EH, Burroughs SG, Boktour M, Saharia A et al (2016) Hepatocellular carcinoma: a review. J Hepatocellular Carcinoma 3:41–53. https://doi.org/10.2147/JHC.S61146
35. Chen Y, Yang F, Lu H, Wang B, Chen Y, Lei D et al (2011) Characterization of fecal microbial communities in patients with liver cirrhosis. Hepatology 54(2):562–572
36. Bajaj JS, Heuman DM, Hylemon PB, Sanyal AJ, White MB, Monteith P, Noble NA, Unser AB, Daita K, Fisher AR, Sikaroodi M, Gillevet PM (2014) Altered profile of human gut microbiome is associated with cirrhosis and its complications. J Hepatol 60(5):940–947. https://doi.org/10.1016/j.jhep.2013.12.019
37. Ren Z, Li A, Jiang J, Zhou L, Yu Z, Lu H, Xie H, Chen X, Shao L, Zhang R, Xu S, Zhang H, Cui G, Chen X, Sun R, Wen H, Lerut JP, Kan Q, Li L, Zheng S (2019) Gut microbiome analysis as a tool towards targeted non-invasive biomarkers for early hepatocellular carcinoma. Gut. 68(6):1014–1023. https://doi.org/10.1136/gutjnl-2017-315084
38. Zheng R, Wang G, Pang Z, Ran N, Gu Y, Guan X, Yuan Y, Zuo X, Pan H, Zheng J, Wang F (2020) Liver cirrhosis contributes to the disorder of gut microbiota in patients with hepatocellular carcinoma. Cancer Med 9(12): 4232–4250. https://doi.org/10.1002/cam4.3045
39. Gérard P (2013) Metabolism of cholesterol and bile acids by the gut microbiota. Pathogens. 3(1):14–24. https://doi.org/10.3390/pathogens3010014
40. Piñero F, Vazquez M, Baré P, Rohr C, Mendizabal M, Sciara M, Alonso C, Fay F, Silva M (2019) A different gut microbiome linked to inflammation found in cirrhotic patients with and without hepatocellular carcinoma. Ann Hepatol 18(3):480–487. https://doi.org/10.1016/j.aohep.2018.10.003
41. Ponziani FR, Bhoori S, Castelli C, Putignani L, Rivoltini L, Del Chierico F et al (2019) Hepatocellular carcinoma is associated with gut microbiota profile and inflammation in nonalcoholic fatty liver disease. Hepatology 69(1):107–120
42. Aly AM, Adel A, El-Gendy AO, Essam TM, Aziz RK (2016) Gut microbiome alterations in patients with stage 4 hepatitis C. Gut Pathog 8(1):42. https://doi.org/10.1186/s13099-016-0124-2
43. Sydor S, Best J, Messerschmidt I, Manka P, Vilchez-Vargas R, Brodesser S et al (2020) Altered microbiota diversity and bile acid signaling in cirrhotic and noncirrhotic NASH-HCC. Clin Transl Gastroenterol 11(3):e00131-e
44. Wu Y-N, Zhang L, Chen T, Li X, He L-H, Liu G-X (2020) Granulocyte-macrophage colony-stimulating factor protects mice against hepatocellular carcinoma by ameliorating intestinal dysbiosis and attenuating inflammation. World J Gastroenterol 26(36):5420–5436. https://doi.org/10.3748/wjg.v26.i36.5420
45. Arumugam M, Raes J, Pelletier E, Le Paslier D, Yamada T, Mende DR et al (2011) Enterotypes of the human gut microbiome. Nature. 473(7346):174–180. https://doi.org/10.1038/nature09944
46. Thorburn Alison N, Macia L, Mackay CR (2014) Diet, metabolites, and "Western-Lifestyle" inflammatory diseases. Immunity. 40(6):833–842. https://doi.org/10.1016/j.immuni.2014.05.014
47. Chen W, Wang S, Wu Y, Shen X, Guo Z, Li Q, Xing D (2020) Immunogenic cell death: a link between gut microbiota and anticancer effects. Microb Pathog 141:103983. https://doi.org/10.1016/j.micpath.2020.103983

29

Identification and expression analysis of antigenic sites of hepatitis C virus genotype 3a NS3 and NS5A genes of local isolate

Sabeen Sabri[1], Muhammad Idrees Khan[2], Shazia Rafique[2], Amjad Ali[3] and Muhammad Saleem Khan[4*]

Abstract

Background: Hepatitis C virus, a silent killer, has infected 71 million people globally. The recombinant viral antigenic proteins might be used in the early diagnosis of HCV infection. The NS3 and NS5A genes of HCV function in HCV replication and influence host cellular factors that are involved in HCV pathogenesis. The current study was designed to select NS3 and NS5A antigenic sites, amplified, cloned, and expressed in order to find out better assays for diagnosis or drug and vaccine development. The antigenic sites within NS3 and NS5A genes were selected and confirmed through sequencing and were cloned. The antigenic recombinant proteins were expressed in bacterial strain *E. coli BL21ply**, and the expression was confirmed by western blotting by using gene-specific and vector-specific antibodies.

Results: Specific antigenic regions within the NS3 and NS5A genes of the HCV 3A genotype were amplified. PCR results showed 328 bp and 747 bp antigenic regions, respectively. The regions were confirmed by DNA sequencing and cloned into a bacterial expression vector. Expression analysis showed 12 kDa and 28 kDa of NS3 and NS5A antigenic recombinant proteins, respectively. Taken together, these studies will help to analyze the genetic variability within the local HCV isolates as these antigenic recombinant proteins were quite important in the screening of HCV-infected patients.

Conclusions: This study might help to enhance the progress in the treatment of HCV infection through the modeling of HCV non-structural genes (NS3 and NS5A) from local isolate, and it might also present the viral genes as potential therapeutic targets.

Keywords: Analysis, Hepatitis C, Genotype, 3a NS3, NS5A, Genes

Background

The basic structural research on designing new therapeutic drugs against the silent killer (HCV) enhances the management of hepatitis C virus infection [1–4]. The prompt and efficient diagnosis of HCV is quite useful for the cure of the disease manifestation [5–8]. Concerning clinical data, it is perceived that antibody response against certain HCV proteins was quite variable. The immunogenicity of hepatitis C proteins varies as some of the proteins are highly immunogenic while others are not [9–11]. The serological diagnosis of HCV is mainly done by using the specific antibody through the enzyme immunoassays (EIAs) [12, 13].

Along with the routine diagnostic tests, some new methods are required for the selection of sequence variants of antigens that can develop antibodies against the diverse genotypes of HCV. Recombinant HCV proteins are most suitable for the study of the antigenic heterogenecity of the proteins. The available data showed that the determined antigenic regions of HCV possess sequence heterogeneity which influences the antigenic properties of these antigenic regions [14]. Keeping this

* Correspondence: SamiiKhan@uo.edu.pk
[4]Department of Zoology, Faculty of Life Sciences, University of Okara, Okara, Punjab 56130, Pakistan
Full list of author information is available at the end of the article

in view, the antigenic sites of NS3 and NS5A genes of HCV genotype 3a from the local isolate were determined, amplified, and cloned into the bacterial expression vector. The antigenic recombinant proteins were expressed in the bacterial strain *E. coli BL21ply**, and the expression was confirmed through western blotting by using gene-specific and vector-specific antibodies.

Methods

Synthesis of cDNA and amplification of NS3 and NS5A genes of HCV3a

After the identification of chronically infected HCV genotype 3a patient from the Division of Molecular Virology and Molecular Diagnostics, the cDNA was synthesized of the extracted RNA as described [15]. The synthesized cDNA was used as a template for the full-length amplification of the NS3 and NS5A genes of HCV 3a genotype of the local isolate using gene-specific primers [15]. The amplified products of NS3 and NS5A were submitted to GeneBank, and accession numbers were obtained.

Identification of antigenic sites within the NS3 and NS5A genes

From the confirmed sequences of NS3 and NS5A genes of HCV 3a genotype, the antigenic sites were selected by using the software Antigenicity Plot ((http://www.bioinformatics.org/JaMBW/3/1/7/). The selected antigenic regions of NS3 and NS5A genes were designated as NS3.1 (nt ~ 328 bp) and NS5A.1 (nt ~ 747 bp) and were used as a template.

Amplification of the NS3.1 and NS5A.1 antigenic sites

To amplify the antigenic sites NS3.1- and NS5A.1-specific primers containing the restriction enzyme, sites were designed. For NS3.1 primers, *HindIII* and *XhoI* restriction enzyme sites were added to the primers while NS5A.1 primer contained *EcoR1* and *HindIII* restriction enzyme sites.

Construction of expression vector containing NS3.1 and NS5A.1 antigenic sites and bacterial transformation

To construct an expression vector containing the NS3.1 and NS5A.1 antigenic regions, both the amplified sites and vector were treated with restriction enzymes. For the construction of the NS3.1 expression vector, the gene and vector were treated with *HindIII* and *XhoI* restriction enzymes. In order to construct the NS5A.1 vector, the amplified antigenic site and vector were treated with *EcoR1* and *HindIII* enzymes. The digested genes were ligated into the digested plasmid to construct the vector expressing the NS3.1 and NS5A.1 antigenic regions of HCV 3a. After the confirmation of correct ligation by sequencing 2 µl of plasmids harboring the antigenic regions (NS3.1 and NS5A.1) of NS3 and NS5A, genes of HCV 3a genotype of the local isolate were transformed into competent BL21 DE3 pLysS bacterial cells by heat shocking for 90 s at 42 °C. LB medium of 500 ml free of antibiotics was added and incubated for 1 h at 37 °C. Selection of transformants of NS3.1 and NS5A.1 was done on LB-agar plates containing kanamycin (25 mg/ml) and chloramphenicol (34 mg/ml) and incubated overnight at 37 °C.

Expression studies of NS3.1 and NS5A.1 antigenic sites

The expression of the antigenic sites of the NS3 and NS5A genes of the HCV 3a genotype was determined by western blotting. Individual pET28 clones NS3.1-28 and NS5A.1-28 was transformed into the bacterial strain by using the heat shock method as mentioned previously; 2 µl of plasmid was transformed into the BL21 (DE3) pLysS, and selection was done on L-agar plates supplemented with chloramphenicol (34 mg/ml) and kanamycin (25 mg/ml). Isolated colonies were selected and inoculated into L-broth supplemented with chloramphenicol and kanamycin and incubated at 37 °C overnight on a shaker.

Western blot analysis

The confirmed clones (colony PCR) were then used for expression analysis. Individual colonies were given induction of 0.5 M IPTG for 4 h. For protein, isolation cells were harvested, and for 1 g of pellet, 10 ml of lysis buffer was added. Thaw the pellet at room temperature. Prepare a protein sample by mixing 65 µl of the sample with 35 µl of 6X protein loading dye. This is the sample of the total extract. Now, add 0.004 g of lysozyme to the remaining extract and mix well. Sonicate (Mixsonic, USA) the lysed cells for 15 s × 4 pulses. Transfer the pellet into a separate tube and wash the pellet with three times with lysis buffer. Now resuspend the pellet 400 µl of 1X PBS. Prepare the protein sample by mixing 65 µl of pellet and 35 µl of 6Xprotein loading dye. Heat shock for 7 minutes in boiling water bath and snap cool on ice for 5 min. Run-on 15% SDS-PAGE gel at 60 V for 90 min. Western blot was performed following [15] using the gene-specific and vector-specific His tag antibodies.

Results

Selected antigenic site of NS3 and NS5A genes

To determine the antigenic regions of the NS3 and NS5A genes, antigenicity plot was used. The full sequence of NS3 and NS5A genes was analyzed for the analysis of the antigenic sites. Figure 1 illustrates the antigenic sites NS3.1 determined in the NS3 gene of the virus. In Fig. 2, the determined antigenic site NS5A.1 of NS5A gene of the virus is shown.

```
NS3.1

ggccgtgaggtgttgttgggacctgctgatgactatcgggagatgggctggcgtctgttggccccgatta
cagcatacgcccagcaaactaggcgtctttttgggactattgtgaccagcttgactggcagggacaagaa
cgtggtggccggcgaagtgcaggtgctttctacggctacccagaccttcctaggtacaacattgggaggg
gttatgtggactgtttaccatggagcaggttcgagaacacttgcgggcgtcaaacatcctgcgctccaaa
tgtacacaaatgtagatcaggacctcgttggatggccagctcctccgggggctaagtctcttgaaccgtg
cacctgcgggtctgcggacttgtacttggttacccgcgaagctgatgtcatccctgctagacgcaggggg
gactccacagcgagcttgctcagtcctaggcctctcgcctgtctcaaaggttcctctggaggtcctgtta
tgtgcccttcgggccacgtagcggggatctttagggctgctgtgtgcaccagaggtgtagcaaaagccct
acagttcataccagtggaaacccttagcacacaggctaggtctccatccttttctgacaattcaactcct
cctgctgttccacagagctatcaagtagggtaccttcatgccccgaccggcagcggtaagagcacaaagg
tcccggccgcttatgtagcacaaggatataatgttctcgtgttgaatccatcagtggcggccacactagg
cttcggctctttcatgtcgcgagcttatgggatcgaccccaacatccgcaccgggaacggcacggttaca
actggtgctaatctgacctattccacctatggtaagtttctcgcggacgggggttgctcgggggagcat
atgatgtgattatctgtgatgagtgtcatgcccaagactctactagcatactgggtataggcacggtcct
agatcaggctgaaacggctggggtgaggctgacggttttagcaacagcaactcccccaggcagcatcatt
gggccccattctaacctcaaagaagtggcccttggttctgaggggagatccctttcttcggcaaggcca
taccgctagccctgctaaggggaaaggcaccttattttttccattccaagaaaaatgtgatgagatg
gcatccaaactcagaggcatggggctcaacgctgaaggagtactacaggggtcttgatgtgtccgtcata
ccaacatcaggagacgttgtagtttgcgctactgacgccctcatgactggattcaccggagacttcgact
ctgtcatagattgcaacgtggctgttgaacagtacgttgatttcagcttggaccccacctttccattga
gactcgcactgctccccaagacgcggtttcccgcagtcaacgtcgtggccgtacgggccgaggtagactc
ggcacgtaccgatatgtcacccccggtgaaagaccgtctgggatgtttgactcggctgttctctgtgagt
gctatgacgcgggctgctcgtggtacgacttgcagcccgccgagaccacagtcagactaagagcttactt
gtccacgccggggttacctgtctgccaagaccacttggaattttgggagagcgtcttcactggactaact
cacatagatgcccactttctatcacagaccaagcagcagggactcaacttcccatacctagctgcctacc
aagccactgtgtgcgctcgcgcgcaagctcctcccccaagttgggacgagacatggaagtgtctcgtgcg
gcttaagccaacactacatggacctacaccccttcgatatcggccggggcctgtccaaaatgaaacctgc
ttgacacaccccatcacaaaatacctcatggcatgcatgtcagccgatctggaagtaaccacc
```

Fig. 1 Full gene sequence of NS3 gene indicating (highlighted) specific antigenic site NS3.1

PCR amplification of antigenic site

To clone the antigenic site regions into the pET-28a vector the determined antigenic regions NS3.1 and NS5A.1 were PCR amplified by utilizing the antigenic site-specific restriction primers. Designed primers for NS3.1- and NS5A.1-specific antigenic sites having a start codon ATG and specific restriction sites were synthesized. Figure 4 revealed the amplified regions of the specific antigenic site NS3.1 of the NS3 gene. The expected band size of NS3.1 was 328 bp which was observed on the gel. In Fig. 3, 747 bp gene band of the NS5A.1 antigenic region was observed. This indicates that the determined antigenic sites were successfully amplified. The PCR amplified products were observed onto 2% agarose gel which is stained with ethidium bromide. Both the amplified products were confirmed by restriction digestion and sequencing.

Cloning of the amplified antigenic sites into the pET-28a vector

To check the expression of the antigenic recombinant clones of NS3.1 and NS5A.1, these amplified antigenic sites were cloned into the pET28a vector. The results were as shown in Fig. 4.

```
NS5A.1
agcgacgattggctacgtaccatctgggactgggtctgcatggtgttgctcgacttcaagacatggctgtctgctaa
gatcatgccattgctccctgggttgcccttcatttcctgtcaaaagggatataagggcgtttggcagggggacggcg
tggtgtccactcgctgtccttgcggagcagtgataaccggtcatgtgaagaacgggtccatgcggcttgcaggacca
cgtacatgtgctaacatgtggcacggcaccttccccatcaacgagtacaccaccggacccagcacaccttgcccatc
acccaactacactcgtgcactgtggcgcgtggctgccaacagctacgtcgaagtgcgacgggtgggagacttccact
acatcacgggggccacagaagatgagctcaagtgtccgtgccaagtgccggctgctgagttctttactgaagtggat
ggggtgagacttcaccgttacgcccctccatgcaggcccctgttgagggatgagatcactttcgtagtagggctgaa
ttcttacgcgatagcatcccaactcccttgtgagcccgaaccggacgtctctgtgctgacctcgatgttgagagacc
cttcccatatcaccgccgagacggcagcgcgccgccttgcacgcgggtcccctccatcagaggcaagctcatccgcc
agtcaactatcggctccatcgttgaaggccacttgccaaacgcataggcctcatcccgacgcgagctggtggacgcc
aacttgtgtttggcgacaagagatgggcagcaacatcacacgggtagagtccgaaacaaaggttgtgattcttgact
cattcgaacctctgagggccgagactgatgacaccgagctctcggtagcagcagagtgtttcaagaaacctcccaag
tatcctccagccctccctatctgggctaggccagactacaaccctccactgttggatcgttggaaatcaccggatta
tgaaccaccaattgttcatgggtgcgccttaccaccacagggtactccaccggtgcctccccctcggaggaaaagaa
caatccagctggacggctccaatgtgtccgcggcgctagctgcgctagcggaaaaatcattcccggcctcaaaaccg
ttggaagcgggtagctcatcctcaggggtcgatacacagtccagcactacttccaaggtgcctccctcttcggagag
agagtccgacacagaatcgtgctcgtccatgcctcctctcgagggggagccgggcgatccagacttgagttgcgact
cttggtccactgttagtgacagcgaggagcagagcgtggtctgctgc
```

Fig. 2 Full gene sequence of NS5A gene indicating (highlighted) specific antigenic site NS5A.1

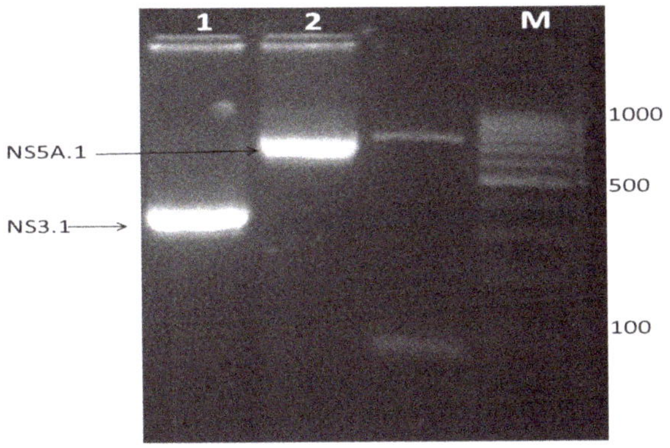

Fig. 3 PCR amplification of antigenic sites (NS3.1 (328 bp) and NS5A.1 (747 bp)) using antigenic restriction site-specific primers. Lane 1: NS3.1-amplified antigenic site (328); lane 2: NS5A.1-amplified antigenic site (747); M: 100 bp marker

Restriction and digestion analysis and sequencing confirmation

The antigenic recombinant clones NS3.1-28 and NS5A.1-28 that showed positive results for plasmid PCR were further confirmed by restriction and digestion analysis. The double digestion of NS3.1-28 clones was done with *HindIII* and *XhoI* restriction enzymes. The results are shown in Fig. 5 confirm the presence of the desired gene of interest with the vector backbone. The restriction and digestion analysis showed an exact product of 328 bp of the NS3.1 region. Lanes 2, 3, 4, and 6 showed positively digested NS3.1-28 antigenic recombinant clones. Figure 6 showed the restriction and digestion analysis of the NS5A.1-28 antigenic recombinant clone. NS5A.1-28 was digested with *EcoRI* and *HindIII* enzyme which gives the required product of 747 bp. The figure shows that lanes 4, 6, and 8 showed positively digested NS5A.1-28 antigenic recombinant vector. These results indicate that the required NS3.1 and NS5A.1 antigenic regions were successfully cloned into the pET28a vector. The dye termination sequencing method was used on an automated sequencer. The sequencing of the positively digested NS3.1-28 and NS5A.1-28 vectors was done by using a T7 vector-specific primer. The results indicate that the amplified antigenic sites NS3.1 and NS5A.1 were successfully ligated in the correct orientation in the pET28a vector. The sequences were BLAST and compared with the known sequences of the 3a genotype. The comparison results indicated that the cloned antigenic sites were of NS3 and NS5A genes of hepatitis C virus genotype 3a of Pakistani isolate.

Production of antigenic recombinant proteins in bacterial cells

The expression of the NS3.1-28 and NS5A.1-28 antigenic replicons was checked in *E. coli* BL21 ply* bacterial strain. The confirmed antigenic recombinant clones were used for expression studies. To characterize the antigenic recombinant protein, the confirmed plasmids NS3.1-28 and NS5A.1-28 were transformed into the *E. coli* BL21 ply* strain. Isolated colonies were selected to check the expression of the antigenic recombinant

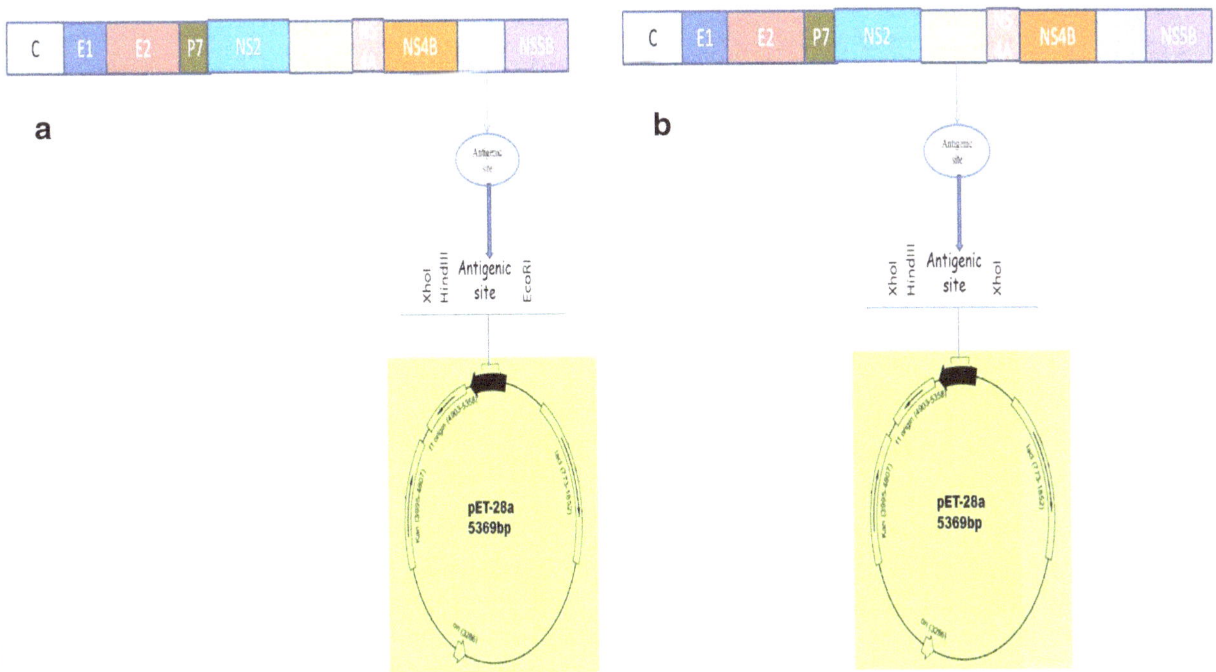

Fig. 4 pet28a constructs of NS3.1 (**a**) and NS5A.1 (**b**) encoding antigenic sites

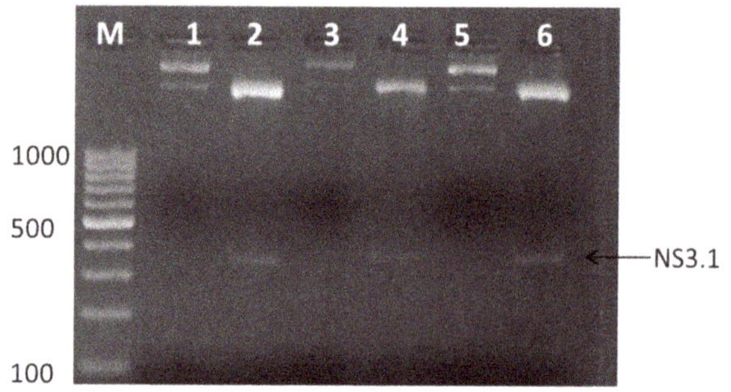

Fig. 5 Restriction and digestion analysis of pet28a vector expressing NS3.1 antigenic sites. Lanes 1, 3, and 5: uncut vectors; lanes 2, 4, and 6: positively NS3.1-digested plasmids; M: 100 bp marker

vectors. The individual colonies were grown overnight in L-broth supplemented with chloramphenicol (34 mg/ml) and kanamycin (25 mg/ml). An induction of 0.5 M IPTG was given for fours. The un-induced culture was used as a control. Protein was extracted after induction, and samples were identified through western blot by using gene-specific as well as vector-specific antibodies. Results shown in Figs. 7 and 8 demonstrated that the expected NS3.1 protein of 12 kDa was observed with both gene and vector-specific antibodies.

The results of NS5A.1 expression were analyzed which showed approximate bands 28 kDa with gene-specific and vector-specific antibodies (Figs. 9 and 10). These results indicated that the amplified antigenic sites of NS3 and NS5A HCV 3a genotype genes were successfully cloned into a bacterial expression vector and expressed well in the bacterial system. These antigenic recombinant proteins were quite important in the screening of HCV-affected patients

Discussion

The antigenic site is the antibody binding region. It is the hydrophobic part on the surface of the protein molecule which serves as a receptor for the antibody molecule. The determination of antigenic sites is important

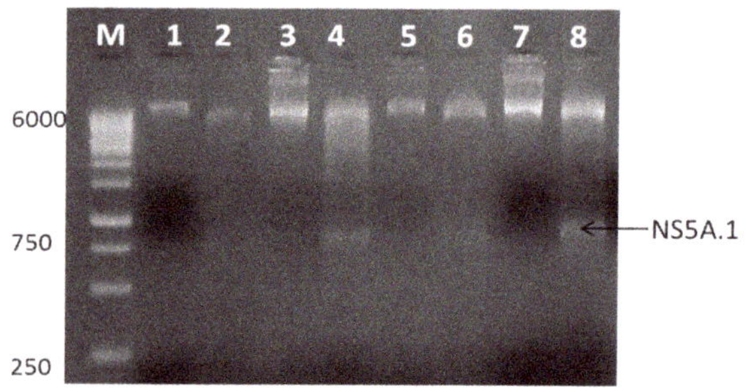

Fig. 6 Restriction and digestion analysis of pet vector expressing NS5A.1 antigenic site. Lanes 1, 3, 5, and 7: uncut plasmids; lanes 4, 6, and 8: positively digested plasmids; M: 1 kb marker

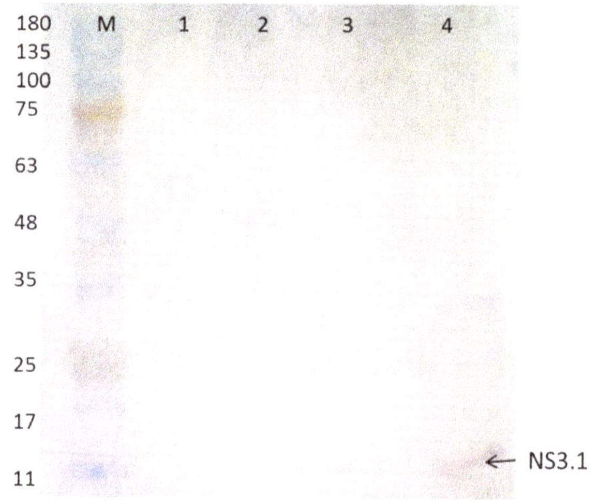

Fig. 7 NS3.1 antigenic recombinant protein expressed in bacterial cells (gene-specific antibodies). Lanes 1–4: NS3.1 protein; lane 4: positive NS3.1; M: prestained protein marker.

because a particular antigen triggers the immune response against a particular pathogen. The study of the antigenic sites of the non-structural genes NS3 and NS5A of hepatitis C virus 3a genotype of local isolate might help in designing specific synthetic peptides and development of prophylactic vaccines or enhancing therapeutic drugs or vaccines against the hepatitis C virus. It may also be used to characterize the defensive response against the hepatitis C virus. The determined antigenic regions might prove useful for the development of new screening methods for HCV as well.

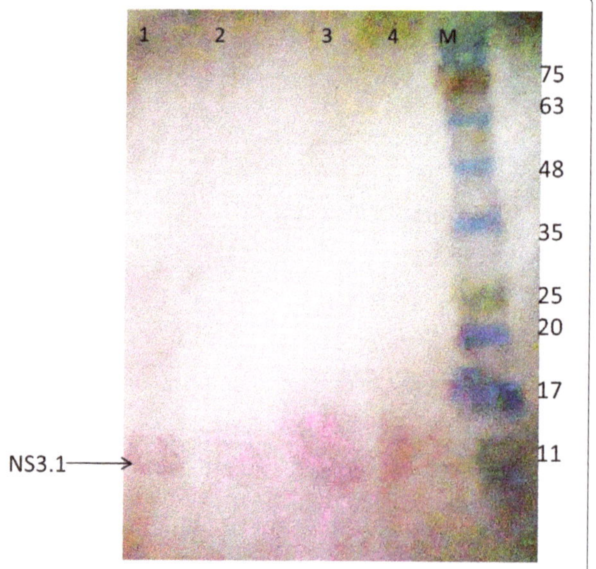

Fig. 8 NS3.1 antigenic site protein expressed in bacterial cells (vector-specific antibodies). Lanes 1–4: NS3.1 protein; M: prestained protein marker

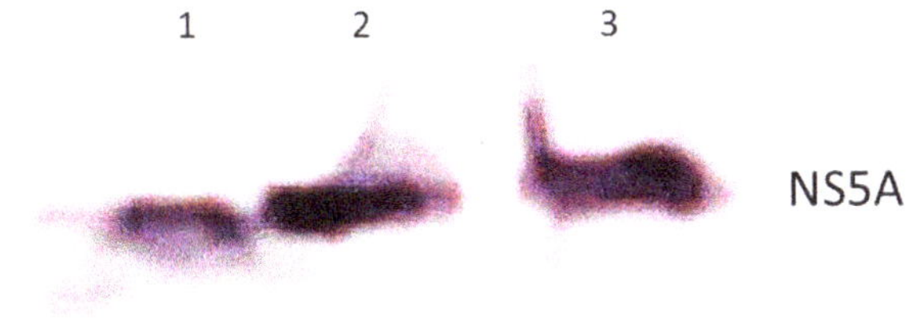

Fig. 9 NS5A.1 antigenic site protein expressed in bacterial cells (gene specific). Lanes 1–3: NS5A.1 antigenic protein

The regimens for HCV management mainly involved an early diagnosis of HCV infection. The quantification of HCV antigens (Ag) has been used for viral detection which also serves as a substitute for viral load estimation [16]. The determination of an appropriate antigenic site or epitope region is a prerequisite for the development of diagnostic approaches, medicines, and therapeutic drugs [17]. To improve the routinely used diagnostic procedures for HCV infection and to thwart the spread of this prevailing infection in the local population, this study was designed to determine the immunogenic or antigenic regions within the HCV non-structural genes (NS3 and NS5A). The determined antigenic regions are of high significance as these are implemented in ELSA-based diagnostics tests for HCV infection which gives more reliable and less false-positive results. The generated recombinant proteins might be used to develop screening assays for HCV infection and to develop certain vaccines. The available data also showed that the immunogenic region within the HCV genes is valuable to establish new screening techniques and the development of new therapeutic drugs [14, 16, 17]. Moreover, these results are also beneficial to analyze the genetic variability within the HCV non-structural genes (NS3 and NS5A) of Pakistani isolate which might be significant in HCV treatment through modeling of the HCV recombinant antigenic proteins.

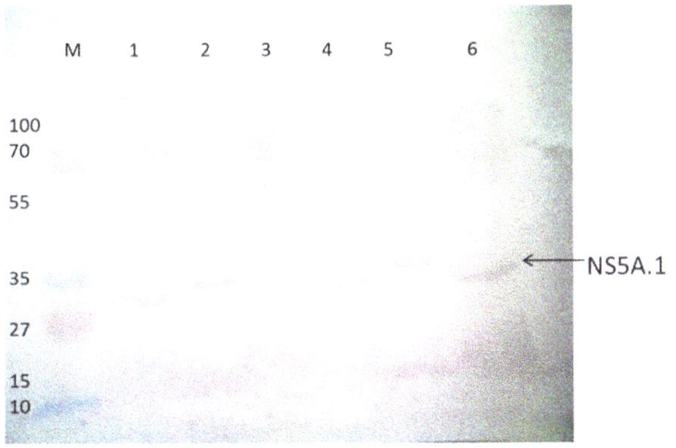

Fig. 10 NS5A.1 antigenic site protein expressed in bacterial cells (vector specific). Lanes 1, 2, 4, and 6: NS5A.1 antigenic protein; M: prestained protein marker

Conclusion

This study could help to enhance the progress in the treatment of HCV infection accompanied by the modeling of HCV non-structural genes (NS3 and NS5A) from a local isolate. It may also help characterize the viral genes as potential therapeutic targets for antiviral drugs or prophylactic vaccines.

Abbreviations

ATG: Adenine thymine guanine (methionine, a start codon); BL21DE3: An *E. coli* strain; cDNA: Complementary deoxyribonucleic acid; DNA: Deoxyribonucleic acid; EIAs: Enzyme immunoassays; ELSA: Ethical, legal and social aspects; HCV: Hepatitis C virus; IPTG: Isopropyl β-D-1-thiogalactopyranoside; LB medium: Luria Bertani medium; MIK: Methyl isobutyl ketone; NS3 gene: Hepatitis C virus non-structural protein 3 (HCV NS3); NS5A: Nonstructural protein 5A (NS5A); PCR: Polymerase chain reaction; RNA: Ribonucleic acid; ss: Single strand/single-stranded; SDS-PAGE: Sodium dodecyl sulfate polyacrylamide gel electrophoresis

Acknowledgements

The authors are thankful to Prof. Dr. Anjum Nasim Sabri for providing valuable suggestions to improve this manuscript.

Authors' contributions

All authors have read and approved the manuscript. SS, MIK, and AA take and analyze the data and format the manuscript. SR and MSK search the different databases for literature-selected literature and finalize the manuscript. The authors read and approved the final manuscript.

Declarations

Ethics approval and consent to participate

This study was approved by the ethical review board of the University of the Punjab, Lahore, Pakistan.

Competing interests

The authors declare that they have no competing interests.

Author details

[1]Department of Microbiology and Molecular Genetics, Faculty of Life Sciences, University of Okara, Okara 56130, Punjab, Pakistan. [2]Centre of Excellence and Molecular Biology, University of the Punjab, Lahore, Pakistan. [3]Department of Biotechnology and Genetic Engineering, Hazara University, Hazara, Pakistan. [4]Department of Zoology, Faculty of Life Sciences, University of Okara, Okara, Punjab 56130, Pakistan.

References

1. Ahmed T, Rahool O, Khattak N, Khan F, Din S, Muhammad Saleem K (2016) Prevalence of hepatitis B virus, hepatitis C virus and HIV in blood donors of different areas of Khyber Pukhtoonkhwa, Pakistan. JBES 9:304–309
2. John A, Ibrahim ZG, Magaji SY, Ede JS, Bello SA (2018) Hepatitis B and C: a twin silent killer. World J Pharm Res 3
3. Shahid I, AlMalki WH, AlRabia MW, Hafeez MH, Ahmed M (2017) Hepatitis C virus infection treatment: recent advances and new paradigms in the treatment strategies. Advances in Treatment of Hepatitis C and B:285
4. Suzuki T, Ishii K, Aizaki H, Wakita T (2007) Hepatitis C viral life cycle. Adv Drug Deliv Rev 59:1200–1212
5. Acosta-Rivero N, Poutou J, Alvarez-Lajonchere L, Guerra I, Aguilera Y, Musacchio A, Rodriguez A, Aguilar JC, Falcon V, Álvarez-Obregon JC (2009) Recombinant in vitro assembled hepatitis C virus core particles induce strong specific immunity enhanced by formulation with an oil-based

adjuvant. Biol Res 42:41–56
6. Agravat AH, Gamit MJ, Dhruva GA, Bhojani KR, Pujara KM (2015) Hepatitis C virus: screening, diagnosis, and interpretation of laboratory assays. Int J Curr Res 7:9
7. Gupta E, Bajpai M, Choudhary A (2014) Hepatitis C virus: screening, diagnosis, and interpretation of laboratory assays. Asian J Transfus Sci 8:19
8. Mehmood S, Raza H, Abid F, Saeed N, Rehan HM, Javed S, Khan MS (2019) National prevalence rate of hepatitis B and C in Pakistan and its risk factors. J Public Health 28:751–764
9. Kaukinen P, Sillanpää M, Nousiainen L, Melén K, Julkunen I (2013) Hepatitis C virus NS2 protease inhibits host cell antiviral response by inhibiting IKKε and TBK1 functions. J Med Virol 85:71–82
10. Rafik M, Bakr S, Soliman D, Mohammed N, Ragab D, ElHady WA, Samir N (2016) Characterization of differential antibody production against hepatitis C virus in different HCV infection status. Virol J 13:116
11. Sillanpää M, Melén K, Porkka P, Fagerlund R, Nevalainen K, Lappalainen M, Julkunen I (2009) Hepatitis C virus core, NS3, NS4B and NS5A are the major immunogenic proteins in humoral immunity in chronic HCV infection. Virol J 6:84
12. Kamili S, Drobeniuc J, Araujo AC, Hayden TM (2012) Laboratory diagnostics for hepatitis C virus infection. Clin Infect Dis 55:S43–S48
13. Richter SS (2002) Laboratory assays for diagnosis and management of hepatitis C virus infection. J Clin Microbiol 40:4407–4412
14. Bian Y, Zhao S, Zhu S, Zeng J, Li T, Fu Y, Wang Y, Zheng X, Zhang L, Wang W (2013) Significance of monoclonal antibodies against the conserved epitopes within non-structural protein 3 helicase of hepatitis C virus. PloS one
15. Sabri S, Idrees M, Rafique S, Ali A, Iqbal M, Studies on the role of NS3 and NS5A non-structural genes of Hepatitis C virus genotype 3a local isolate in apoptosis. Int J Infect Dis 2014;25:38–44
16. Florea D, Neaga E, Nicolae I, Maxim D, Popa M, Otelea D (2014) Clinical usefulness of HCV core antigen assay for the management of patients with chronic hepatitis C. J Gastrointestin Liver Dis 23:393–396
17. Rechkina E, Denisova G, Masalova O, Lideman L, Denisov D, Lesnova E, Ataullakhanov R, Gur'ianova S, Kushch A (2006) Epitope mapping of antigenic determinants of hepatitis C virus proteins by phage display. Mol Biol (Mosk) 40:357–368

30

B-type natriuretic peptide (BNP) in HCV-positive Egyptian patients: the impact of HCV eradication on plasma BNP levels

Ali Nada[1], Aliaa Sabry[1], Naglaa S. Elabd[2*], Azza M. Abdu Allah[3], Nada Elnaidany[4] and Mohamed Abbasy[1]

Abstract

Background: Chronic hepatitis C virus (HCV) infection represents a major health-related burden in Egypt. HCV is considered as a major cardiovascular risk factor. BNP (B-type natriuretic peptide) has been determined as a credible diagnostic and prognostic cardiac biomarker. We aimed to assess plasma BNP in HCV-positive Egyptian patients prior and after HCV eradication by direct-acting antiviral agents (DAAs) therapy. Eighty-nine chronic HCV-positive patients were enrolled in our prospective research. They were provided with DAAs therapy in the form of sofosbuvir and daclatasvir without or with ribavirin for 12 weeks. History, clinical evaluation, and laboratory assessment: CBC, liver and kidney function tests, viral markers (HCVAb, HBVsAg, and HIVAb) by ELISA, HCV RNA by real-time PCR, and BNP by ELISA were assessed. FIB-4 and aspartate aminotransferase-to-platelet ratio index (APRI) scores were ranked.

Results: Plasma BNP displayed a non-significant ($p = 0.124$) increase of its serum mean values in post eradication of HCV than its baseline values. Baseline BNP exhibited a significant positive correlation with FIB4 ($r = 0.411$, $P < 0.001$) and APRI score ($r = 0.418$, $p < 0.001$) with a considerably negative correlation with platelets ($r = -0.274$, $p = 0.009$), in addition to higher pretreatment BNP values in cirrhotic than in non-cirrhotic patients ($p < 0.001$), while non-significant relations were found regarding sex, BMI, and drug regimen (with or without ribavirin) ($p = 0.950$, 0.845, and 0.738, respectively). Additionally, plasma BNP values considerably decreased post-treatment in patients presented with higher baseline BNP values and more advanced liver disease (higher FIB4, APRI, and the presence of liver cirrhosis).

Conclusion: Our findings propose on the one side, the necessity of cardiac monitoring during chronic HCV infection and, on the other, the valuable impacts of HCV eradication on HCV-associated cardiac morbidities.

Keywords: BNP, HCV Patients, DAAs therapy

Background

About 185 million subjects are hepatitis C virus (HCV) infected, with an assessed 2.8% rise over the last decade globally. HCV has been evaluated to be the driving cause of worldwide cases of cirrhosis and hepatocellular carcinoma (HCC). HCV prevalence estimations differ greatly worldwide- and region-specific [1, 2]; however, the most noteworthy predominance has been recorded in China, Nigeria, Pakistan, Egypt, India, and Russia those together deemed for more than half of the overall infections [3].

In Egypt, chronic HCV infection is considered as a major health burden that influences about 14.7% of the Egyptian population [4]. Egypt's prevalence of active HCV infection is diverse regarding the region, with 8% being the highest in Menoufia. As stated by the reports of 2015 survey, other governorates with a rate of about ≥ 5% involved Menya, Dakhalia, Gharbia, Behera, Sharkia, Damietta, Beni Suef, and Fayoum [5]. However, a groundbreaking reduction of the HCV epidemic in Egypt has occurred with genotype 4-effective DAAs recently introduced to the treatment protocol; combinations of DAAs

* Correspondence: naglaa_elabd@yahoo.com
[2]Tropical Medicine Department, Faculty of Medicine- Menoufia University, Menoufia, Egypt
Full list of author information is available at the end of the article

have been documented to show high rates of sustained virological response (SVR) as well as a pan-genotypic clinical efficacy in HCV genotypes [6].

The availability of high effectiveness, clear applicability, and acceptable side effect profile of all-oral, direct-acting antiviral drugs encouraged HCV treatment in clinical practice [7]. Sofosbuvir (SOF), the first high-resistance barrier nucleotide NS5B polymerase inhibitor, was affirmed for interferon-free eradication of HCV infection in Europe and the USA at the beginning of 2014 [8].

In addition to the well-known deleterious impacts on the structure and function of the liver, chronic HCV infection is linked to other severe extra-hepatic manifestations. Moreover, chronic HCV infection has been related to enhanced incidence of (CAD) coronary artery disease [9], increased hazard of carotid artery plaques as well as carotid intima-media thickening [10] and cerebrovascular events, like stroke [11]. This indicates that chronic HCV infection could be likelihood deemed to be a cardiovascular hazard factor.

N-terminal proBNP (NT-proBNP) and brain natriuretic peptides or B-type natriuretic peptide (BNP) are predominantly natriuretic hormones produced by the heart ventricles. In general population, both biomarkers were identified as accurate diagnostic and prognostic cardiac markers that correlate with congestive heart failure (CHF) symptoms and the intensity of systolic and diastolic dysfunction [12].

The clinical cardiovascular diseases' presentations are gone before by an asymptomatic phase that can be lengthy and insidious, but cardiac biomarkers can be vital in detecting pathological developments during this period that can lead to clinical cardiac events. Biomarkers are valuable tools for risk stratification of patients for disease progression and for tracking the outcome of diseases in response to therapies. So in this study, we pursued to assess plasma BNP in HCV-positive Egyptian patients before and after sofosbuvir and daclatasvir with or without ribavirin therapy and to clear out the impact of HCV eradication on its levels.

Methods

The present work is a prospective research that was carried out on 89 chronic HCV participants. Patients were treatment-naive chronic HCV patients attended for HCV treatment clinic at the National Liver Institute (NLI) or outpatient clinic of Tropical Medicine Department, Faculty of Medicine, Menoufia University from August 2019 and December 2020. Patients were diagnosed by finding out HCV antibodies then assured by real-time PCR. They consisted of 26 males and 63females.

Patients included in this study were chosen as specified by the following criteria: age more than 18 years, positive HCV antibodies by ELISA that were assured by PCR for HCV RNA, treatment-naïve, and, additionally, patients with Child–Pugh score $\leq$ 8. All patients with HBV (hepatitis B virus) or HIV (human immunodeficiency virus) co-infection, renal impairment, hepatocellular carcinoma or any extra-hepatic malignancy, patients with DM or uncontrolled hypertension, cardiac patients, renal diseases, hyperthyroidism, and obese patients (BMI > or = 30) as well as pregnant females were precluded from the study.

For all patients, history was assessed together with detailed clinical evaluation including estimating BMI. Imaging valuation was performed for all participants by abdominal ultrasound. Laboratory evaluations, including complete blood count, liver function tests (prothrombin time and international normalized ratio (INR), alanine transaminase (ALT), aspartate transaminase (AST), serum total and direct bilirubin, and serum albumin), were investigated. Serum creatinine, fasting blood sugar, lipid profile, and α-fetoprotein were estimated. HCV antibodies, HBVsAg, and HIV antibodies were done by ELISA. HCV RNA level was quantitatively estimated by real-time PCR with a threshold for detection level 15 IU/mL. Plasma B-type natriuretic peptide (BNP) was assessed by ELISA. Upper GIT endoscopy was done when indicated.

For all participants, we calculated aspartate aminotransferase-to-platelet ratio index (APRI) as well as FIB-4 scores. APRI was estimated utilizing the subsequent formula: (AST/upper limit of normal)/platelet count (platelets $\times 10^9$ /L) $\times$ 100 [13], and FIB-4 score was estimated utilizing: age (y) $\times$ AST (IU/L)/platelet count ($\times 10^9$/L) $\times\sqrt{}$ALT (IU/L) formula [14].

Ethical approval

For all participants, an explanation about the study was provided together with informed consents obtained from each one before being enlisted in the study. The study was carried out after approval from the National Liver Institute Ethical Committee and according to the Helsinki Declaration.

HCV patients received DAAs therapy in the form of sofosbuvir 400 mg/day and daclatasvir 60 mg/day with or without ribavirin for 12 weeks according to the approved treatment recommendation (EASL) [15] and the national guidelines. During DAAs therapy, patients' follow-up was performed via clinical examination with lab re-evaluation including CBC and liver and kidney function tests at 4, 8, and 12 weeks of starting receiving DAAs therapy. RT-PCR was performed at the fourth week and at the end of treatment (EOT) and additionally, to determine SVR12, repeated 12 weeks after stopping treatment.

Sampling

Under entirely aseptic conditions and by means of venipuncture, 8 ml of venous blood was withdrawn from everyone included in the study following 8 h of fasting. In a sterile tube, 4 ml was left to clot and subsequently centrifuged at 3000 rpm for 15 min obtaining serum that is utilized to measure serum biochemical tests including ALT, AST, albumin, total bilirubin, fasting blood glucose (FBG), creatinine, AFP, and BNP. For the residual 4 ml of blood, 2 ml was obtained in citrated tubes for assessment of INR, and 2 ml was placed in EDTA tubes for estimation of platelets count, leukocytes, and hemoglobin, in addition to PCR for quantitative assessment of HCV.

Laboratory methods

Viral marker including HCVAb, HBVsAg, and HIVAb were performed utilizing "ECLIA" by Cobas 411 analyzers (Roche Diagnostics, Germany); furthermore, QIAGEN viral RNA Mini Extraction Kit was utilized in nucleic acid extraction for HCV real-time PCR. On Synchron CX9 autoanalyzer, biochemical tests for estimation of ALT, AST, albumin, total bilirubin, fasting blood glucose, and creatinine were performed by making use of kit provided by Beckman (Beckman Instrument Inc., Fullerton, CA, USA).

BNP assessment

Measurement of plasma BNP was carried out by the ELISA method, utilizing the kit provided by Sunred, China, Catalogue No. 201-12-1288 kit using a double-antibody sandwich enzyme-linked immunosorbent assay (ELISA).

Ultrasound of the abdomen

Liver assessment was performed in axial and longitudinal views while the patient was supine and in left lateral decubitus with estimation of the size and patency size of the portal vein (PV). Additionally, we examined patients in the supine as well as the right lateral decubitus for assessment of spleen size in bipolar diameter.

Statistical data analysis

Data of this study were supplied to the computer and analyzed utilizing IBM SPSS software package version 20.0. (Armonk, NY: IBM Corp). The Kolmogorov-Smirnov was used to verify the normality of variables distribution. Comparisons between groups for categorical variables were assessed using Marginal Homogeneity. Test used to analyze the significance between the different stages: Paired t test was assessed for comparison between two periods for normally distributed quantitative variables, while Wilcoxon signed ranks test was assessed for comparison between two periods for abnormally distributed quantitative variables. Kruskal Wallis test was used to compare different groups. For not normally distributed quantitative variables, the Mann Whitney test to compare between two groups was performed. For correlation between quantitative variables, Spearman coefficient was utilized. At the 5% level, significance of the gained results was judged.

Results

This study was carried out on 89 patients with chronic HCV participants, of which there were 26 (29.2%) males and 63 (70.8%) females, with age ranging between 27 and 65 with a mean age of 50.1 ± 9.9. All studied patients received treatment for 12 weeks (63 patients (70.8%) received SOF + DAC and 26 (29.2%) patients received SOF+DAC+RIB) and none of them needed dose modifications; in addition, they showed undetected HCV RNA in week 4, (EOT) end of treatment, and 12 weeks after stopping treatment (SVR12). The basic clinical, laboratory, imaging, and endoscopic data are presented in Table 1.

Comparisons of the assessed parameters prior and after treatment revealed that BMI was not significantly changed pre- and post-treatment (p = 0.446). Comparing laboratory investigations before and after treatment showed that ALT (p <0.001) and AST (p <0.001) were considerably decreased post-treatment; however, total bilirubin showed to have slightly increased and INR did not change post-treatment. CBC showed a non-significant decrease in platelet count and WBCs (p = 0.111 and 0.072, respectively) with significantly lower hemoglobin concentration (p < 0.001). In addition, FIB4 (p = 0.003) was considerably decreased where FIB4 < 1.45, 1.45–3.25, and >3.25 was 48.3%, 47.2%, and 4.5%, respectively, prior treatment, while, 57.3%, 42.7%, and 0%, respectively, post-treatment. Also, APRI score (p = 0.033) significantly differ with lower values post-treatment where APRI score < 0.5, 0.5–1.5, and >1.5 was 51.7%, 43.8%, and 4.5, respectively, prior treatment, while 58.4%, 41.6%, and 0%, respectively, as displayed in Table 2.

Estimation of the plasma BNP variations in studied patients prior and post eradication of HCV showed a non-significant (p = 0.124) increase of its plasma mean values in post-treatment than prior treatment 24.4 ± 25.6 and 21.4 ± 23.9, respectively (Table 2 and Fig. 1a).

Table 3 demonstrated correlation analysis, utilizing spearman coefficient, between pretreatment BNP levels and studied parameters where our results displayed significant positive correlations between BNP and FIB4 (r = 0.411, p < 0.001 and) and also with APRI score (r = 0.418, p < 0.001) together with a significant negative correlation between BNP and platelets (r = – 0.274, p = 0.009) as presented in Fig. 1b. However, no association was observed with other laboratory or imaging finding

Table 1 Distribution of the studied cases according to different clinical parameters (n = 89)

	No. (%)
Sex	
Male	26 (29.2%)
Female	63 (70.8%)
Age (years)	
Mean ± SD.	50.1 ± 9.9
Median (min.–max.)	50 (27–65)
BMI (kg/m^2)	
Mean ± SD.	26.9 ± 2
Median (min.–max.)	27.1(22.9–29.9)
HCV PCR	
Mean ± SD.	918883.5 ± 1228408
Median (min.–max.)	336000 (5592–5330000)
Liver echogenicity	
Normal	61 (68.5%)
Cirrhotic	28 (31.5%)
Spleen (US)	
Normal	79 (88.8%)
Enlarged	10 (11.2%)
FIB4 score	
Mean ± SD.	1.7 ± 0.9
Median (min.–max.)	1.5 (0.6–5.2)
APRI score	
Mean ± SD.	0.6 ± 0.4
Median (min.–max.)	0.5 (0.1–1.9)
Type of drugs	
SOF + DAC	63(70.8%)
SOF + DAC + RIB	26(29.2%)

SD standard deviation, *BMI* body mass index, *APRI score* aspartate aminotransferase-to-platelet ratio index score, *SOF* sofosbuvir, *DAC* daclatasvir, *RIB* ribavirin

and with studying the correlation analysis between post-treatment BNP levels with the same parameters, and a non-significant correlation was found.

Additionally, we observed that higher pretreatment BNP values were detected in patients with liver cirrhosis (mean was 31.9 ± 38.4) than in patients with normal liver echogenicity (mean was 16.6 ± 9.9) by US (p < 0.001). Furthermore, BNP levels increased with increasing FIB4 where its mean values were 13.7 ± 4.4, 22.7 ± 11.3, and 91.2 ± 85.8, respectively, with FIB4 < 1.45, 1.45–3.25, and > 3.25, respectively, and also with increasing APRI score where its mean values were 14.5 ± 5.1, 19.9 ± 6.3, and 115.1 ± 58.2, respectively, with APRI score < 0.5, 0.5–1.5, and > 1.5 respectively (Fig. 1c, d). No significant relations were found regarding sex, grade of BMI, and drug regimen (with or without ribavirin) (p = 0.950, 0.845, and 0.738, respectively. Also, we perceived that post-treatment BNP levels were not significantly related to the sex, BMI, the drug regimen, liver echogenicity, and FIB4 or APRI scores as presented in Table 4.

Interestingly, after calculating delta BNP that represent the change of BNP after HCV eradication (BNP after – BNP before treatment), we observed that delta BNP was not significantly correlated to age (r = 0.128 and p = 0.234), as well as being not related to sex, BMI, or drug regimen (p = 0.620, 0.150, and 0.698, respectively) (Fig. 2b). However, it was considerably related to liver echogenicity (p = 0.001) where delta BNP was – 12.8 ± 39.1 in patients with cirrhotic liver and 10.2 ± 34.7 in patients with normal liver echogenicity (Fig. 2a). Similarly, it was significantly related to FIB4 score (p <0.001), delta BNP in patients with FIB4 > 3.25 was – 67.6 ± 91.8 while that in < 1.45 FIB4 patients was 16.1 ± 38.5. Furthermore, delta BNP was considerably related to APRI score (p < 0.001) as delta BNP values in patients with APRI score > 1.5 and < 0.5, respectively, were – 96.3 ± 58.7 and 12.6 ± 37.5, respectively (Table 5 and Fig. 2c, d)

Discussion

Around 399,000 individuals die every year from HCV or from complications linked to its chronic infection including liver cirrhosis, liver failure, or hepatocellular carcinoma (HCC). Six major HCV genotypes have been identified in the Middle East and Africa including Egypt, HCV genotype 4 is the most prevalent [15].

Besides the widely known harmful effects of HCV on the liver structure and function, its chronic infection is connected with different extra-hepatic manifestations, such as glomerulonephritis, non-Hodgkin B cell lymphoma, mixed cryoglobulinemia, pulmonary fibrosis, autoimmune diseases, and ocular and dermatological diseases, whose mechanisms blamed in its pathogenesis are persistent immune system stimulation in addition to the tropism of the HCV virus for other tissues [16].

Moreover, chronic HCV has been also associated with higher risk of cardiovascular diseases. In reality, some authors have been hypothesized that chronic HCV infection could take part in the atheromatous process basically by means of increased oxidative stress, chronic inflammation, and insulin resistance (IR) as well as replication of HCV virus on the pre-existing plaques. Furthermore, few studies have investigated the potential hazardous effects of HCV infection on both right and left heart; nevertheless, the findings are conflicting. Hypertrophic and dilated cardiomyopathies have been depicted as extra-hepatic morbidity linked to chronic HCV; however, their true frequency is quiet unknown [17].

Compared to interferon-based therapy (IBT), DAAs have demonstrated outstanding efficacy safety and

Table 2 Comparison between pre and post-treatment according to different clinical and laboratory parameters

	Pre (n = 89)	Post (n = 89)	Test of sig.	P
BMI (kg/m^2)				
18.5–24.9	22(24.7%)	18(20.2%)	MH = 2.828	0.157
25.0–29.9	67(75.3%)	71(79.8%)		
Mean ± SD.	26.9 ± 2	26.8 ± 2.1	Z = 0.763	0.446
Median (min.–max.)	27.1(22.9–29.9)	27.1(20.7–29.4)		
Total bilirubin				
Mean ± SD.	0.9 ± 0.2	1.2 ± 0.2	Z = 6.922*	< 0.001*
Median (nin.–max.)	0.8 (0.6–1.6)	1.2 (0.7–1.6)		
INR				
Mean ± SD.	1.1 ± 0.1	1.1 ± 0.1	Z = 1.068	0.286
Median (min.–max.)	1 (1–1.4)	1 (1–1.3)		
ALT				
Mean ± SD.	49.3 ± 28.6	36.4 ± 7.6	Z = 7.237*	< 0.001*
Median (min.–max.)	45 (14–199)	36 (16–50)		
AST				
Mean ± SD.	44.7 ± 18	34.3 ± 7.3	Z = 7.003*	< 0.001*
Median (min.–max.)	43 (15–100)	34 (17–60)		
Creatinine				
Mean ± SD.	0.9 ± 0.2	1.0 ± 0.2	Z = 1.866	0.062
Median (min.–max.)	0.9 (0.6–1.4)	0.9 (0.6–1.6)		
FIB4				
< 1.45	43 (48.3%)	51 (57.3%)	MH = 28.0*	0.003*
1.45–3.25	42 (47.2%)	38 (42.7%)		
> 3.25	4 (4.5%)	0 (0%)		
Mean ± SD.	1.7 ± 0.9	1.6 ± 0.6	Z = 2.199*	0.028*
Median (min.–max.)	1.5 (0.6–5.2)	1.4 (0.7–3.0)		
APRI				
< 0.5	46 (51.7%)	52 (58.4%)	MH = 37.0*	0.033*
0.5 –1.5	39 (43.8%)	37 (41.6%)		
> 1.5	4 (4.5%)	0 (0%)		
Mean ± SD.	0.6 ± 0.4	0.5 ± 0.2	Z = 4.464*	< 0.001*
Median (min.–max.)	0.5 (0.1–1.9)	0.4 (0.1–0.9)		
HB				
Mean ± SD.	13.5 ± 1.4	12.6 ± 1.2	t = 7.009*	< 0.001*
Median (min.–max.)	13.7 (9–16)	12.6 (10–15.0)		
Platelet count				
Mean ± SD.	209 ± 65.3	199.3 ± 61.9	Z = 1.592	0.111
Median (min.–max.)	202 (83–478)	198 (101–417)		
WBCs				
Mean ± SD.	6.7 ± 1.8	6.1 ± 1.4	Z = 1.802	0.072
Median (min.–max.)	6.3 (3.6–10.3)	5.9(4.5–9.3)		
BNP level TTT				
Mean ± SD.	21.4 ± 23.9	24.4 ± 25.6	Z=1.536	0.124
Median (min.–max.)	16 (0.7–165.5)	18.4 (8.7–180.7)		
Delta BNP level	3 ± 37.5			

MH marginal homogeneity test, *t* paired *t* test, *Z* Wilcoxon signed ranks test, *SD* standard deviation, *p* p value for comparing between *pre* and *post*
BMI body mass index, *INR* international normalized ratio, *ALT* alanine aminotransferase, *AST* aspartate aminotransferase, *HB* hemoglobin concentration, *WBCs* white blood cells, *APRI score* aspartate aminotransferase-to-platelet ratio index score, *BNP* B-type natriuretic peptide, *delta BNP* BNP after – BNP before treatment
*Statistically significant at $p < 0.05$

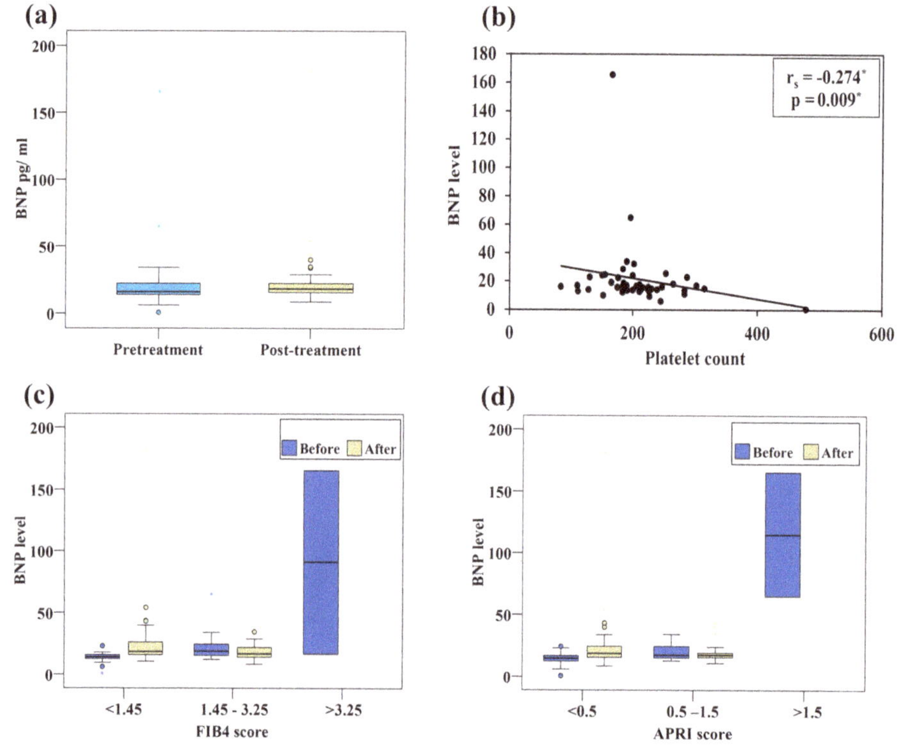

Fig. 1 **a** Comparison between plasma BNP levels pretreatment and post-treatment. **b** Correlation between plasma BNP levels and platelet count. **c** Relation between plasma BNP levels and pretreatment FIB4 score. **d** Relation between plasma BNP levels and pretreatment APRI score

Table 3 Correlation between BNP (before and after treatment) level and different laboratory parameters

	BNP level			
	Before (basal)		After	
	r_s	p	r_s	p
Age	– 0.131	0.222	0.184	0.085
Total bilirubin	0.134	0.210	0.0	1.000
Serum albumin	– 0.022	0.836	0.025	0.813
INR	0.064	0.553	0.045	0.672
ALT	0.052	0.627	– 0.142	0.185
AST	0.126	0.240	– 0.197	0.065
FIB4	0.531	<0.001*	– 0.071	0.506
APRI	0.474	<0.001*	– 0.174	0.102
HB	0.151	0.158	0.166	0.120
Platelet count	– 0.274	0.009*	– 0.098	0.361
WBC	0.023	0.831	– 0.098	0.361

r_s Spearman coefficient
INR international normalized ratio, *ALT* alanine aminotransferase, *AST* aspartate aminotransferase, *APRI score* aspartate aminotransferase-to-platelet ratio index score, *HB* hemoglobin concentration, *WBCs* white blood cells, *BNP* B-type natriuretic peptide
*Statistically significant at $p < 0.05$

revolutionized paradigms for HCV towards wider approaches for cure [18]. It has been shown that HCV virologic cure invariably diminish liver inflammation, indicated by improved aminotransferase levels and decreased rates of liver fibrosis progression. SVR also contributes to regression of liver cirrhosis and improves the clinical signs of portal hypertension as well as end-stage liver disease in some patients. Additionally, it has been reported eradication of HCV was linked with general improvement in extra-hepatic comorbidities such as cryoglobulinemia, insulin sensitivity, and non-Hodgkin's lymphoma [19]. However, few studies have investigated the effects of the DAAs on cardiovascular biomarkers after HCV elimination.

The aim of our study was to investigate plasma B-type natriuretic peptide (BNP) in chronic HCV Egyptian patients prior and after sofosbuvir and daclatasvir with or without ribavirin therapy and to highlight the effect of HCV eradication on plasma BNP levels.

The present study was performed on 89 chronic HCV participants; they received DAAs therapy in the form of sofosbuvir 400 mg/day and daclatasvir 60 mg/day with or without ribavirin for 12 weeks. All patients showed undetected HCV RNA in week 4, end of treatment (EOT), and SVR12. We observed that achieving SVR12 was associated with lowering ALT and AST levels, besides lowering of FIB-4 and

Table 4 Relation between BNP (before and after treatment) level and different parameters

	N	BNP level			
		Before		After	
		Median(min.–max.)	Mean ± SD.	Median(min.–max.)	Mean ± SD.
Sex					
Male	26	14.8(6.1–34)	18.2 ± 7.5	16.5(22.3 ± 12)	22.3 ± 12
Female	63	16.2(0.7–165.5)	22.8 ± 28	18.5(8.7–180.7)	25.2 ± 29.5
U(*p*)		812.0(0.950)		742.0(0.487)	
BMI					
18.5–24.9	22	15.8(6.1–84.8)	20.3 ± 15.4	16.9(13.4–23.9	17.1 ± 3.1
25.0–29.9	67	16.2(0.7–165.5)	21.8 ± 26.2	18.6(8.7–180.7)	26.2 ± 28.4
U(*p*)		716.50(0.845)		464.50(0.075)	
Type drug					
SOF + AC	63	15.8(0.7–64.8)	18.8 ± 10.6	18.6(10.8–180.7)	26.2 ± 27.9
SOF + DAC + RIB	26	16.9(6.1–165.5)	27.7 ± 40.9	16.7(8.7–43.4)	20 ± 9.7
U(*p*)		782.0(0.738)		668.0(0.173)	
FIB4					
< 1.45	43	14.2(0.7–22.9)	13.7 ± 4.4	18.8(10.8–180.7)	28.9 ± 32.9
1.45–3.25	42	19.2(12.5–64.8)	22.7 ± 11.3	17.5(8.7–34.5)	18.4 ± 6
> 3.25	4	91.2(16.9–165.5)	91.2 ± 85.8	–	–
H(p)		27.925*(<0.001*)		760.0(0.083)	
APRI					
< 0.5	46	14.8(0.7–241)	14.5 ± 5.1	18.8(8.7–180.7)	27.5 ± 32.5
0.5–1.5	39	17.6(12.8–34)	19.9 ± 6.3	17.1(10.8–43.4)	20.1 ± 8.8
> 1.5	4	115.1(64.8–165.5)	115.1 ± 58.2	–	–
H(p)		24.899*(<0.001*)		807.0(0.197)	
Liver echogenicity					
Cirrhosis	28	23.5(6.1–165.5)	31.9 ± 38.4	17.2(8.7–34.5)	19.1 ± 6.5
Normal	61	14.8(0.7–64.8)	16.6 ± 9.9	18.6(10.8–180.7)	26.8 ± 30.4
U(*p*)		336.0(<0.001*)		746.0(0.340)	

U Mann Whitney test, *H* H for Kruskal Wallis test, *p* p value for association between different categories
BMI body mass index, *SOF* sofosbuvir, *DAC* daclatasvir, *RIB* ribavirin, *APRI score* aspartate aminotransferase-to-platelet ratio index score
*Statistically significant at $p \leq 0.05$

APRI scores, and this was agreed with previous reports [20].

BNP as well as other structurally linked peptides, which are C-type natriuretic peptide (CNP), atrial natriuretic peptide (ANP), and urodilatin, is a member of the natriuretic peptide family. The natriuretic peptides possess a typical biochemical structure consisting of a 17 amino acid ring together with a bridge of disulfide in-between two molecules of cysteine. It was found that the ventricular myocardium is considered to be the main source of BNP synthesis and secretion. ANP is stowed in granules, and after stimulation, it could be released immediately, while only little amounts of BNP are stowed in granules and the implied mechanism for the organization of BNP secretion is speedy gene expression accompanied by de novo synthesis of the peptide. It was reported that BNP is synthesized as a prohormone (proBNP) containing 108 amino acids. When proBNP is released in the circulation, it is cleaved to egalitarian proportions into the biologically active 32 amino acid BNP, which represents the C-terminal part and a 76 amino acid N-terminal part that is biologically inactive [21].

Myocardial wall stress was notified to be the crucial stimulus for increasing the synthesis and secretion of BNP and NT-proBNP. Additionally, other stimulating agents like cytokines, myocardial ischaemia, and endocrine (paracrine) modulation by other neurohormones are also essential [21].

We displayed noteworthy outcomes, where overall plasma BNP changes in studied HCV patients prior and post eradication of HCV showed a non-significant difference of its plasma mean values in post-treatment compared to prior treatment indicating, to some extent, the

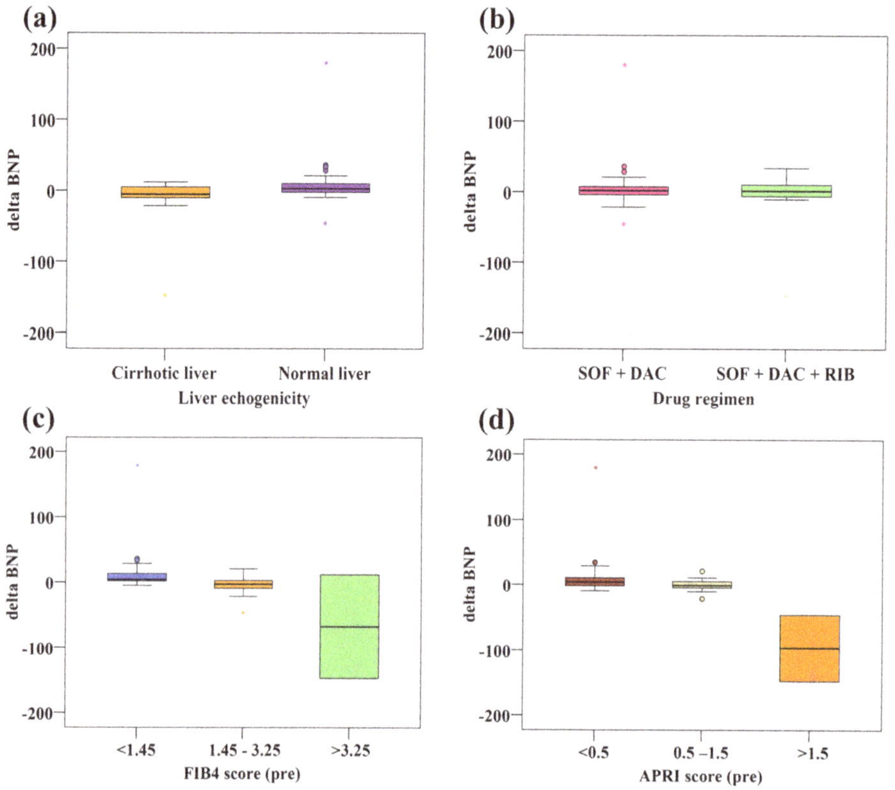

Fig. 2 **a** Relation between delta BNP and echogenicity of the liver. **b** Relation between delta BNP and drug regimen (with and without ribavirin). **c** Relation between delta BNP and pretreatment FIB4 score. **d** Relation between delta BNP and pretreatment APRI score

cardiovascular safety of used drugs. These results were in accordance with previous literature, where mean values of BNP were found to be not changed before and 3 months after HCV eradication [22].

In a former study, it was stated that plasma BNP offers prognostic details in chronic heart failure patients as well as in patients with asymptomatic or symptomatic left ventricular dysfunction [23]. Furthermore, it has been shown that plasma NT-proBNP independently foretells long-term death risk due to congestive heart failure [12]. In the general population, both biomarkers were identified as accurate diagnostic and prognostic cardiac markers that correlate with both CHF symptoms and the severity of systolic and diastolic dysfunction [24]. Moreover, these biomarkers have been shown to be associated with the extent of circulatory dysfunction in patients with liver cirrhosis [25].

In the present study we noticed a non-significant relation found between BNP levels and BMI. These results disagree with those of Wang and his colleagues who have elucidated a consistent inverse relationship between circulating BNP levels and BMI [26]. This difference can be attributed to the difference in the population samples as they classified the patients as obese defined as having a BMI of 30 or greater and non-obese with BMI less than 30. We planned in our study to exclude patients with BMI equal or more than 30 to evade the influence of obesity on BNP levels.

Our study demonstrated significant positive correlations among BNP levels and FIB4 and APRI scores together with a considerable negative correlation among BNP levels and platelets. Additionally, we observed that higher baseline BNP levels were detected in patients with liver cirrhosis than in patients with normal liver echogenicity.

A body of evidence suggests that the impact of HCV-associated inflammation on cardiovascular risk could be higher in patients with more liver damage. The profibrogenic and proinflammatory environment driving liver fibrogenesis in HCV patients may likewise be systemically activated, over and above enhancing the development of cardiovascular lesions [27]. Consistent with these data, a cohort study has found that chronic HCV patients with higher liver stiffness values had a substantial hazard for development of cardiovascular events compared to those with lower stiffness values [28]. Additionally, Maruyama and his colleagues have reported that in chronic HCV patients a considerable link was present between myocardial injury and both the severity of necroinflammatory activity and subsequent liver

Table 5 Relation between delta BNP and different parameters

	N	delta in BNP		Test of sig.	*p*
		Median (min.–max.)	Mean ± SD.		
Sex					
Male	26	1.7(− 21–35.9)	4.2 ± 14.1	*U* = 764.0	0.620
Female	63	1.9(− 147.1–180)	2.5 ± 43.7		
BMI (pre)					
18.5–24.9	22	− 1.2(− 45.4–10.4)	− 3.5 ± 14.2	*U* = 585.0	0.150
25.0–29.9	67	3.2(− 147.1–180.0)	5.1 ± 42.3		
Normal liver					
No	28	− 5.4(− 147.1–11.9)	− 12.8 ± 39.1	*U* = 492.0*	0.001*
Yes	61	2.8(− 45.4–180)	10.2 ± 34.7		
Type drug					
SOF + DAC	63	1.9(− 45.4–180)	7.4 ± 34.6	*U* = 776.0	0.698
SOF + DAC + RIB	26	1.5(− 147.1–33.9)	− 7.7 ± 42.6		
FIB4 (pre)					
< 1.45	43	3.9(− 5–180)	16.1 ± 38.5	*H* = 18.428*	< 0.001*
1.45–3.25	42	− 2.9(− 45.4–20.7)	− 3.7 ± 13.1		
> 3.25	4	− 67.6(− 147.1–11.9)	− 67.6 ± 91.8		
APRI (pre)					
< 0.5	46	3.9(− 9.5–180)	12.6 ± 37.5	*H* = 15.741*	< 0.001*
0.5–1.5	39	− 1(− 21–35.9)	1.8 ± 12.8		
> 1.5	4	− 96.3(− 147.1–− 45.4)	− 96.3 ± 58.7		

U Mann Whitney test, *H H* for Kruskal Wallis test, *p p* value for association between different categories
BMI body mass index, *SOF* sofosbuvir, *DAC* daclatasvir, *RIB* ribavirin, *APRI score* aspartate aminotransferase-to-platelet ratio index score
*Statistically significant at $p \leq 0.05$

damage [29]. Several factors were also suggested to mediate the link between HCV infection and risk of CVD development including augmented oxidative stress, modified iron homeostasis, activation of immunological, and/or inflammatory processes leading to a disrupted cytokine imbalance as well as induction of hepatic steatosis, a risk factor in insulin sensitivity and related metabolic abnormalities [30].

To the best of our knowledge, there were no considerable data available demonstrating the correlations between the change in BNP levels and the severity of liver disease. In our study, we observed that delta BNP was considerably related to liver echogenicity where BNP was significantly decreased in patients with advanced liver disease as determined by pretreatment presence of liver cirrhosis and higher FIB4 or APRI scores than its baseline values before starting treatment, as we previously reported that these patients showed baseline higher BNP levels. These results reflected the beneficial cardiac effects of HCV eradication as one of its extra-hepatic manifestations.

It was formerly illustrated by Dalbeni and his colleagues that HCV is accountable for cardiac and vascular remodeling via direct cytotropic toxicity in addition to an indirect immune-mediated mechanism, most likely both are eliminated when HCV is eradicated. Moreover, they found that in participants with a detectable high cytokines concentration, they observed a significant decrease of TNF-α [17]. TNF-α has been considered to be a potent proinflammatory molecule, which is associated with cardio-toxic effect, is secreted via the activated monocytes and macrophages in response to diverse infections. It stimulates the release of acute phase proteins in the liver driving lymphocyte and endothelial activation [31]; however, Dalbeni et al. found non-significant differences in mean values of both HS-TnT and NT-proBNP as cardiac biomarkers between pretreatment and post-treatment [17]. The difference in the results of cardiac biomarkers and those we obtained may be related to the biomarker used as well as they did not calculate the delta BNP for correlating it with baseline levels or degree of liver disease

Conclusion

Our findings propose on the one side the necessity of cardiac monitoring during chronic HCV infection and, on the other, the valuable impacts of HCV eradication on HCV-associated cardiac morbidities. In spite of our finding of a non-significant change of plasma BNP levels in post eradication of HCV compared to its baseline values, we noticed that plasma BNP values were considerably decreased post-treatment in patients presented with higher baseline BNP values and more advanced liver disease (higher FIB4, APRI, and the presence of liver cirrhosis). Given the burden of chronic hepatitis C virus infection both nationally and internationally, there is an imperative requirement to assess the worth of cardiac biomarkers that may potentially help define cardiovascular benefits of HCV eradication among HCV-infected patients more precisely and by long-term follow-up.

We acknowledge that the results were analyzed with a relatively small cohort; therefore, to implement a practical policy in real-life settings, studies with larger cohorts are a must with long-term follow-up.

Abbreviations

BNP: B-type natriuretic peptide; HCV: Hepatitis C virus; HBV: Hepatitis B virus; HIV: Human immunodeficiency virus; HCC: Hepatocellular carcinoma; SVR: Sustained virological response; CAD: Coronary artery disease; CHF: Congestive heart failure; INR: International normalized ratio; ALT: Alanine transaminase; AST: Aspartate transaminase; APRI: Aspartate aminotransferase-to-platelet ratio index; EOT: End of treatment; ELISA: Enzyme-linked immunosorbent assay

Acknowledgements

Not applicable.

Authors' contributions

All authors contributed in the conception and designing of the work. NE and AN were the major contributors in writing and revision of the manuscript. AA contributed in the interpretation of the laboratory data including BNP. AN, AS, NE, and MA contributed in the collection of clinical data about HCV patients. NE corrected and edited the manuscript. The authors have read and approved the final manuscript.

Declarations

Ethics approval and consent to participate

The study was carried out after approval from the National Liver Institute Ethical Committee, Menoufia University, Egypt, with ethics committee reference number NLI IRB 00003413. For all participants, an explanation about the study was provided together with informed written consent was obtained from each one before enlisted in the study.

Competing interests

The authors declare that they have no competing interests.

Author details

[1]Hepatology, Gastroenterology Department, National Liver Institute, Menoufia University, Menoufia, Egypt. [2]Tropical Medicine Department, Faculty of Medicine- Menoufia University, Menoufia, Egypt. [3]Medical Biochemistry and Molecular Biology Department, Faculty of Medicine-Menoufia University, Menoufia, Egypt. [4]Faculty of Pharmacy, MSA University, 6th of October City, Egypt.

References

1. Mohd Hanafiah K, Groeger J, Flaxman AD, Wiersma ST (2013) Global epidemiology of hepatitis C virus infection: new estimates of age specific antibody to HCV seroprevalence. Hepatology (Baltimore, Md) 57(4):1333–1342
2. Petruzziello A, Marigliano S, Loquercio G, Cozzolino A, Cacciapuoti C (2016) Global epidemiology of hepatitis C virus infection: an up-date of the distribution and circulation of hepatitis C virus genotypes. World J Gastroenterol 22(34):7824–7840
3. Gower E, Estes C, Blach S, Razavi-Shearer K, Razavi H (2014) Global epidemiology and genotype distribution of the hepatitis C virus infection. J Hepatol 61(1 Suppl):S45–S57
4. Elgharably A, Gomaa AI, Crossey MM, Norsworthy PJ, Waked I, Taylor-Robinson SD (2016) Hepatitis C in Egypt - past, present, and future. Int J Gen Med 10:1–6
5. Egypt Health Issues Survey (2015) Ministry of health and population [Egypt], El-Zanaty and associates [Egypt], and ICF International. Ministry of Health and Population and ICF International, Cairo and Rockville
6. Omran D, Alboraie M, Zayed RA, Wifi MN, Naguib M, Eltabbakh M, Abdellah M, Sherief AF, Maklad S, Eldemellawy HH, Saad OK, Khamiss DM, El Kassas M (2018) Towards hepatitis C virus elimination: Egyptian experience, achievements and limitations. World J Gastroenterol 24(38):4330–4340
7. Welzel TM, Dultz G, Zeuzem S (2014) Interferon-free antiviral combination therapies without nucleosidic polymerase inhibitors. J Hepatol 61(1 Suppl): S98–S107. https://doi.org/10.1016/j.jhep.2014.08.014 [Cross Ref] [PubMed] [Google Scholar]
8. Sovaldi (sofosbuvir) prescribing information. Foster City: Gilead Sciences, 2014. http://www.gilead.com/~/media/Files/pdfs/medicines/liver-disease/sovaldi/sovaldi_pi.pdf. [Google Scholar]
9. Vassalle C, Masini S, Bianchi F, Zucchelli GC (2004) Evidence for association between hepatitis C virus seropositivity and coronary artery disease. Heart. 90:565–566
10. Ishizaka N, Ishizaka Y, Takahashi E et al (2002) Association between hepatitis C virus seropositivity, carotid-artery plaque, and intima-media thickening. Lancet (London, England) 359:133–135
11. Liao C-C, Su T-C, Sung F-C, Chou W-H, Chen T-L (2012) Does hepatitis C virus infection increase risk for stroke? A population-based cohort study. PLoS One 7:e31527
12. Doust JA, Glasziou PP, Pietrzak E, Dobson AJ (2004) A systemic review of the diagnostic accuracy of naturetic peptides for heart failure. Arch Intern Med 164(18):1978–1984 [PubMed] [Google Scholar]
13. Wai CT, Greenson JK, Fontana RJ et al (2003) A simple noninvasive index can predict both significant fibrosis and cirrhosis in patients with chronic hepatitis C. Hepatology 38:518–526 [PubMed] [Google Scholar]
14. Sterling RK, Lissen E, Clumeck N et al (2006) APRICOT Clinical Investigators. Development of a simple noninvasive index to predict significant fibrosis in patients with HIV/HCV coinfection. Hepatology 43:1317–1325 [PubMed] [Google Scholar]
15. Doss W, Shiha G, Hassany M, Soliman R, Fouad R, Khairy M, Samir W, Hammad R, Kersey K, Jiang D, Doehle B, Knox SJ, Massetto B, McHutchison JG, Esmat G (2015) Sofosbuvir plus ribavirin for treating Egyptian patients with hepatitis C genotype 4. J Hepatol 63(3):581–585. https://doi.org/10.1016/j.jhep.2015.04.023 Epub 2015 May 1. PMID: 25937436
16. Rosenthal E, Cacoub P (2015) Extrahepatic manifestations in chronic hepatitis C virus carriers. Lupus. 24:469–482
17. Dalbeni A, Romano S, Bevilacqua M, Piccoli A, Imbalzano E, Mantovani A, Benati M, Montagnana M, Donato A, Torin G, Monaco C, Cattazzo F, Tagetti A, Paon V, Ieluzzi D, Iogna Prat L, Roccarina D, Ribichini F, Capra F, Minuz P, Fava C (2020) Beneficial effects of DAAs on cardiac function and structure in hepatitis C patients with low-moderate liver fibrosis. J Viral Hepat 27(11): 1214–1221. https://doi.org/10.1111/jvh.13355 Epub 2020 Aug 13. PMID: 32593212
18. Afdhal NH, Zeuzem S, Schooley RT, Thomas DL, Ward JW et al (2013) The new paradigm of hepatitis C therapy: integration of oral therapies into best practices. J Viral Hepat 20:745–760 DOI PubMed PMC
19. Hsu Y-C, Ho HJ, Huang Y-T et al (2015) Association between antiviral treatment and extrahepatic outcomes in patients with hepatitis C virus infection. Gut. 64:495–503

20. Tada T, Kumada T, Toyoda H, Mizuno K, Sone Y, Kataoka S et al (2017) Improvement of liver stiffness in patients with hepatitis C virus infection who received direct-acting antiviral therapy and achieved sustained virological response. J Gastroenterol Hepatol 32:1982–1988
21. Weber M, Hamm C (2006) Role of B-type natriuretic peptide (BNP) and NT-proBNP in clinical routine. Heart 92(6):843–849. https://doi.org/10.1136/hrt.2005.071233 PMID: 16698841; PMCID: PMC1860679
22. Alaarag AF, Hamam AM, Amin OA (2021) The safety of the directly acting antiviral treatment for hepatitis C virus according to the Egyptian National Program Protocol in patients with midrange ejection fraction. Glob Heart 16:3. https://doi.org/10.5334/gh.906
23. Tsutamoto T, Wada A, Maeda K et al (1999) Plasma brain natriuretic peptide level as a biochemical marker of morbidity and mortality in patients with asymptomatic or minimally symptomatic left ventricular dysfunction. Comparison with plasma angiotensin II and endothelin-1. Eur Heart J 20(24): 1799–1807 Cross ref CAS PubMed Web of Science® Google Scholar
24. Clerico A, Emdin M (2004) Diagnostic accuracy and prognostic relevance of the measurement of cardiac naturetic peptides: a review. Clin Chem 50(1): 33–50 Crossref, CAS, PubMed, Web of Science®, Google Scholar
25. Henriksen JH, Gotze JP, Fuglsang S, Christensen E, Bendtsen F, Moller S (2003) Increased circulating pro-brain natriuretic peptide (proBNP) and brain natriuretic peptide (BNP) in patients with cirrhosis: relation to cardiovascular dysfunction and severity of disease. Gut 52(10):1511–1517 Crossref, CAS, PubMed, Web of Science®, Google Scholar
26. Wang TJ, Larson MG, Levy D, Benjamin EJ, Leip EP, Wilson PW, Vasan RS (2004) Impact of obesity on plasma natriuretic peptide levels. Circulation 109(5):594–600 [PubMed] [Ref list]
27. Petta S (2017) Hepatitis C virus and cardiovascular: a review. J Adv Res 8(2): 161–168. https://doi.org/10.1016/j.jare.2016.06.001
28. Cacoub P, Gragnani L, Comarmond C, Zignego AL (2014) Extrahepatic manifestations of chronic hepatitis C virus infection. Dig Liver Dis 46(suppl 5):S165–S173 [PubMed] [Google Scholar]
29. Maruyama S, Koda M, Oyake N, Sato H, Fujii Y, Horie Y (2013) Myocardial injury in patients with chronic hepatitis C infection. J Hepatol 58:11–15 [PubMed] [Google Scholar]
30. Badawi A, Di Giuseppe G, Arora P (2018) Cardiovascular disease risk in patients with hepatitis C infection: results from two general population health surveys in Canada and the United States (2007-2017). PLoS One 13(12):e0208839. Published 2018 Dec 12. https://doi.org/10.1371/journal.pone.0208839
31. Tracey KJ, Cerami A (1994) Tumor necrosis factor: a pleiotropic cytokine and therapeutic target. Annu Rev Med 45:491–503

Permissions

All chapters in this book were first published by Springer; hereby published with permission under the Creative Commons Attribution License or equivalent. Every chapter published in this book has been scrutinized by our experts. Their significance has been extensively debated. The topics covered herein carry significant findings which will fuel the growth of the discipline. They may even be implemented as practical applications or may be referred to as a beginning point for another development.

The contributors of this book come from diverse backgrounds, making this book a truly international effort. This book will bring forth new frontiers with its revolutionizing research information and detailed analysis of the nascent developments around the world.

We would like to thank all the contributing authors for lending their expertise to make the book truly unique. They have played a crucial role in the development of this book. Without their invaluable contributions this book wouldn't have been possible. They have made vital efforts to compile up to date information on the varied aspects of this subject to make this book a valuable addition to the collection of many professionals and students.

This book was conceptualized with the vision of imparting up-to-date information and advanced data in this field. To ensure the same, a matchless editorial board was set up. Every individual on the board went through rigorous rounds of assessment to prove their worth. After which they invested a large part of their time researching and compiling the most relevant data for our readers.

The editorial board has been involved in producing this book since its inception. They have spent rigorous hours researching and exploring the diverse topics which have resulted in the successful publishing of this book. They have passed on their knowledge of decades through this book. To expedite this challenging task, the publisher supported the team at every step. A small team of assistant editors was also appointed to further simplify the editing procedure and attain best results for the readers.

Apart from the editorial board, the designing team has also invested a significant amount of their time in understanding the subject and creating the most relevant covers. They scrutinized every image to scout for the most suitable representation of the subject and create an appropriate cover for the book.

The publishing team has been an ardent support to the editorial, designing and production team. Their endless efforts to recruit the best for this project, has resulted in the accomplishment of this book. They are a veteran in the field of academics and their pool of knowledge is as vast as their experience in printing. Their expertise and guidance has proved useful at every step. Their uncompromising quality standards have made this book an exceptional effort. Their encouragement from time to time has been an inspiration for everyone.

The publisher and the editorial board hope that this book will prove to be a valuable piece of knowledge for researchers, students, practitioners and scholars across the globe.

List of Contributors

Rania Nabil Bedair, Gehan M. Magour, Eman M. Amar and Ahmed Mostafa Awad
Chemical Pathology Department, Medical Research Institute, Alexandria University, Alexandria, Egypt

Said Ahmed Ooda
Department of Experimental and Clinical Internal Medicine, Medical Research Institute, University of Alexandria, Alexandria, Egypt

Heba M. Adel Abou Zaghla, Aziza Ahmed El Sebai, Ayat Fawzy Ahmed and Azza Abdel Rahman Saab
Clinical Pathology, Ain Shams University, Cairo, Egypt

Nahla Mohamed Teama, Waleed Anwar Abdel-Mohsen and Sarah Mohamed El Sayed
Department of Internal Medicine and Nephrology, Faculty of Medicine, Ain Shams University, Ramsis 38 Street, Abassia, Cairo 11211, Egypt

Ossama Ashraf Ahmed and Ahmed Mohamed ElGhandour
Department of Internal Medicine and Gastroenterology, Faculty of Medicine, Ain Shams University, Cairo, Egypt

Mohy-Eldin Abd-Elfattah and Mohammed Elkheer
Bioorganic Chemistry Department, Faculty of Science, Suez Canal University, Sheikh Zayed City, Ismailia 42524, Egypt

Mary Naguib
Clinical Pathology Department, National Liver Institute, Menoufia University, Shibin El Kom, Egypt

Eman Abdelsameea and Ali Nada
Hepatology and Gastroenterology Department, National Liver Institute, Menoufia University, Shibin El Kom, Egypt

Inas E L-Khedr Mohamed, Kadry Mohamed EL-Saeed and Christina Alphonse Anwar
Gastro-enterology and Hepatology Faculty of Medicine, Ain Shams University, Cairo, Egypt

Mahmoud Hassan Al-Sadik
Abbassia Fever Hospital, Cairo, Egypt

Asmaa M. Elbrolosy and Emad M. Eed
Department of Medical Microbiology and Immunology, Faculty of Medicine, Menoufia University, Shibin El Kom, Egypt

Moamena S. Elhamouly and Naglaa S. Elabd
Department of Tropical Medicine, Faculty of Medicine, Menoufia University, Shibin El Kom, Egypt

Gamalat A. El Gedawy
Department of Clinical Biochemistry and Molecular Diagnostics, National Liver Institute, Menoufia University, Shibin El Kom, Egypt

Mai Abozeid
Department of Hepatology and Gastroenterology, National Liver Institute, Menoufia University, Shibin El Kom, Egypt

Nancy Abdel Fattah Ahmed
Mansoura Specialized Medical Hospital, Internal Medicine Department Hepatology & Gastroenterology Unit, Faculty of Medicine, Mansoura University, Mansoura, Egypt

Ahmed Shawky Hassan Ali and Islam Abd El-Hamid El-Zayyadi
Specialized Medical Hospital, Internal Medicine Department, Faculty of Medicine, Mansoura University, Mansoura, Egypt

Rizk Ahmed El Baz
Genetic Unit, Pediatric Hospital, Faculty of Medicine, Mansoura University, Mansoura, Egypt

Amira Isaac, Basant Elmarashly, Kadry El Saeed, Rasha Samir Mohamed and Eslam Safwat
Department of Internal Medicine, Gastroenterology and Hepatology Unit, Faculty of Medicine, Ain Shams University, Cairo 11566, Egypt

Shereen Abdelmonem Ibrahim
Department of Clinical Pathology, Faculty of Medicine, Ain Shams University, Cairo 11566, Egypt

Reham A. Aboelwafa and Marwa A. Gamaleldin
Clinical Pathology Department, Faculty of Medicine, Alexandria University, Alexandria, Egypt

Marwa A. Saad
Internal medicine department, Faculty of Medicine, Alexandria University, Alexandria, Egypt

Nermine Ehsan and Dina Sweed
Pathology Department, National Liver Institute, Menofia University, Shibin El-Kom 32511, Egypt

Maha Elsabaawy
Hepatology and Gastroenterology Department, National Liver Institute, Menofia University, Shibin El-Kom, Egypt

Helmy Elshazly, Hasan Zaghlah, El-Sayed Tharwa and Ahmed Abuamer
Hepatology and Gastroenterology Department, National Liver Institute, Menoufia University, Menoufia, Egypt

Dina Nor-Eldin
Tanta Fever Hospital, Tanta, Gharbiah, Egypt

Reem El Sheemy
Tropical Medicine Department, Faculty of Medicine, Minia University, Minya, Egypt

Mohamed El Kassas
Endemic Medicine Department, Faculty of Medicine, Helwan University, Ain Helwan, Cairo 11795, Egypt

Ayman El-Shayeb, Sawsan El-Mallah, Samar El-Hewely and Doaa Elwazzan
Tropical Medicine Department, Faculty of Medicine, Alexandria University, Alexandria, Egypt

Akram Deghady
Clinical Pathology Department, Faculty of Medicine, Alexandria University, Alexandria, Egypt

Ayman El Shayeb, Essam Saeed Bedewy, Sahar Badawy and Nermeen Abdeen
Tropical Medicine Department, Faculty of Medicine, Alexandria University, Alexandria, Egypt

Akram Deghedy
Clinical Pathology Department, Faculty of Medicine, Alexandria University, Alexandria, Egypt

Iman S. Naga
Department of Microbiology, Medical Research Institute, University of Alexandria, Alexandria, Egypt

Amel Abdel Fattah Kamel, Hadeer Muhammad Fath Elbab and Rania Mohamed El-Sharkawy
Department of Chemical Pathology, Medical Research Institute, University of Alexandria, Alexandria, Egypt

Elsayed Ghoneem, Ahmed Saleh and Shahira Aly El-Etreby
Department of Internal Medicine, Hepatology & Gastroenterology Unit, Faculty of Medicine, Mansoura University, Mansoura, Egypt

Metwaly Ibrahim Mortada and Mayada A. Ghannam
Department of Clinical Pathology, Hematology Unit, Faculty of Medicine, Mansoura University, Mansoura, Egypt

Shaimaa El-Ashwah and Noha Eisa
Department of Clinical Hematology, Oncology Center Mansoura University (OCMU), Faculty of Medicine, Mansoura University, Mansoura, Egypt

Amira Isaac, Khaled Hamdy Abd El-Mageed, Hany Haroun Kaisar, Hany Samir Rasmy, Ramy Samir Abd Elhamid Ghait, Ibrahim Magdy Ibrahim and George Safwat Riad
Internal Medicine Department, Hepatology and Gastroenterology Department, Faculty of medicine, Ain Shams University, Cairo, Egypt

Waleed Mohamed Serag
Faculty of Science, Suez University, Suez, Egypt

Basem Eysa Elsayed
National Hepatology and Tropical Medicine Research Institute, Cairo, Egypt

Sadia Rafique, Muhammad Wajid, Ahmad Waheed and Ali Umar
Department of Zoology, Faculty of Life Sciences, University of Okara, Okara 56130, Pakistan

Rabia Unar
Jinnah Post Graduate Medical Center Hospital, Karachi, Pakistan

Rasha Eletreby, Ahmed Fouad, Mostafa Al Bassiouni, Naglaa Zayed, Ayman Yosry and Zeinab Abdellatif
Endemic Medicine and Hepatogastroentrology Departement, Faculty of Medicine, Cairo University, Cairo, Egypt

Maged Abd Elraouf
Gynecology and Obstetrics Department, Faculty of Medicine, Cairo University, Cairo, Egypt

Mona Nasser
Clinical and Chemical Pathology Department, Faculty of Medicine, Beni-Suef University, Beni-Suef, Egypt

Walaa M. Hashem, Ossama A. Ahmed and Ahmed Mansour
Gastroenterology, Hepatology and Internal Medicine Department, Ain Shams University, Cairo, Egypt

Manal Hamdy El-Sayed
Department of Paediatrics and Clinical Research Center, Ain Shams University, Cairo, Egypt

Hany M. Dabbous, Mohamed Kamal Shaker and Ahmed Fouad Sherief
Tropical Medicine Department, Ain Shams University, Cairo, Egypt

Mary Gamal Naguib
Clinical Haematology and Internal Medicine Department, Ain Shams University, Cairo, Egypt

Shereen Abdel-Monem Ibrahim
Department of Clinical Pathology, Ain Shams University, Cairo, Egypt

Marwa Ahmed Sakr, Khaled Abdel Hamid Mohamed, Mohamed Hassan Fouad and Ahmed Samir Allam
Department of Internal Medicine, Faculty of Medicine, Ain Shams University, Cairo, Egypt

Ahmed Mohamed Hussein
Department of Radiology, Faculty of Medicine, Ain Shams University, Cairo, Egypt

Nadia Abdel Ataay Abdelkader, Ahmed Fouad Sherief, Doaa Mahmoud Kandil, Mohammed Soliman Gado and Amira Mahmoud Al Balakosy
Tropical Medicine Department, Faculty of Medicine, Ain Shams University, 38 Abbassia street, Postal code, Cairo 1181, Egypt

Osama Ashraf Ahmed
Internal Medicine Department, Faculty of Medicine, Ain Shams University, Cairo, Egypt

Ouafa Kallala, Saoussen Kacem, Imene Fodha and Trabelsi Abdelhalim
Research Laboratory or "Epidemiology and Immunogenetics of Viral Infections" (LR14SP02), Sahloul University Hospital, University of Sousse, Sousse, Tunisia
Faculty of Pharmacy, University of Monastir, Avicenne Street, Monastir, Tunisia

Bruno Pozzetto
GIMAP EA3064, Faculté de Médecine, Université de Saint-Etienne/Université de Lyon, Lyon, France
Laboratoire des Agents infectieux et d'Hygiène, CHU de Saint-Etienne, Saint-Priest-en-Jarez, France

Essam Mohamed Bayoumy, Wesam Ahmed Ibrahim, Moataz Mohamed Sayed and Mohamed Magdy Salama
Division of Gastroenterology and Hepatology, Department of Internal Medicine, Faculty of Medicine, Ain Shams University, Cairo, Egypt

Ashraf Bekheet Salama
Division of Gastroenterology and Hepatology, Department of Internal Medicine, Faculty of Medicine, Ain Shams University, Cairo, Egypt
Tanta University, Tanta, Egypt

Nahla Mohamed Teama
Division of Nephrology, Department of Internal Medicine, Faculty of Medicine, Ain Shams University, Ramsis Street 38, Abbasia, Cairo 11566, Egypt

Maissa El Raziky, Hanan Abdel Hafez and Aisha Elsharkawy
Department of Endemic Medicine, Faculty of Medicine, Cairo University, Cairo 11562, Egypt

Tarek Ahmed Moneer
National Tropical Medicine & Hepatology Institute, Cairo, Egypt

Suzan M. EL-Sheikh and Sahar A. Sharaf
Department of Clinical and Chemical Pathology, Faculty of Medicine, Cairo University, Cairo, Egypt

Rabab M. Maher
Fellow of Tropical Medicine, Cairo University Student Hospital, Cairo, Egypt

Khaled Mohieldeen, Soraya Abdel Fatah Hamoda, Abdurrahman Najeeb and Walid Ismail Ellakany
Tropical Medicine Department, Faculty of Medicine, Alexandria University, Alexandria, Egypt

Shwikar Mahmoud Ahmed
Medical Microbiology and Immunology Department, Faculty of Medicine, Alexandria University, Alexandria, Egypt

Sabeen Sabri
Department of Microbiology and Molecular Genetics, Faculty of Life Sciences, University of Okara, Okara 56130, Punjab, Pakistan

Muhammad Idrees Khan and Shazia Rafique
Centre of Excellence and Molecular Biology, University of the Punjab, Lahore, Pakistan

Amjad Ali
Department of Biotechnology and Genetic Engineering, Hazara University, Hazara, Pakistan

Muhammad Saleem Khan
Department of Zoology, Faculty of Life Sciences, University of Okara, Okara, Punjab 56130, Pakistan

Aliaa Sabry and Mohamed Abbasy
Hepatology, Gastroenterology Department, National Liver Institute, Menoufia University, Menoufia, Egypt

Azza M. Abdu Allah
Medical Biochemistry and Molecular Biology Department, Faculty of Medicine- Menoufia University, Menoufia, Egypt

Nada Elnaidany
Faculty of Pharmacy, MSA University, 6th of October City, Egypt

Index

www.ingramcontent.com/pod-product-compliance
Lightning Source LLC
LaVergne TN
LVHW081037210926
848485LV00004B/1046
* 9 7 8 1 6 4 6 4 7 5 6 2 9 *